Irritable Bowel Syndrome

Guest Editor

WILLIAM D. CHEY, MD

GASTROENTEROLOGY CLINICS OF NORTH AMERICA

www.gastro.theclinics.com

March 2011 • Volume 40 • Number 1

SAUNDERS an imprint of ELSEVIER, Inc.

W.B. SAUNDERS COMPANY

A Division of Elsevier Inc.

Elsevier Inc. • 1600 John F. Kennedy Blvd., Suite 1800 • Philadelphia, Pennsylvania 19103-2899
http://www.theclinics.com

GASTROENTEROLOGY CLINICS OF NORTH AMERICA Volume 40, Number 1
March 2011 ISSN 0889-8553, ISBN-13: 978-1-4557-0450-7

Editor: Kerry Holland
Developmental Editor: Jessica Demetriou

Gastroenterology Clinics of North America (ISSN 0889-8553) is published quarterly by Elsevier Inc., 360 Park Avenue South, New York, NY 10010-1710. Months of issue are March, June, September, and December. Business and Editorial Offices: 1600 John F. Kennedy Blvd., Suite 1800, Philadelphia, PA 19103-2899. Customer Service Office: 6277 Sea Harbor Drive, Orlando, FL 32887-4800. Periodicals postage paid at New York, NY and additional mailing offices. Subscription prices are $282.00 per year (US individuals), $142.00 per year (US students), $458.00 per year (US institutions), $310.00 per year (Canadian individuals), $558.00 per year (Canadian institutions), $392.00 per year (international individuals), $195.00 per year (international students), and $558.00 per year (international institutions). Foreign air speed delivery is included in all *Clinics* subscription prices. All prices are subject to change without notice. **POSTMASTER**: Send address changes to *Gastroenterology Clinics of North America*, Elsevier Health Sciences Division, Subscription Customer Service, 3251 Riverport Lane, Maryland Heights, MO 63043. Telephone: 1-800-654-2452 (U.S. and Canada); 314-447-8871 (outside U.S. and Canada). Fax: 314-447-8029. E-mail: journalscustomerservice-usa@elsevier.com (for print support); journalsonlinesupport-usa@elsevier.com (for online support).

Reprints. For copies of 100 or more, of articles in this publication, please contact the Commercial Reprints Department, Elsevier Inc., 360 Part Avenue South, New York, New York 10010-1710. Tel. (212) 633-3813, Fax: (212) 462-1935, E-mail: reprints@elsevier.com.

Gastroenterology Clinics of North America is also published in Italian by Il Pensiero Scientifico Editore, Rome, Italy; and in Portuguese by Interlivros Edicoes Ltda., Rua Commandante Coelho 1085, 21250 Cordovil, Rio de Janeiro, Brazil.

Gastroenterology Clinics of North America is covered in *MEDLINE/PubMed (Index Medicus)*, *Excerpta Medica*, *Current Contents/Clinical Medicine*, *Science Citation Index*, *ISI/BIOMED*, and *BIOSIS*.

Printed and bound by CPI Group (UK) Ltd, Croydon, CR0 4YY

Transferred to Digital Print 2011

Contributors

GUEST EDITOR

WILLIAM D. CHEY, MD, AGAF, FACG, FACP
Professor of Medicine; Director, GI Physiology Laboratory; Co-Director, Michigan
Bowel Control Program, Division of Gastroenterology, University of Michigan Health
System, Ann Arbor, Michigan

AUTHORS

NIKHIL AGARWAL, MD
VA Greater Los Angeles Healthcare System, David Geffen School of Medicine, University
of California, Los Angeles, Los Angeles, California

BROOKS D. CASH, MD, FACP, FACG, AGAF
Chief of Medicine, and Gastroenterology Service, National Naval Medical Center;
and Professor of Medicine, Uniformed Services University of the Health Sciences,
Bethesda, Maryland

CHRISTOPHER CHANG, MD, PhD
GI Motility Program, Cedars-Sinai Medical Center, Los Angeles, California

LIN CHANG, MD, AGAF
Professor of Medicine in Residence, Division of Digestive Disease, Department of
Medicine; VA Greater Los Angeles Healthcare System, David Geffen School of Medicine;
Co-Director, UCLA Center for Neurovisceral Sciences and Women's Health, Center for
Neurobiology of Stress, University of California, Los Angeles, Los Angeles, California

WILLIAM D. CHEY, MD, AGAF, FACG, FACP
Professor of Medicine; Director, GI Physiology Laboratory; Co-Director, Michigan Bowel
Control Program, Division of Gastroenterology, University of Michigan Health System,
Ann Arbor, Michigan

ROK SEON CHOUNG, MD
Assistant Professor of Medicine, Division of Gastroenterology and Hepatology, Mayo
Clinic, Rochester, Minnesota

DOUGLAS A. DROSSMAN, MD
Professor of Medicine and Psychiatry, Co-Director, UNC Center for Functional GI and
Motility Disorders, University of North Carolina, Chapel Hill, North Carolina

SHANTI ESWARAN, MD
Clinical Lecturer, Division of Gastroenterology, University of Michigan Health System,
Ann Arbor, Michigan

ALEXANDER C. FORD, MD, MRCP
Senior Lecturer, University of Leeds, Leeds Gastroenterology Institute, Leeds General
Infirmary, Leeds, United Kingdom

DAVID L. FURMAN, MD
Gastroenterology Service, National Naval Medical Center, Bethesda, Maryland

MADHUSUDAN GROVER, MD
Instructor in Medicine, Division of Gastroenterology and Hepatology, Mayo Clinic, Rochester, Minnesota

WILLIAM L. HASLER, MD
Professor of Internal Medicine, Division of Gastroenterology, University of Michigan Health System, Ann Arbor, Michigan

ANTHONY LEMBO, MD
Associate Professor of Medicine, Division of Gastroenterology, Department of Medicine, Beth Israel Deaconess Medical Center, Boston, Massachusetts

G. RICHARD LOCKE III, MD
Professor of Medicine, Division of Gastroenterology and Hepatology, Mayo Clinic, Rochester, Minnesota

SUMA MAGGE, MD
Fellow in Gastroenterology, Division of Gastroenterology, Department of Medicine, Beth Israel Deaconess Medical Center, Boston, Massachusetts

MONTHIRA MANEERATTANAPORN, MD
Research Fellow in Neurogastroenterology and Functional Bowel Disorders, Division of Gastroenterology, University of Michigan Health System, Ann Arbor, Michigan; Clinical Lecturer, Division of Gastroenterology, Siriraj Hospital, Mahidol University, Bangkok, Thailand

PAUL MOAYYEDI, MB ChB, PhD, MPH, FRCP, FRCPC, AGAF, FACG
Director, Division of Gastroenterology, Farncombe Family Digestive Health Research Institute; Professor of Medicine, Department of Medicine, McMaster University Medical Centre, Hamilton, Ontario, Canada

MARK PIMENTEL, MD, FRCP(C)
Director, GI Motility Program, Cedars-Sinai Medical Center, Los Angeles, California

EAMONN M.M. QUIGLEY, MD, FRCP, FACP, FACG, FRCPI
Department of Medicine, Alimentary Pharmabiotic Centre, Cork University Hospital, University College Cork, Cork, Ireland

RICHARD J. SAAD, MD
Assistant Professor of Medicine, Division of Gastroenterology, University of Michigan Health System, Michigan

YURI A. SAITO, MD, MPH
Assistant Professor of Medicine, Division of Gastroenterology and Hepatology, Mayo Clinic, Rochester, Minnesota

BRENNAN M.R. SPIEGEL, MD, MSHS
VA Greater Los Angeles Healthcare System, David Geffen School of Medicine, University of California, Los Angeles, Los Angeles, California

ROBIN C. SPILLER, MD
Professor of Gastroenterology; Director of the NIHR Biomedical Research Unit;
Head of Nottingham Digestive Diseases Centre, University Hospital, Nottingham,
United Kingdom

JAN TACK, MD, PhD
Professor of Medicine, Department of Gastroenterology, University Hospital
Gasthuisberg, University of Leuven, Herestraat, Leuven, Belgium

Contents

Irritable bowel syndrome (IBS) is a common functional gastrointestinal (GI) disorder. Because not everyone needs to seek care, population-based studies are needed to truly understand the epidemiology of IBS. About 10% of the population has IBS at any one time and about 200 people per 100,000 will receive an initial diagnosis of IBS over the course of a year. IBS patients are more frequently younger in age, and a female predominance has been observed in Western countries and tertiary care settings. IBS patients commonly report overlapping upper GI, as well as a variety of non-GI, complaints.

Irritable bowel syndrome (IBS) is a highly prevalent condition with a large health economic burden of illness marked by impaired health-related quality of life (HRQOL), diminished work productivity, and high expenditures. Clinicians should routinely screen for diminished HRQOL by performing a balanced biopsychosocial history rather than focusing just on bowel symptoms. HRQOL decrements should be acknowledged and addressed when making treatment decisions.

The pathogenesis of symptoms in irritable bowel syndrome (IBS) is multifactorial and varies from patient to patient. Disturbances of motor function in the small intestine and colon and smooth-muscle dysfunction in other gut and extraintestinal regions are prominent. Abnormalities of sensory function in visceral and somatic structures are detected in most patients with IBS, which may relate to peripheral sensitization or altered central nervous system processing of afferent information. Contributions from psychosocial disturbances are observed in patients from tertiary centers and primary practice. Proof of causation of symptom genesis for most of these factors is limited.

Irritable bowel syndrome (IBS) is a common disorder that has been shown to aggregate in families and to affect multiple generations, but not in a manner consistent with a major Mendelian effect. Relatives of an individual with IBS are 2 to 3 times as likely to have IBS, with both genders being affected.

To date, more than 100 genetic variants in more than 60 genes from various pathways have been studied in a number of candidate gene studies, with several positive associations reported. These findings suggest that there may be distinct, as well as shared, molecular underpinnings for IBS and its subtypes.

Irritable bowel syndrome (IBS) is the most common gastrointestinal condition, affecting 10% to 20% of adults in developed countries. Over the last few years, growing evidence has supported a new hypothesis for IBS based on alterations in intestinal bacterial composition. This article reviews the evidence for a bacterial concept in IBS and begins to formulate a hypothesis of how these bacterial systems could integrate in a new pathophysiologic mechanism in the development of IBS. Data suggesting an interaction between this gut flora and inflammation in the context of IBS is also presented.

Medical students are taught that 90% of all diagnoses are made through careful assessment of the patients' symptoms. Clinicians now rely heavily on techniques such as endoscopy or radiology before making a definitive diagnosis of organic disease. Most gastroenterologists would require endoscopic confirmation before labeling a patient as having peptic ulcer disease and would make a diagnosis of Crohn disease based on small bowel radiology or colonoscopy. However, the most common causes of symptoms of the gastrointestinal tract are functional. It is important that clinicians obtain a thorough history so that the disorder of the patient can be accurately defined.

This article discusses the diagnostic criteria and processes applicable to irritable bowel syndrome (IBS). The authors describe the various diagnostic criteria with a focus on the Rome criteria for IBS and the judicious application of historical information such as alarm features and the yield of various diagnostic modalities such as blood, stool, breath, and endoscopic tests.

A "biomarker" (biological marker) is an indicator of a bodily function that can be objectively measured. A wide range of possible biomarkers for IBS have been considered but at present only gut transit measured using radio-isotope markers meet the criteria of reproducibility and availability. While barostat studies perform reasonably in expert centers, to do them reproducibly requires considerable effort and standardization. This makes them unsuitable for widespread use. However radio-isotope tests are expensive and of limited availability so the search for other more convenient markers including blood and stool tests is still an important goal for the future.

After years of inattention, there is a growing body of evidence to suggest that dietary constituents at least exacerbate symptoms and perhaps contribute to the pathogenesis of the irritable bowel syndrome (IBS). Although patients with IBS self-report food allergies more often than the general population, the evidence suggests that true food allergies are relatively uncommon. Less clearly defined food intolerances may be an important contributor to symptoms in IBS patients. This article reviews the literature supporting a causal link between food and the symptoms of IBS as well as the evidence supporting dietary interventions as a means of managing IBS symptoms.

Gut-acting therapies are common therapies for irritable bowel syndrome (IBS). Most of these peripheral acting agents are primarily targeted at individual symptoms. The evidence supporting the use of these agents in IBS is largely anecdotal. Serotonergic agents and the chloride channel activator lubiprostone have shown efficacy in treating symptoms of IBS. The clinical evidence supporting the use of these agents is based on data from high-quality clinical trials. The use of serotonergic agents for IBS in the United States is limited to the 5-hydroxytryptamine-3 antagonist alosetron in the treatment of women with severe IBS with diarrhea refractory to traditional therapy.

Irritable bowel syndrome (IBS) and other functional gastrointestinal (GI) disorders typically defy traditional diagnostic methods based on structural abnormalities, and has led to the emergence of the discipline of neurogastroenterology or the study of the "brain-gut axis," which is based on dysregulation of neuroenteric pathways as a key pathophysiological feature of IBS. Centrally acting treatments can influence these pathways and improve the clinical manifestations of pain and bowel dysfunction associated with this disorder. To successfully implement these treatment strategies, it is important to recognize their dual effects on brain and gut, understanding the nature and severity of the GI symptoms and their psychosocial concomitants, and applying them within the context of the patient's understanding of their value.

Several recent observations have raised the possibility that disturbances in the gut microbiota and/or a low-grade inflammatory state may contribute to symptomatology and the etiology of irritable bowel syndrome (IBS). Consequent on these hypotheses, several therapeutic categories have found their way into the armamentarium of those who care for IBS sufferers. These agents include probiotics, prebiotics, antibiotics, and anti-inflammatory agents.

The irritable bowel syndrome (IBS) is a symptom-based disorder defined by the presence of abdominal pain and altered bowel habits. Clinical presentations of IBS are diverse, with some patients reporting diarrhea, some constipation, and others a mixture of both. Like the varied clinical phenotypes, the pathogenesis of IBS is also diverse. IBS is not a single disease entity, but rather likely consists of several different disease states. This fact has important implications for the choices and efficacy of IBS treatment. This article reviews the IBS drugs that have reached phase II or III clinical trials.

Irritable bowel syndrome (IBS) is a common chronic gastrointestinal disorder, characterized by chronic or recurrent abdominal pain and bloating. Complementary and alternative medicine (CAM) is a diverse group of medical treatments that are not commonly considered to be a part of conventional medicine yet frequently used together with conventional medicine. CAM is widely used, particularly for chronic medical conditions that are difficult to treat. Because only a limited number of treatments are available for IBS, many patients choose CAM. This article reviews current evidence supporting the use of CAM in IBS, with a focus on prebiotics, acupuncture, and herbal medicines.

ISSUE OF RELATED INTEREST

Gastrointestinal Endoscopy Clinics of North America, January 2009
(Volume 19, Issue 1)
Gastrointestinal Motility and Neurogastroenterology
Richard W. McCallum, MD, FACP, FACG, *Guest Editor*

THE CLINICS ARE NOW AVAILABLE ONLINE!

Access your subscription at:
www.theclinics.com

Preface

Irritable Bowel Syndrome

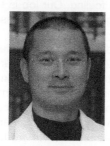

William D. Chey, MD, AGAF
Guest Editor

It is with great pride that I introduce this issue of *Gastroenterology Clinics of North America*, which presents state-of-the-art clinical reviews on Irritable Bowel Syndrome or IBS. It has been more than 5 years since *Gastroenterology Clinics* last reviewed this prevalent but vexing disorder. In that period of time, much has been learned about a variety of topics relevant to IBS. A search of the term "irritable bowel syndrome" on ISI Web of Knowledge, limited to GI specialty journals, yields over 1,800 published articles over the past 5 years. In the following pages, the world's leading experts summarize and place into clinical perspective much of the most important emerging evidence on IBS.

Throughout this issue of *Gastroenterology Clinics*, our esteemed group of contributors describes IBS as a symptom-based condition consisting of abdominal pain, bloating, and altered bowel habits. Although factually accurate, this statement in so many ways understates why a reader should care about IBS. It is really all that flows from this symptom cluster that makes IBS worthy of the health system's, and indeed society's, attention. IBS is a remarkable example of a condition that is greater than the sum of its parts. After all, we have therapies that work relatively well for individual symptoms of IBS such as diarrhea or constipation. Unfortunately, to many affected individuals, it is the totality and complexity of symptoms that are so problematic. Although often disdained by physicians and ridiculed by unaffected members of the general public, IBS can be a very serious condition that dramatically affects all aspects of an affected person's life. Putting the personal consequences of IBS aside, the financial consequences to the health system, employers, and society at large provide a mandate for better understanding the root causes and the best ways to manage IBS.

Patients and providers remain fearful and frustrated when it comes to IBS. Why? The answer can in part be found in the oft-used quote by the late American poet and essayist, Ralph Waldo Emerson, who coined the phrase, "Fear always springs from ignorance." Patients and providers remain uncomfortable with symptom-based conditions such as IBS where there are theories but no universal truths regarding

Gastroenterol Clin N Am 40 (2011) xiii–xiv
doi:10.1016/j.gtc.2011.01.002
0889-8553/11/$ – see front matter © 2011 Elsevier Inc. All rights reserved.

gastro.theclinics.com

pathogenesis, and management remains largely empiric and often ineffective. Readers of this issue of *Gastroenterology Clinics* will find new concepts and strategies to apply to their patients with IBS. Through this update, we hope to move the conversation on IBS toward the thoughts of President Barack Obama, who said, "…we're going to break through the fear and the frustration people are feeling. Our job is to make sure that even as we make progress, that we are also giving people a sense of hope and vision for the future."

In the following pages, comprehensive reviews by the world's leading authorities will provide readers with the latest information on a wide variety of topics relevant to IBS, including epidemiology, burden to illness, a review of traditional and cutting edge concepts regarding pathogenesis, evidence-based recommendations concerning diagnosis, practical recommendations regarding nonmedical and medical management strategies, and a look at what the future holds with regard to biomarkers and emerging therapies. I am greatly indebted to each of the authors for their invaluable contributions to this issue of *Gastroenterology Clinics*. My coauthors and I very much hope that this issue of *Gastroenterology Clinics* furthers the process of demystifying IBS and helps providers to better care for their patients with this misunderstood disorder.

William D. Chey, MD, AGAF
Division of Gastroenterology
University of Michigan Health System
3912 Taubman Center, SPC 5362
Ann Arbor, MI 48109-5362, USA

E-mail address:
wchey@med.umich.edu

Epidemiology of IBS

Rok Seon Choung, MD, G. Richard Locke III, MD*

KEYWORDS

- Irritable bowel syndrome • Epidemiology
- Overlap • Natural history

Irritable bowel syndrome (IBS) is a common functional gastrointestinal disorder (FGID) that manifests as abdominal pain or discomfort and diarrhea or constipation, or both.[1–3] The definition of IBS has evolved over time, from a diagnosis of exclusion to the symptom-based diagnostic criteria including Manning, Rome I, Rome II, and Rome III criteria. IBS is one of the most common disorders affecting the gastrointestinal (GI) tract. IBS accounts for 10% to 15% of primary care visits and 25% to 50% of gastroenterology referral visits.[4] Data from the National Disease and Therapeutic Index (NDTI) showed that IBS accounts for 2.6 million office-based visits and 3.5 million all-location physician visits.[5] However, a limited proportion of subjects suffering from IBS seek medical attention for this condition.[6] Thus, knowledge of IBS epidemiology depends on research in the general population. This review addresses the comprehensive epidemiology in terms of prevalence, incidence, overlap, and natural history of one of the most common GI disorders, IBS.

PREVALENCE

For chronic conditions, the best way to estimate how commonly they occur is to report the number of people with the condition at any given time, the prevalence. In general, IBS is considered a highly prevalent FGID. However, IBS epidemiology varies considerably according to the definition used. Many population-based surveys have estimated the prevalence of IBS using the responses of surveys that record bowel symptoms. The prevalence rates in these studies have varied between 3 and 32 per hundred.[4,5,7,8] Why do the prevalence rates from these IBS-specific symptom surveys vary tenfold? Although this may represent true differences in populations, it more likely reflects differences in the IBS definition. For example, the earlier Manning criteria are more generous and less restrictive than the recent Rome criteria.[9–11] Higher prevalence rates are identified using a threshold of 2 of 6 Manning criteria.[10] Lower prevalence rates are identified using more specific criteria, whether by increasing the threshold of Manning criteria necessary to make the diagnosis or using the Rome criteria. In a direct comparison, prevalence using standard Rome criteria is

Division of Gastroenterology and Hepatology, Mayo Clinic, 200 First Street Southwest, Rochester, MN 55905, USA
* Corresponding author.
E-mail address: locke.giles@mayo.edu

Gastroenterol Clin N Am 40 (2011) 1–10
doi:10.1016/j.gtc.2010.12.006
0889-8553/11/$ – see front matter © 2011 Elsevier Inc. All rights reserved.

gastro.theclinics.com

comparable to using a threshold of 3 of 6 Manning criteria.[10] Moreover, Mearin and colleagues[12] studied the differences between the Rome I and Rome II criteria, and found that only 31% of those meeting Rome I criteria met Rome II criteria for IBS. Those not meeting the Rome II definition met other FGIDs, such as functional constipation, functional diarrhea, or functional bloating. Recently, the symptom based diagnostic Rome III criteria for IBS has been developed and used, clinically and in research. The epidemiology of IBS may be difficult to interpret given these changing definitions.

The major IBS prevalence studies in Western countries are summarized in **Table 1**. The range of prevalence is from 3% to 32%, with most studies reporting results between 5% and 15% depending on the definition applied.[4,7–9,11,13–26] In a comprehensive review of the epidemiology of IBS in North America in 2002,[27] the prevalence estimates for IBS in the United States ranged from 3% to 20%. In addition, this study showed that the prevalence decreased slightly with age, and the prevalence in women was slightly higher (2:1 female to male predominance). However, this study was performed before the development of the Rome II criteria. In more recent studies of the epidemiology of IBS in the United States or Canada using Rome II criteria, the prevalence of IBS has been estimated as from 5% to 12%. In another systemic review of IBS in 2007, which was based on 13 studies in European Union nations, the prevalence of IBS was approximately 4% based on Rome II criteria. In addition, there was a 2:1 female:male predominance.

Table 2 summarizes the major epidemiologic studies in Asian countries. The prevalence of IBS by the Rome II criteria in Asia has been reported to range from 1% to 22%.[28–41] Across Asia, the prevalence of IBS is higher in the younger age groups. Of note, the female predominance reported in the West has not been reported in some Asian countries. It is noteworthy that a higher prevalence of IBS in males has been reported in some Asian countries.

Based on Rome III criteria, the prevalence of IBS has been estimated to range from 10% to 18% in the general population of Western countries,[25,26] whereas the prevalence of IBS reported from Asian countries has been from 1% to 9%.[41–43] The prevalence of IBS does decrease slightly with age,[14,44] although new-onset symptoms may occur in the elderly. Also among the elderly, Talley and colleagues[44] showed that the prevalence of IBS was found to increase with age from 8% among those aged 65 to 74 years to more than 12% for those older than 85. However, more and better data are needed.

Overall, the prevalence of IBS has been reported as between 2% and 15% from Western or Asian countries, with IBS patients more frequently younger in age. Female predominance is more prevalent in Western countries or tertiary hospital care settings. Of course, comparison across countries is made difficult because of language and cultural differences. Even in the same study, questionnaires need to be developed and validated for each language, and even then one's threshold to endorse symptoms may vary.

Regarding IBS bowel habit subtypes, one systemic review[45] reported that population-based studies from the United States (Manning) found similar distributions among constipation predominant IBS (IBS-C), diarrhea predominant IBS (IBS-D), and IBS alternating between diarrhea and constipation (IBS-A), while European studies (Rome I, Rome II, or self-reporting) showed either IBS-C or IBS-A as the most prevalent subtypes. For example, in one study approximately 16% of the IBS patients had IBS-C, 21% had IBS-D, and 63% had IBS-A.[21] Whether the agreement between subtyping of IBS patients based on Rome II versus Rome III criteria is good or poor[46,47] is controversial. Very few data by IBS subgroup based on the recent Rome III classification system are available.

Table 1
Prevalence of irritable bowel syndrome in Western countries

First Author,[Ref.] Country	Year	N	Case Definition	% IBS Overall	Men	Women
Talley,[4] USA	1987	835	Manning 2	15.8	15.8	18.2
			Manning 3	12.8	12.1	13.6
Hahn,[13] USA	1989	42392	Manning 2	3	—	—
			Rome I	12		
Drossman,[14] USA	1990	5430	Rome I	9.4	7.7	14.5
Saito,[15] USA	1992	643	Manning 3	15.7	13.5	17.7
			Rome I	8.4	8.4	8.4
Mearin,[9] Spain	2001	2000	Manning	10.3		
			Rome I	12.1		
			Rome II	3.3	1.9	4.6
Brommelaer,[16] France	2002	8221	Manning	2.5	1.7	3.1
			Rome I	2.1	1.4	2.8
			Rome II	1.1	0.9	1.3
Thompson,[17] Canada	2002	1149	Rome II	12.1	8.7	15.2
Boyce,[18] Australia	1997	2910	Manning	13.6		
			Rome I	4.4	4.4	9.1
Jones,[7] England	1992	1620	Manning	21.6	18.7	24.3
Agreus,[19] Sweden	1988	1290	Rome I	12.5	—	—
Wilson[20] UK	2003	4807	Rome II	8.1	—	—
Hungin,[21] Europe (UK, France, Germany, Italy, Holland, Belgium, Spain, Switzerland)	2003	41984	Overall	9.6	7.1	12
			Manning	6.5		
			Rome I	4.2		
			Rome II	2.9		
Kennedy,[22] UK	1998	3179	Manning 3	17.2	10.5	22.9
Icks,[7] Germany	2002	1281	Patient report	12.5	—	—
Kay,[8] Denmark	1994	4581	Symptom criteria	6.6	5.6	7.7
Heaton,[24] UK	1992	1896	Manning 3	9.5	5.0	13.0
			Manning 2	21.6	18.7	24.3
Hillila,[11] Finland	2004	3650	Manning 2	16.2	13.1	19.2
			Manning 3	9.7	8.3	11.2
			Rome I	5.5	5.1	6.1
			Rome II	5.1	5.1	5.3
Jung,[25] USA	2004	2273	Rome III	11	8	14
Olafsdottir,[26] Iceland	1996	1336	Manning 2	31	—	—
	2006	799	Rome III	10		
			Manning 2	32		
			Rome II	5.0		
			Rome III	13		

INCIDENCE

Incidence of IBS is not easy to estimate, because IBS may develop slowly and people may not seek care.[48] From a population-based study in the United States, which was based on 2 surveys sent to a random sample of population about 1 year apart, the IBS onset rate was 9%. However, in another study based on physician-based IBS diagnosis in the same population, the incidence rate of clinically diagnosed IBS was

Table 2
Prevalence of irritable bowel syndrome in Asian countries

First Author,[Ref.] Country	Year	N	Case Definition	% IBS Overall	% IBS Men	% IBS Women
Gwee,[28] Singapore	1998	2276	Manning 2	11	9.5	12.6
			Rome I	10.4	9.0	11.7
			Rome II	8.6	7.8	9.4
Xiong,[29] South China	2002	4178	Manning	11.5	9.7	13.0
			Rome II	5.7	5.0	6.3
Lau,[30] Hong Kong	1996	1298	Rome II	3.7	3.6	3.8
Ho,[31] Singapore	1990	696	Manning	2.3	—	—
Kwan,[32] Hong Kong	2000	1797	Rome II	6.6	—	—
Danivat,[33] Thailand	1988	1077	Manning	4.4	—	—
Masud,[34] Bangladesh	2000	2426	Rome I	8.5	5.8	10.7
Rajendra,[35] Malaysia	2000	949	Rome II	14	—	—
Ghoshal,[36] India	2005	7285	Clinical	4.2	4.3	4.0
Han,[37] Korea	2004	1066	Rome II	6.6	7.1	6.0
Husain,[38] Pakistan	2006	880	Rome II	13.3	13.1	13.4
Lu,[39] Taiwan	2001	2865	Rome II	22.1	21.8	22.8
Miwa,[40] Japan	2006	10000	Rome III	13.1	10.7	15.5
Sorouri,[41] Iran	2006	18180	Rome III	1.1	0.6	1.5

much lower, 196 cases per 100,000 person-years.[49] A study from Europe showed a similar annual incidence rate of IBS, about 200 to 300 per 100,000 people.[50] Symptoms may come and go and change over time.[51] Thus, the coming and going of IBS may not represent a brand new case. Therefore, the 9% onset rate may have occurred in people who had IBS at some time in the past. Similarly, many people with IBS in the community do not seek care. The incidence of a clinical diagnosis of IBS is likely an underestimate. Nonetheless, if only half seek care, the observed incidence can be doubled to 400 per 100,000 per year and then multiplied by a 20-year disease duration to get a prevalence of 12%, which is in keeping with the data. Moreover, IBS may develop in a higher proportion of patients with certain conditions, such as an acute episode of infectious gastroenteritis. From a systematic review of postinfectious IBS, the incidence rate of IBS in patients with acute GI infection has been reported to be 10% (95% confidence interval: 9.4–85.6).[52]

Overlap with Other Functional Gastrointestinal Disorders

Patients with IBS seeking health care commonly report other GI and/or extraintestinal complaints. Because of how commonly it occurs, it is possible that IBS overlaps with other intestinal or extraintestinal diseases simply due to chance. However, many population-based and clinical studies[14,22,25,53–56] have reported the associations with other diseases, specifically other FGIDs. For example, a community study[22] in the United Kingdom showed that IBS, gastroesophageal reflux disease (GERD), and symptomatic bronchial hyperresponsiveness occurred more frequently together than expected; in subjects with IBS, 47% had GERD. Also, in a United States community study, Jung and colleagues[25] showed that IBS and GERD occurred together more commonly than expected by chance; the prevalence of IBS-GERD overlap was 4% of the population. Finally, a recent systematic review[57] of the overlap of GERD and IBS using the population-based studies and clinical studies suggested that there is a strong overlap between GERD and IBS that exceeds the individual presence of each condition. A recent systematic review evaluated the relationship between dyspepsia and IBS using 19 eligible studies (13 population-based and 6 clinical studies).[58] The analysis showed that the degree of overlap between the two conditions varied from 15% to 42%, depending on diagnostic criteria used for each, and individuals with dyspepsia had an eightfold increase in prevalence of IBS compared with the population. Thus, the demonstration of significant overlap with other FGIDs raises the question as to whether these disorders should be considered a more common clinic entity or not. Locke and colleagues[53] showed in a community based study that 4% to 9% of the population had any 2 GI symptom complexes and 1% to 4% of the population had 3 GI symptom complexes. Many other studies also have shown overlap of pairs of FGIDs. Although many possibilities exist, the mechanism behind this overlap is not yet clear.

Overlap with Extraintestinal Disorders

At least one subset of IBS patients also suffer with non-GI symptoms. IBS patients make 2 or 3 times as many non-GI health care visits as control subjects.[14,59] Non-GI nonpsychiatric disorders documented to be associated with IBS in a detailed literature review included chronic fatigue syndrome (51%), chronic pelvic pain (50%), and temporomandibular joint disorders (64%).[60] In referred patients with IBS, psychiatric disorders have also been reported to be very common, leading some to argue that IBS is a part of the psychiatric disease spectrum and not a unique condition.[61,62] Whitehead and colleagues[60] performed a study comparing the comorbidities between 3153 patients with IBS and age- and gender-matched controls in a health maintenance organization. They found that psychiatric disorders, especially major depression, anxiety, and somatoform disorders, occur in up to 94% in IBS patients. The investigators argued that the elevated incidence of non-GI disorders might occur in a subset because patients with IBS are hypervigilant and consult much more readily for problems than those without IBS, although this remains to be established. Some of the burden of extraintestinal comorbid conditions may also be explained by somatization or other psychiatric disorders coexisting with IBS,[62] but this could not account for at least two-thirds of patients with IBS.[60] In fact, there has been a recent movement to overhaul the classification of somatoform disorder.[63] Thus, in the future much can be learned about the prevalence and epidemiology of IBS with regard to overlap or comorbid conditions, which may help lead to a more appropriate classification scheme and management.

NATURAL HISTORY OF IBS

IBS is considered a chronic stable disorder that may wax and wane for years. However, data regarding the natural history of the IBS are limited. Early studies of the natural history of IBS had shown that about half of IBS patients improved over 2 to 5 years of follow-up.[64-66] In a community-based study, Talley and colleagues[67] evaluated the natural history of IBS by surveying one cohort 2 times over 1 year. The prevalence of IBS on the first and second surveys was similar. However, 9% of people without symptoms on the first survey developed IBS symptoms on the second survey, and 38% of those with IBS had their symptom disappear during the 18-month period between surveys. Thus, the overall prevalence of IBS appears to be relatively stable over 12 to 20 months. Another 7-year follow-up study in Sweden showed the natural history of IBS and other FGIDs.[68] The results showed substantial symptom fluctuation among the GI symptom complexes with increasing prevalence of IBS over a 7-year period. Further, a recent long-term follow-up study from Olmsted County evaluated the transitions amongst FGIDs over 12 years.[51] Halder and colleagues[51] showed the substantial transition among the categories, with about one-third of subjects with IBS developing another FGID. In a systematic review on the natural history of IBS based on 14 longitudinal observational studies of clinic-based IBS patients, El-Serag and colleagues[69] showed that approximately 30% to 50% of patients had unchanged symptoms, and concluded that IBS, a chronic disorder, is a stable diagnosis.

In general, it has been assumed that IBS is not associated with any increase in mortality. In a study from Mayo Clinic, 112 subjects first diagnosed with IBS in the period 1961 to 1963 were followed up for a mean of 29 years, and the observed survival was not different from expected.[70] However, these data might be underpowered to detect any mortality from IBS. Recently, one additional study from the Olmsted County community evaluated survival in IBS.[71] In this study a total of 4176 respondents from randomly selected cohorts of Olmsted County residents were followed between 1988 and 1993 to assess the survival over 20 years. No association between survival and IBS was detected in more than 30,000 person-years of follow-up. Of note, better survival also was not observed in this study. Whether no survival benefits or harm despite excessive health care use reflects a balance between excess risk exposure and benefits of frequent health care visits is uncertain.

SUMMARY

This article summarizes the epidemiology of IBS. The emphasis is placed on population-based data because many people with IBS never seek health care, and no obvious diagnostic test exists for confirming this disease; therefore, symptom-based diagnostic criteria may be used.

Several surveys from a variety of Western and Asian populations have been done to assess the prevalence of this disorder. Rates have varied depending on the definition used, with Manning being the most generous definition. Overall, IBS affects about 10% of the population. The annual incidence rate of IBS is 200 per 100,000 people. Moreover, IBS frequently overlaps with other FGIDs, and symptoms change over time among FGIDs. However, studies of the natural history of IBS with overlapping FGIDs are still in their infancy, and better understanding of these will be important in determining the efficacy of future therapeutic interventions.

REFERENCES

1. Longstreth GF. Definition and classification of irritable bowel syndrome: current consensus and controversies. Gastroenterol Clin North Am 2005;34(2):173–87.
2. Thompson WG. Irritable bowel syndrome: pathogenesis and management. Lancet 1993;341(8860):1569–72.
3. Longstreth GF, Thompson WG, Chey WD, et al. Functional bowel disorders. Gastroenterology 2006;130(5):1480–91.
4. Talley NJ, Zinsmeister AR, Van Dyke C, et al. Epidemiology of colonic symptoms and the irritable bowel syndrome. Gastroenterology 1991;101(4):927–34.
5. Sandler RS. Epidemiology of irritable bowel syndrome in the United States. Gastroenterology 1990;99(2):409–15.
6. Drossman DA, Camilleri M, Mayer EA, et al. AGA technical review on irritable bowel syndrome. Gastroenterology 2002;123(6):2108–31.
7. Jones R, Lydeard S. Irritable bowel syndrome in the general population. Br Med J 1992;304(6819):87–90.

8. Kay L, Jorgensen T, Jensen KH. The epidemiology of irritable bowel syndrome in a random population: prevalence, incidence, natural history and risk factors. J Intern Med 1994;236(1):23–30.

9. Mearin F, Badia X, Balboa A, et al. Irritable bowel syndrome prevalence varies enormously depending on the employed diagnostic criteria: comparison of Rome II versus previous criteria in a general population. Scand J Gastroenterol 2001;36(11):1155–61.

10. Saito YA, Talley NJ, Melton LJ, et al. The effect of new diagnostic criteria for irritable bowel syndrome on community prevalence estimates. Neurogastroenterol Motil 2003;15(6):687–94.

11. Hillila MT, Farkkila MA. Prevalence of irritable bowel syndrome according to different diagnostic criteria in a non-selected adult population. Aliment Pharmacol Ther 2004;20(3):339–45.

12. Mearin F, Roset M, Badia X, et al. Splitting irritable bowel syndrome: from original Rome to Rome II criteria. Am J Gastroenterol 2004;99(1):122–30.

13. Hahn BA, Saunders WB, Maier WC. Differences between individuals with self-reported irritable bowel syndrome (IBS) and IBS-like symptoms. Dig Dis Sci 1997;42(12):2585–90.

14. Drossman DA, Li Z, Andruzzi E, et al. U.S. householder survey of functional gastrointestinal disorders. Prevalence, sociodemography, and health impact. Dig Dis Sci 1993;38(9):1569–80.

15. Saito YA, Locke GR, Talley NJ, et al. A comparison of the Rome and Manning criteria for case identification in epidemiological investigations of irritable bowel syndrome. Am J Gastroenterol 2000;95(10):2816–24.

16. Bommelaer G, Poynard T, Le Pen C, et al. Prevalence of irritable bowel syndrome (IBS) and variability of diagnostic criteria. Gastroenterol Clin Biol 2004;28 (6–7 Pt 1):554–61.

17. Thompson WG, Irvine EJ, Pare P, et al. Functional gastrointestinal disorders in Canada: first population-based survey using Rome II criteria with suggestions for improving the questionnaire. Dig Dis Sci 2002;47(1):225–35.

18. Boyce PM, Koloski NA, Talley NJ. Irritable bowel syndrome according to varying diagnostic criteria: are the new Rome II criteria unnecessarily restrictive for research and practice? Am J Gastroenterol 2000;95(11):3176–83.

19. Agreus L, Svardsudd K, Nyren O, et al. Irritable bowel syndrome and dyspepsia in the general population: overlap and lack of stability over time. Gastroenterology 1995;109(3):671–80.

20. Wilson S, Roberts L, Roalfe A, et al. Prevalence of irritable bowel syndrome: a community survey. Br J Gen Pract 2004;54(504):495–502.

21. Hungin AP, Whorwell PJ, Tack J, et al. The prevalence, patterns and impact of irritable bowel syndrome: an international survey of 40,000 subjects. Aliment Pharmacol Ther 2003;17(5):643–50.

22. Kennedy TM, Jones RH, Hungin AP, et al. Irritable bowel syndrome, gastro-oesophageal reflux, and bronchial hyper-responsiveness in the general population. Gut 1998;43(6):770–4.

23. Icks A, Haastert B, Enck P, et al. Prevalence of functional bowel disorders and related health care seeking: a population-based study. Z Gastroenterol 2002; 40(3):177–83.

24. Heaton KW, O'Donnell LJ, Braddon FE, et al. Symptoms of irritable bowel syndrome in a British urban community: consulters and nonconsulters. Gastroenterology 1992;102(6):1962–7.

25. Jung HK, Halder S, McNally M, et al. Overlap of gastro-oesophageal reflux disease and irritable bowel syndrome: prevalence and risk factors in the general population. Aliment Pharmacol Ther 2007;26(3):453–61.

26. Olafsdottir LB, Gudjonsson H, Jonsdottir HH, et al. Stability of the irritable bowel syndrome and subgroups as measured by three diagnostic criteria—a 10-year follow-up study. Aliment Pharmacol Ther 2010;32(5):670–80.

27. Saito YA, Schoenfeld P, Locke GR 3rd. The epidemiology of irritable bowel syndrome in North America: a systematic review. Am J Gastroenterol 2002; 97(8):1910–5.

28. Gwee KA, Wee S, Wong ML, et al. The prevalence, symptom characteristics, and impact of irritable bowel syndrome in an Asian urban community. Am J Gastroenterol 2004;99(5):924–31.

29. Xiong LS, Chen MH, Chen HX, et al. A population-based epidemiologic study of irritable bowel syndrome in South China: stratified randomized study by cluster sampling. Aliment Pharmacol Ther 2004;19(11):1217–24.

30. Lau EM, Chan FK, Ziea ET, et al. Epidemiology of irritable bowel syndrome in Chinese. Dig Dis Sci 2002;47(11):2621–4.

31. Ho KY, Kang JY, Seow A. Prevalence of gastrointestinal symptoms in a multiracial Asian population, with particular reference to reflux-type symptoms. Am J Gastroenterol 1998;93(10):1816–22.

32. Kwan AC, Hu WH, Chan YK, et al. Prevalence of irritable bowel syndrome in Hong Kong. J Gastroenterol Hepatol 2002;17(11):1180–6.

33. Danivat D, Tankeyoon M, Sriratanaban A. Prevalence of irritable bowel syndrome in a non-Western population. Br Med J (Clin Res Ed) 1988;296(6638):1710.

34. Masud MA, Hasan M, Khan AK. Irritable bowel syndrome in a rural community in Bangladesh: prevalence, symptoms pattern, and health care seeking behavior. Am J Gastroenterol 2001;96(5):1547–52.

35. Rajendra S, Alahuddin S. Prevalence of irritable bowel syndrome in a multi-ethnic Asian population. Aliment Pharmacol Ther 2004;19(6):704–6.

36. Ghoshal UC, Abraham P, Bhatt C, et al. Epidemiological and clinical profile of irritable bowel syndrome in India: report of the Indian Society of Gastroenterology Task Force. Indian J Gastroenterol 2008;27(1):22–8.

37. Han SH, Lee OY, Bae SC, et al. Prevalence of irritable bowel syndrome in Korea: population-based survey using the Rome II criteria. J Gastroenterol Hepatol 2006;21(11):1687–92.

38. Husain N, Chaudhry IB, Jafri F, et al. A population-based study of irritable bowel syndrome in a non-Western population. Neurogastroenterol Motil 2008;20(9):1022–9.

39. Lu CL, Chen CY, Lang HC, et al. Current patterns of irritable bowel syndrome in Taiwan: the Rome II questionnaire on a Chinese population. Aliment Pharmacol Ther 2003;18(11–12):1159–69.

40. Miwa H. Prevalence of irritable bowel syndrome in Japan: Internet survey using Rome III criteria. Patient Prefer Adherence 2008;2:143–7.

41. Sorouri M, Pourhoseingholi MA, Vahedi M, et al. Functional bowel disorders in Iranian population using Rome III criteria. Saudi J Gastroenterol 2010;16(3): 154–60.

42. Park DW, Lee OY, Shim SG, et al. The differences in prevalence and sociodemographic characteristics of irritable bowel syndrome according to Rome II and Rome III. J Neurogastroenterol Motil 2010;16(2):186–93.

43. Dong YY, Zuo XL, Li CQ, et al. Prevalence of irritable bowel syndrome in Chinese college and university students assessed using Rome III criteria. World J Gastroenterol 2010;16(33):4221–6.

44. Talley NJ, O'Keefe EA, Zinsmeister AR, et al. Prevalence of gastrointestinal symptoms in the elderly: a population-based study. Gastroenterology 1992;102(3): 895–901.

45. Guilera M, Balboa A, Mearin F. Bowel habit subtypes and temporal patterns in irritable bowel syndrome: systematic review. Am J Gastroenterol 2005;100(5): 1174–84.

46. Dorn SD, Morris CB, Hu Y, et al. Irritable bowel syndrome subtypes defined by Rome II and Rome III criteria are similar. J Clin Gastroenterol 2009;43(3):214–20.

47. Ersryd A, Posserud I, Abrahamsson H, et al. Subtyping the irritable bowel syndrome by predominant bowel habit: Rome II versus Rome III. Aliment Pharmacol Ther 2007;26(6):953–61.

48. Cremonini F, Talley NJ. Irritable bowel syndrome: epidemiology, natural history, health care seeking and emerging risk factors. Gastroenterol Clin North Am 2005;34(2):189–204.

49. Locke GR 3rd, Yawn BP, Wollan PC, et al. Incidence of a clinical diagnosis of the irritable bowel syndrome in a United States population. Aliment Pharmacol Ther 2004;19(9):1025–31.

50. Ruigomez A, Wallander MA, Johansson S, et al. One-year follow-up of newly diagnosed irritable bowel syndrome patients. Aliment Pharmacol Ther 1999; 13(8):1097–102.

51. Halder SL, Locke GR 3rd, Schleck CD, et al. Natural history of functional gastrointestinal disorders: a 12-year longitudinal population-based study. Gastroenterology 2007;133(3):799–807.

52. Thabane M, Kottachchi DT, Marshall JK. Systematic review and meta-analysis: The incidence and prognosis of post-infectious irritable bowel syndrome. Aliment Pharmacol Ther 2007;26(4):535–44.

53. Locke GR 3rd, Zinsmeister AR, Fett SL, et al. Overlap of gastrointestinal symptom complexes in a US community. Neurogastroenterol Motil 2005;17(1):29–34.

54. Koloski NA, Talley NJ, Boyce PM. Epidemiology and health care seeking in the functional GI disorders: a population-based study. Am J Gastroenterol 2002; 97(9):2290–9.

55. Corsetti M, Caenepeel P, Fischler B, et al. Impact of coexisting irritable bowel syndrome on symptoms and pathophysiological mechanisms in functional dyspepsia. Am J Gastroenterol 2004;99(6):1152–9.

56. Talley NJ, Holtmann G, Agreus L, et al. Gastrointestinal symptoms and subjects cluster into distinct upper and lower groupings in the community: a four nations study. Am J Gastroenterol 2000;95(6):1439–47.

57. Nastaskin I, Mehdikhani E, Conklin J, et al. Studying the overlap between IBS and GERD: a systematic review of the literature. Dig Dis Sci 2006;51(12):2113–20.

58. Ford AC, Marwaha A, Lim A, et al. Systematic review and meta-analysis of the prevalence of irritable bowel syndrome in individuals with dyspepsia. Clin Gastroenterol Hepatol 2010;8(5):401–9.

59. Levy RL, Whitehead WE, Von Korff MR, et al. Intergenerational transmission of gastrointestinal illness behavior. Am J Gastroenterol 2000;95(2):451–6.

60. Whitehead WE, Palsson OS, Levy RR, et al. Comorbidity in irritable bowel syndrome. Am J Gastroenterol 2007;102(12):2767–76.

61. Whitehead WE, Palsson O, Jones KR. Systematic review of the comorbidity of irritable bowel syndrome with other disorders: what are the causes and implications? Gastroenterology 2002;122(4):1140–56.

62. Henningsen P, Zipfel S, Herzog W. Management of functional somatic syndromes. Lancet 2007;369(9565):946–55.

63. Kroenke K. Physical symptom disorder: a simpler diagnostic category for somatization-spectrum conditions. J Psychosom Res 2006;60(4):335–9.
64. Waller SL, Misiewicz JJ. Prognosis in the irritable-bowel syndrome. A prospective study. Lancet 1969;2(7624):754–6.
65. Svendsen JH, Munck LK, Andersen JR. Irritable bowel syndrome—prognosis and diagnostic safety. A 5-year follow-up study. Scand J Gastroenterol 1985; 20(4):415–8.
66. Chaudhary NA, Truelove SC. The irritable colon syndrome. A study of the clinical features, predisposing causes, and prognosis in 130 cases. Q J Med 1962;31: 307–22.
67. Talley NJ, Weaver AL, Zinsmeister AR, et al. Onset and disappearance of gastro-intestinal symptoms and functional gastrointestinal disorders. Am J Epidemiol 1992;136(2):165–77.
68. Agreus L, Svardsudd K, Talley NJ, et al. Natural history of gastroesophageal reflux disease and functional abdominal disorders: a population-based study. Am J Gastroenterol 2001;96(10):2905–14.
69. El-Serag HB, Pilgrim P, Schoenfeld P. Systemic review: natural history of irritable bowel syndrome. Aliment Pharmacol Ther 2004;19(8):861–70.
70. Owens DM, Nelson DK, Talley NJ. The irritable bowel syndrome: long-term prognosis and the physician-patient interaction. Ann Intern Med 1995;122(2):107–12.
71. Chang JY, Locke GR 3rd, McNally MA, et al. Impact of functional gastrointestinal disorders on survival in the community. Am J Gastroenterol 2010;105(4):822–32.

The Effect of Irritable Bowel Syndrome on Health-Related Quality of Life and Health Care Expenditures

Nikhil Agarwal, MD, Brennan M.R. Spiegel, MD, MSHS*

KEYWORDS

• Irritable bowel syndrome • Health-related quality of life
• Health care expenditures

Irritable Bowel Syndrome (IBS) is a multisymptom condition defined by abdominal pain, abdominal discomfort, and abnormalities in stool form and frequency.[1] IBS is a highly prevalent condition that can affect patients physically, psychologically, socially, and economically. Understanding the IBS burden of illness serves several purposes. For patients, it emphasizes that they are not alone, and that many others suffer from IBS and share the same disease-related experiences. For health care providers, it offers an opportunity to improve their treatment of IBS patients, who comprise a large portion of their medical practice. By better understanding the IBS illness experience, providers are better equipped to intervene and implement treatments tailored to each patient's symptoms and health-related quality of life (HRQOL) decrement. For researchers and drug-approval authorities, IBS is approached as a condition with a prevalence and HRQOL impact that matches other major diagnoses such as diabetes, hypertension, or kidney disease.[2,3] For employers and health care insurers, the overwhelming direct and indirect expenditures related to IBS are revealed, providing a business rationale to ensure that IBS is treated effectively. This article will summarize data regarding the burden of illness of IBS, including: the prevalence of IBS and its subtypes, the age of onset and gender distribution, the effect on HRQOL, and the economic burden of IBS, including direct and indirect expenditures and related clinical predictors.

Department of Gastroenterology, Veterans Affairs Greater Los Angeles Healthcare System, David Geffen School of Medicine at University of California Los Angeles, 11301 Wilshire Boulevard, Building 115, Room 215, Los Angeles, CA 90073, USA
* Corresponding author.
E-mail address: bspiegel@mednet.ucla.edu

Gastroenterol Clin N Am 40 (2011) 11–19
doi:10.1016/j.gtc.2010.12.013
0889-8553/11/$ – see front matter. Published by Elsevier Inc.

PREVALENCE OF IBS

It is estimated that the prevalence of IBS in North America and Europe ranges from 1% to over 20%.[4,5] This wide range indicates that IBS prevalence depends on many variables, including the case-finding definition employed (eg, Manning criteria vs Rome criteria), the characteristics of the source population (eg, primary care vs specialty clinic), and the study methods and sampling frame of the studies. To refine the prevalence estimate, it is worth evaluating the studies that specifically employ consensus-based Rome definitions (the gold standard) and draw upon patients from the general adult community (ie, not exclusively from primary or specialty care). Four eligible studies evaluating 32,638 North American subjects meet these criteria.[6–9] When comparing these studies, the IBS prevalence varied from 5% to 10%, with a pooled prevalence of 7% (95% confidence interval [CI] 6% to 8%).[6–9] Previous reviews indicate that IBS patients are divided evenly among the three major subgroups (IBS-diarrhea, IBS-constipation, and IBS-mixed).[10] However, the true prevalence of IBS subtypes in North America remains unclear; one study suggested that IBS with diarrhea is the most common subtype,[7] whereas another indicated that mixed-type IBS is most common.[8]

DEMOGRAPHIC PREDICTORS OF IBS

Demographic predictors of IBS include gender, age, and socioeconomic status. The odds of having IBS are higher in women than men (pooled odds ratio [OR] 1.46; 95% CI 1.13 to 1.88).[6–9] However, IBS is now recognized to be a key component of the Gulf War syndrome, a multisymptom complex affecting soldiers (a predominantly male population was engaged in the Gulf War).[11–13] Patients under the age of 50 years are more commonly diagnosed with IBS, although 2% to 6% of patients are 50 years or older.[6–8] These data suggest that the pretest likelihood for IBS is higher in younger patients, but that patients of all ages may be diagnosed with the condition. This review identified two studies that report IBS prevalence by income strata,[7,9] both of which revealed a graded decrease in IBS prevalence with increasing income. Eight percent to 16% of people earning less than $20,000 annually carry the diagnosis, compared with only 3% to 5% of people earning greater than $75,000.[6,8]

HRQOL OF IBS

Several studies have compared HRQOL in IBS patients with HRQOL in healthy controls or patients with non-IBS medical disorders, and these have been summarized in a previous systematic review.[2] Data consistently reveal that patients with IBS score lower on all 8 scales of the SF-36 HRQOL questionnaire compared with normal non-IBS cohorts. IBS patients have the same physical HRQOL as patients with diabetes, and a lower physical HRQOL compared with patients who have depression or gastroesophageal reflux disease.[2,3] Also, mental HRQOL scores on the SF-36 were lower in patients with IBS than in those with chronic renal failure, an organic condition characterized by considerable physical and psychological disability. The health utility of severe IBS, where utility is a measure of HRQOL on a scale of 0 (death) to 1 (perfect health), was found to be 0.7.[14] This utility is similar to that of Class 3 congestive heart failure (CHF) and rheumatoid arthritis.[14]

This HRQOL decrement in IBS patients can be severe enough to raise the risk of suicidal behavior is some cases.[15,16] The relationship between IBS and suicidality appears to be independent of comorbid psychiatric diseases such as depression. However, studies examining this relationship were performed in tertiary care referral populations. Therefore, the HRQOL decrement and suicidality risk documented in these cohorts may not be applicable to community-based populations. Regardless, IBS unquestionably has a negative impact on HRQOL, and failing to recognize this impact could undermine the physician–patient relationship and lead to dissatisfaction with care. Given that HRQOL decrements are common in IBS, it is recommended that routine screening for diminished HRQOL in IBS patients be performed. Treatment of IBS should be initiated when the symptoms are found to reduce functional status and diminish overall HRQOL. Furthermore, clinicians should remain alert to the potential for suicidal behavior in patients with severe IBS symptoms, and initiate timely interventions if suicide forerunners are identified.

Accurate measurement of HRQOL requires a thorough and often time-consuming evaluation of biologic, psychologic, and social health domains. In the setting of a busy outpatient clinic, this may be a practical limitation. To help providers gain better insight into their patients' HRQOL, a concise list of factors known to predict HRQOL in IBS might be helpful, which providers then could use to question patients routinely in a timely manner. Several studies have identified predictors of HRQOL in IBS,[17–20] the most consistent of which is the severity of the predominant bowel symptom. Data from several studies indicate that in patients with IBS, HRQOL decreases in parallel with increasing symptom severity.[18,19,21] Therefore, it is important to identify and gauge the severity of the predominant symptom of patients with IBS. Studies have shown that the impact of physical HRQOL symptoms in IBS is associated with an increase in the duration of symptom flares and the presence of abdominal pain (as opposed to discomfort).[19] Mental HRQOL symptoms are associated with abnormalities in sexuality, mood, and anxiety.[19] Each of these domains shares a common association with symptoms of chronic stress and vital exhaustion, including tiring easily, feeling low in energy, and experiencing sleep difficulties.[19] Patients acknowledge that these symptoms prompt avoidance of socially vulnerable situations (eg, being away from restrooms) and activities (eg, eating out for dinner). In contrast, HRQOL is not strongly determined by the presence of specific gastrointestinal (GI) symptoms (eg, diarrhea, constipation, bloating, dyspepsia), degree of previous GI evaluation (eg, previous flexible sigmoidoscopy or colonoscopy), or common demographic characteristics (eg, gender, age, marital status).[19]

These findings suggest that in addition to the physiologic epiphenomena used to gauge HRQOL (eg, stool frequency, stool characteristics, subtype of IBS), it may be more efficient to assess HRQOL by gauging global symptom severity, addressing symptom-related fears and concerns, and identifying and eliminating factors contributing to vital exhaustion in IBS. This process may occur through teaching coping mechanisms and relaxation skills, developing a greater sense of self-efficacy by encouraging control over IBS symptoms, promoting lifestyle modifications to reduce symptoms (ie, diet, exercise, quitting smoking), and encouraging patients to recognize their own limitations. When combined with standard medical therapies, these approaches yield improved overall HRQOL.[20,22,23] In short, treating bowel-related symptoms of IBS is important, but may not be sufficient, to impact overall HRQOL. In addition to treating symptoms, providers should attempt to positively modify the cognitive interpretation of IBS symptoms (ie, acknowledge and address the emotional context in which symptoms occur).

MEASURING HRQOL IN IBS

Measuring HRQOL can provide useful information for various clinical and research purposes. For example, it can provide insight not only to a patient's physical symptoms and burden of illness, but also provide information about emotional well being, social functioning, and other emotions and behaviors. Originally, the SF-36 question-naire was used to measure HRQOL in IBS patients. However, given that the SF-36 is a generic instrument, the need for a syndrome-specific questionnaire arose. Multiple IBS-targeted HRQOL questionnaires have been developed and validated including the IBS-QOL,[24–26] IBSQOL, and IBS HRQOL. **Table 1** shows these instruments in comparison to the generic SF-36 questionnaire. The information provided across HRQOL domains could be useful to develop targeted therapy. For example, if an IBS patient has a low HRQOL related to poor emotional well being as measured by the IBS-QOL, then the clinician might address coping mechanisms or initiate pharma-cotherapy with a selective serotonin reuptake inhibitor (SSRI) based on this information.

None of these interventions can occur if providers fail to measure overall HRQOL. Administering a full HRQOL instruments would provide abundant, useful information; however, it may not be practical in a busy clinic. To assist with clinic-based HRQOL assessments, a short HRQOL questionnaire has been developed specifically for use in everyday clinical practice. The idea is that the questionnaire can be administered in the waiting room, and a nurse can quickly score the results and put it on the doctor's intake sheet like a vital sign. This type of information may be much more valuable in IBS than the typical vital signs, like temperature, blood pressure, heart rate, and respiratory rate. Based on previous research, including interviews with patients, experts, and the authors' own database studies, the authors created a questionnaire with only 4 questions, which is shown in **Fig. 1**.[27] Most patients fill out the questionnaire in less than 1 minute, and a nurse can score it in under 30 seconds using a simple algorithm. The score ranges between 0 and 100, where 100 is the worst score, and 0 is the best score. This questionnaire is called the BEST

Table 1
Comparative properties of disease-targeted HRQOL measures in IBS

Scales	HRQOL Measures			
	SF-36	IBS-QOL	IBSQOL	IBS-HRQOL
Physical functioning	10	7	3	6
Physical role limitations	4	0	3	0
Bodily pain	2	0	0	0
General health perception	5	0	0	0
Energy/fatigue	4	0	3	6
Social functioning	2	7	3	0
Emotional role limitations	4	0	3	0
Emotional well being	5	8	3	6
Sexual function	0	2	3	0
Food avoidance	0	3	3	0
Health worry	0	3	3	0
Body image	0	4	0	0
Bowel symptoms	0	0	0	8
Sleep	0	0	3	0

Measures are listed in reference to their included scales and are presented in comparison with the generic SF-36 health survey. Numbers indicate the item total in each subscale.
Abbreviations: HRQOL, health-related quality of life; IBS, irritable bowel syndrome.

How bad have your bowel symptoms been, on average, over the last 4 weeks?

___ **None**: No symptoms

___ **Mild**: symptoms can be ignored

___ **Moderate**: symptoms cannot be ignored

___ **Severe**: symptoms affect your lifestyle

___ **Very Severe**: symptoms markedly affect lifestyle

Consider the following statement: *"I feel like my bowel symptoms mean there is something seriously wrong with my body."*

Does this statement describe the way you have felt over the past 4 weeks?

___ No, not at all

___ Yes, slightly

___ Yes, somewhat

___ Yes, quite a bit

___ Yes, a great deal

How frequently have your bowel symptoms made you feel tense or "wound up" over the past 4 weeks?

___ Most of the time

___ A lot of the time

___ From time to time, occasionally

___ Not at all

Consider the following statement: *"Because of my bowel symptoms, I can no longer enjoy the things I used to enjoy."*

Does this statement describe the way you have felt over the past 4 weeks?

___ No, not at all

___ Yes, slightly

___ Yes, somewhat

___ Yes, quite a bit

___ Yes, a great deal

Fig. 1. The BEST Questionnaire to measure health-related quality of life in the office setting. The answers to these questions can be scored along a scale from 0 (best) to 100 (worst) using a standard scoring algorithm, and the score can be given to the doctor as a sort of snapshot vital sign for how the patient is feeling. This information might help direct the doctor to help make treatment decision, and is designed to provide information that many doctors fail to obtain during a standard patient interview.

score, because the 4 questions spell out BEST (not necessarily because this is the best way to measure HRQOL):

"How Bad are your bowel symptoms?"
"Can you still Enjoy the things you used to enjoy?"
"Do you feel like your bowel symptoms mean there's something Seriously wrong?"
"Do your bowel symptoms make you feel Tense?"

Data indicate that the BEST score is an excellent stand-in for the IBS-QOL, a highly validated research questionnaire that is useful for research purposes, but onerous for everyday clinical practice (**Fig. 2**).[27] The data suggest that BEST could provide a quick snap-shot of overall HRQOL without having to burden the patient with multiple or long

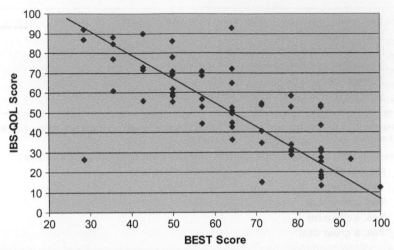

Fig. 2. The 4-question BEST score compared with the 34-question irritable bowel syndrome quality of life (IBS-QOL) score. These data are from a study of 58 people with IBS designed to evaluate their BEST scores compared with their IBS-QOL scores. The graph shows that as the BEST increases, the IBS-QOL score decreases, and that the 2 are closely related. This suggests that the BEST score, which was purposefully designed to be used in the office setting, could possibly be used as a stand-in for the longer IBS-QOL for doctors who are otherwise unwilling to use longer research-oriented questionnaires in their office. (*From* Spiegel BMR, Naliboff, Mayer E, et al. Development and initial validation of a concise point-of-care IBS severity index: the 4-item BEST questionnaire. Gastroenterology 2006;130:S1040.)

questionnaires. Future research will aim to better understand how this score works over multiple follow-up visits, and to better understand how having this information can improve not only provider decision-making, but also the overall patient–provider relationship.

Ultimately, the purpose of having questionnaires like BEST is to improve patient care by bridging the gap between providers and their patients. If doctors can learn what questions to ask, and if patients can provide the right information, then this exchange might be more valuable than any vital sign or individual symptoms.

RESOURCE USE IN IBS

Patients with IBS consume a disproportionate amount of resources. Burden of illness studies estimate that there are 3.6 million physician visits in the United States annually for IBS, and that IBS care consumes over $20 billion in both direct and indirect expenditures.[28] Moreover, patients with IBS consume over 50% more health care resources than matched controls without IBS.[29,30] These data suggest that the economic burden of IBS stems not only from the high prevalence of the disease, but also from the disproportionate use of resources it causes.

Despite the implementation and use of guidelines reinforcing these data,[10] much of the cost of care in IBS arises from sequential and redundant diagnostic tests, invasive procedures, and abdominal operations.[31] For example, patients with IBS are three times more likely than matched controls to undergo cholecystectomy[31,32] despite knowledge that IBS symptoms will almost invariably persist following the surgery. Similarly, nearly 25% of colonoscopies performed in patients younger than 50 years of age are for IBS symptoms.[33] Yet data indicate that colonoscopy has a low diagnostic yield in IBS, and that negative examinations fail to improve intestinal symptoms, do not augment HRQOL, and are unlikely to provide additional reassurance compared with not performing colonoscopy.[34,35] Resource use in IBS is also driven by the presence of comorbid somatization, a trait found in up to one-third of IBS patients that is characterized by the propensity to overinterpret normal physiologic processes.[36,37] Patients with somatization typically report a barrage of seemingly unrelated physical complaints (eg, back pain, tingling, headaches, temporomandibular joint pain, muscle aches) that may, in fact, be linked to underlying psychosocial distress.[36,37] These patients are sometimes misclassified as having several underlying organic conditions, and subsequently undergo sequential diagnostic tests in chase of the symptoms.[38] There is a linear and highly significant relationship between levels of somatization and the amount of diagnostic testing in IBS, suggesting that providers should remain aware of somatization in IBS, and aggressively treat or refer somatization patients to an experienced specialist rather than performing potentially unnecessary diagnostic tests.[38]

In addition to direct costs of care, IBS patients engender significant indirect costs of care as a consequence of both missing work and suffering impaired work performance while on the job. Employees with IBS are absent 3% to 5% of the workweek, and report impaired productivity 26% to 31% of the week,[39–41] rates that exceed those of non-IBS control employees by 20%.[40] This is equivalent to 14 hours of lost productivity per 40-hour workweek. Compared with IBS patients who exhibit normal work productivity, patients with impaired productivity have more extraintestinal comorbidities (eg, chronic fatigue syndrome, fibromyalgia, interstitial cystitis), and more disease-specific fears and concerns.[41] In contrast, the specific profile of individual bowel symptoms do not undermine work productivity,[41] suggesting that enhancing work productivity in patients with IBS may require treatments that improve both GI and non-GI symptom frequency and intensity, while also modifying the cognitive and behavioral responses to bowel symptoms and the contexts in which they occur. In other words, it may be inadequate to treat bowel symptoms alone without simultaneously addressing the emotional context in which the symptoms occur.

IBS BURDEN OF ILLNESS: SUMMARY

Overall, data indicate that IBS is a common condition with a large health economic burden of illness marked by HRQOL decrements, diminished work productivity, and high expenditures. Clinicians should routinely screen for diminished HRQOL by performing a balanced biopsychosocial history rather than focusing just on bowel symptoms. HRQOL decrements should be acknowledged and addressed when making treatment decisions. Patients with severe HRQOL decrements should be screened for suicidal ideation, and identification of suicide forerunners must prompt timely intervention and appropriate referral. When faced with IBS patients reporting multiple and seemingly unrelated somatic complaints, clinicians should consider the possibility of underlying somatization, and should aim to address somatization in lieu of performing costly and potentially unhelpful tests, procedures, and operations.

REFERENCES

1. Longstreth GF, Thompson WG, Chey WD, et al. Functional bowel disorders. Gastroenterology 2006;130:1480–91.
2. El-Serag HB, Olden K, Bjorkman D. Health-related quality of life among persons with irritable bowel syndrome: a systematic review. Aliment Pharmacol Ther 2002; 16:1171–85.

3. Gralnek IM, Hays RD, Kilbourne A, et al. The impact of irritable bowel syndrome on health-related quality of life. Gastroenterology 2000;119:654–60.
4. Saito YA, Schoenfeld P, Locke GR 3rd. The epidemiology of irritable bowel syndrome in North America: a systematic review. Am J Gastroenterol 2002;97: 1910–5.
5. Systematic review on the management of irritable bowel syndrome in the European Union. Eur J Gastroenterol Hepatol 2007;19(Suppl 1):S11–37.
6. Saito YA, Talley NJ, Melton LJ, et al. The effect of new diagnostic criteria for irritable bowel syndrome on community prevalence estimates. Neurogastroenterol Motil 2003;15:687–94.
7. Andrews EB, Eaton SC, Hollis KA, et al. Prevalence and demographics of irritable bowel syndrome: results from a large Web-based survey. Aliment Pharmacol Ther 2005;22:935–42.
8. Hungin AP, Chang L, Locke GR, et al. Irritable bowel syndrome in the United States: prevalence, symptom patterns, and impact. Aliment Pharmacol Ther 2005;21:1365–75.
9. Minocha A, Johnson WD, Abell TL, et al. Prevalence, sociodemography, and quality of life of older versus younger patients with irritable bowel syndrome: a population-based study. Dig Dis Sci 2006;51:446–53.
10. Brandt LJ, Chey WD, Foxx-Orenstein AE, et al. An evidence-based position statement on the management of irritable bowel syndrome. Am J Gastroenterol 2009; 104(Suppl 1):S1–35.
11. Dunphy RC, Bridgewater L, Price DD, et al. Visceral and cutaneous hypersensitivity in Persian Gulf War veterans with chronic gastrointestinal symptoms. Pain 2003;102:79–85.
12. Gray GC, Reed RJ, Kaiser KS, et al. Self-reported symptoms and medical conditions among 11,868 Gulf War-era veterans: the Seabee Health Study. Am J Epidemiol 2002;155:1033–44.
13. Hunt SC, Richardson RD. Chronic multisystem illness among Gulf War veterans. JAMA 1999;282:327–8 [author reply: 328–9].
14. Spiegel B, Harris L, Lucak S, et al. Developing valid and reliable health utilities in irritable bowel syndrome: results from the IBS PROOF Cohort. Am J Gastroenterol 2009;104:1984–91.
15. Miller V, Hopkins L, Whorwell PJ. Suicidal ideation in patients with irritable bowel syndrome. Clin Gastroenterol Hepatol 2004;2:1064–8.
16. Spiegel B, Schoenfeld P, Naliboff B. Systematic review: the prevalence of suicidal behaviour in patients with chronic abdominal pain and irritable bowel syndrome. Aliment Pharmacol Ther 2007;26:183–93.
17. Hahn BA, Kirchdoerfer LJ, Fullerton S, et al. Patient-perceived severity of irritable bowel syndrome in relation to symptoms, health resource utilization, and quality of life. Aliment Pharmacol Ther 1997;11:553–9.
18. Naliboff BD, Balice G, Mayer EA. Psychosocial moderators of quality of life in irritable bowel syndrome. Eur J Surg Suppl 1998;583:57–9.
19. Spiegel BM, Gralnek IM, Bolus R, et al. Clinical determinants of health-related quality of life in patients with irritable bowel syndrome. Arch Intern Med 2004; 164:1773–80.
20. van der Veek PP, van Rood YR, Masclee AA. Clinical trial: short- and long-term benefit of relaxation training for irritable bowel syndrome. Aliment Pharmacol Ther 2007;26:943–52.
21. Lembo A, Ameen VZ, Drossman DA. Irritable bowel syndrome: toward an understanding of severity. Clin Gastroenterol Hepatol 2005;3:717–25.

22. Shaw G, Srivastava ED, Sadlier M, et al. Stress management for irritable bowel syndrome: a controlled trial. Digestion 1991;50:36–42.
23. Spiegel BMR, Naliboff B, Mayer E, et al. The effectiveness of a model physician–patient relationship versus usual care in irritable bowel syndrome: a randomized controlled trial. Gastroenterology 2006;130:A773.
24. Patrick DL, Drossman DA. Comparison of IBS-36 and IBS-QOL instruments. Am J Gastroenterol 2002;97:3204 [author reply: 3204–5].
25. Patrick DL, Drossman DA, Frederick IO, et al. Quality of life in persons with irritable bowel syndrome: development and validation of a new measure. Dig Dis Sci 1998;43:400–11.
26. Drossman DA, Patrick DL, Whitehead WE, et al. Further validation of the IBS-QOL: a disease-specific quality-of-life questionnaire. Am J Gastroenterol 2000; 95:999–1007.
27. Spiegel BMR, Naliboff, Mayer E, et al. Development and initial validation of a concise point-of-care IBS severity index: the 4-item BEST questionnaire. Gastroenterology 2006;130:S1040.
28. Everhart JE, Ruhl CE. Burden of digestive diseases in the United States part 2: lower gastrointestinal diseases. Gastroenterology 2009;136(3):741–54.
29. Talley NJ, Gabriel SE, Harmsen WS, et al. Medical costs in community subjects with irritable bowel syndrome. Gastroenterology 1995;109:1736–41.
30. Longstreth GF, Wilson A, Knight K, et al. Irritable bowel syndrome, health care use, and costs: a US managed care perspective. Am J Gastroenterol 2003;98:600–7.
31. Longstreth GF. Avoiding unnecessary surgery in irritable bowel syndrome. Gut 2007;56:608–10.
32. Longstreth GF, Yao JF. Irritable bowel syndrome and surgery: a multivariable analysis. Gastroenterology 2004;126:1665–73.
33. Lieberman DA, Holub J, Eisen G, et al. Utilization of colonoscopy in the United States: results from a national consortium. Gastrointest Endosc 2005;62:875–83.
34. Spiegel BM, Gralnek IM, Bolus R, et al. Is a negative colonoscopy associated with reassurance or improved health-related quality of life in irritable bowel syndrome? Gastrointest Endosc 2005;62:892–9.
35. Chey WD, Nojkov B, Rubenstein JH, et al. The yield of colonoscopy in patients with nonconstipated irritable bowel syndrome: results from a prospective, controlled US trial. Am J Gastroenterol 2010;105:859–65.
36. Whitehead WE, Palsson O, Jones KR. Systematic review of the comorbidity of irritable bowel syndrome with other disorders: what are the causes and implications? Gastroenterology 2002;122:1140–56.
37. Miller AR, North CS, Clouse RE, et al. The association of irritable bowel syndrome and somatization disorder. Ann Clin Psychiatry 2001;13:25–30.
38. Spiegel BM, Kanwal F, Naliboff B, et al. The impact of somatization on the use of gastrointestinal health care resources in patients with irritable bowel syndrome. Am J Gastroenterol 2005;100:2262–73.
39. Pare P, Gray J, Lam S, et al. Health-related quality of life, work productivity, and health care resource utilization of subjects with irritable bowel syndrome: baseline results from LOGIC (Longitudinal Outcomes Study of Gastrointestinal Symptoms in Canada), a naturalistic study. Clin Ther 2006;28:1726–35 [discussion: 1710–1].
40. Dean BB, Aguilar D, Barghout V, et al. Impairment in work productivity and health-related quality of life in patients with IBS. Am J Manag Care 2005;11:S17–26.
41. Spiegel BMR, Harris L, Lucak S, et al. Predictors of work productivity in irritable bowel syndrome (IBS): results from the PROOF cohort. Gastroenterology 2008; 134:AB157.

Traditional Thoughts on the Pathophysiology of Irritable Bowel Syndrome

William L. Hasler, MD

KEYWORDS

- Pathophysiology • Irritable bowel syndrome • Sensory function
- Psychosocial disturbances

Although much research over the past decade has focused on pathogenic roles of inflammation or altered enteric microbiota in irritable bowel syndrome (IBS), an enormous body of literature published beginning in the 1940s has extensively characterized traditional factors believed to be involved in the genesis of symptoms, including motor, sensory, central nervous system (CNS), and psychological abnormalities. More recent investigations using modern methods and studying IBS subsets well defined by validated clinical surveys have provided more detailed delineation of peripheral sensorimotor and central factors in relation to dominant symptom profiles. Because IBS is a heterogeneous disorder, it is likely that these distinct traditional factors participate to varying degrees in different patients. Furthermore, it is probable that many of the novel pathogenic inflammatory or infectious factors currently being studied also elicit symptoms by influencing gut motor and sensory function or information processing in the CNS.

MOTOR DYSFUNCTION

Disturbances of motor activity in several gastrointestinal and extraintestinal sites have been characterized in the different IBS subtypes; however, their roles in symptom pathogenesis for the most part are unproved. Several mediators have been proposed to contribute to motor dysfunction in IBS.

Small Intestinal Motor Abnormalities

Small intestinal motor function frequently is disturbed in IBS; however, the relevance of these defects to symptom induction is unproved. Small intestinal transit is generally

---

Disclosures: Dr Hasler has no conflicts of interest to report.
Division of Gastroenterology, University of Michigan Health System, 3912 Taubman Center, 5362, Ann Arbor, MI 48109, USA
E-mail address: whasler@umich.edu

reported as delayed in patients with constipation-predominant IBS (C-IBS) and accelerated in patients with diarrhea-predominant (D-IBS), although some large studies have not observed this association.[1] On magnetic resonance imaging (MRI), orocecal transit is accelerated in D-IBS, with associated reductions in terminal ileal diameter, possibly reflecting increased intestinal tone.[2] Likewise, ileocolonic transit measured scintigraphically is accelerated postprandially in D-IBS.[3]

Abnormalities of phasic small bowel contractile activity have been characterized in different subtypes of IBS. During fasting, a stereotypic pattern known as the migrating motor complex (MMC) cycles every 90 to 120 minutes to clear the proximal gut of undigested food residue. After consuming a caloric meal, small bowel motility converts to a fed pattern characterized by irregular phasic contractions that persist for up to 4 hours. Decreases in MMC amplitude and prolonged periodicity in patients with C-IBS and reductions in MMC cycle length in D-IBS have been reported.[4,5] MMC propagation velocities reportedly are accelerated in IBS. Exaggerated jejunal fed responses, including increases in postprandial contractile frequencies, are seen in some patients with IBS although some studies have observed reduced fed amplitudes in C-IBS.[4,5] In both subtypes, the duration of the fed pattern is shorter than in healthy controls.[5] Retrograde duodenal and jejunal contractions are prominent in many patients with IBS, especially postprandially, and are reported to correlate with diarrhea in some cases.[6] Discrete clustered contractions consisting of bursts of phasic contractions occurring every minute in the duodenum or jejunum, and prolonged propagated contractions consisting of intense ileal complexes that evacuate the ileum, may occur more commonly in patients with IBS than in healthy volunteers.[4,5] In some individuals, clustered contractions and prolonged propagated small intestinal contractions are associated with symptom exacerbations.[4,5] However, such clusters also are observed in other gut motor disorders such as chronic intestinal pseudoobstruction (CIP) and in healthy individuals, indicating that these patterns are not specific for IBS.[7] The report of small bowel myenteric neuronal damage in individuals with severe IBS raises the possibility that some cases may fall along a spectrum that includes conditions with greater morbidity such as CIP.[8] Small intestinal phasic contractile responses to other stimuli also may be modified in IBS. Cholecystokinin evokes high-amplitude ileal contractions in patients with D-IBS, whereas neostigmine induces discrete clustered contractions in both IBS subtypes. Conversely, reductions in duodenal motor responses to colonic distention are blunted in IBS.

Colonic Motor Abnormalities

Colonic motor abnormalities are prevalent in IBS, but correlate imperfectly with symptomatic bowel disturbances. In general, colon transit is accelerated in D-IBS and delayed in C-IBS.[9-11] However, recent surveys observed abnormal colon transit in only 30% and 32% of patients with functional gastrointestinal disorders.[1,12] Symptoms correlating with colonic transit in IBS include abnormalities of stool form, frequency, and ease of passage.[13]

IBS has been associated with altered colonic myoelectric activity as well as phasic and tonic contractile function. In contrast to the stomach and small intestine, the colon shows no dominant myoelectric pacemaker activity. Rather, short spike bursts of 5 to 15 seconds underlie short-duration mixing contractions, whereas long spike bursts 15 to 60 seconds in duration are associated with contractions that show some propulsive characteristics. Early investigations observing abnormal 3-cycle-per-minute myoelectric rhythms in IBS were not confirmed by subsequent studies; such dysrhythmias instead were attributed to psychiatric factors in affected patients.[14,15] High-amplitude propagated contractions (HAPCs) occurring infrequently throughout the day produce propulsive mass fecal movements, including those that precede defecation. In some older studies, no differences in phasic colonic motility were observed between patients with IBS and healthy controls. However, using wireless motility capsules, increases in colonic contractile activity were noted in C-IBS compared with healthy controls that are greater in the latter phases of colonic transit (**Fig. 1**).[16] Other recent investigations observe that patients with D-IBS have more frequent HAPCs versus healthy volunteers, whereas patients with C-IBS show fewer such complexes.[9,10,17] In 1 investigation, 90% of HAPCs were associated with painful episodes.[17] Others also have correlated HAPCs with pain reports.[18] In normal volunteers, meal ingestion evokes increased myoelectric and motor activity, known as the gastrocolonic response, which peaks 20 to 30 minutes after eating. Patients with IBS may show exaggerated gastrocolonic responses lasting up to 3 hours, especially after high-fat meals.[14,17,19] Rectal compliance has been reported to be reduced in some but not all studies in IBS.[9,20–22] Colon tone in IBS measured by barostat methods is increased at baseline, is either unaffected or reduced after meal ingestion, and is blunted in response to colonic distention.[23,24] One recent study observed a caloric dependence to abnormal tonic responses to meals in D-IBS, with reduced tone with 250-kcal meals and normalization of the response after consuming 1000 kcal of nutrients.[23] As in the small bowel, IBS is associated with exaggerated colon motor responsiveness to exogenous stimulation, including abnormally prolonged and intense colonic contractions after colorectal balloon inflation, cholinergic stimulation, cholecystokinin administration, and colonic perfusion of deoxycholic acid.[9,17,24] Recent investigations suggest evidence of dyssynergic defecation in some C-IBS cases, with affected patients having prolonged balloon expulsion times.[25] This finding raises the possibility that many of the distal gut symptomatic and functional disturbances in IBS may relate to anorectal outlet dysfunction rather than colon wall abnormalities.

Motor Abnormalities in Other Regions

IBS also is associated with motor dysfunction of other gut and extraintestinal regions. Decreased lower esophageal sphincter pressures and abnormal esophageal body

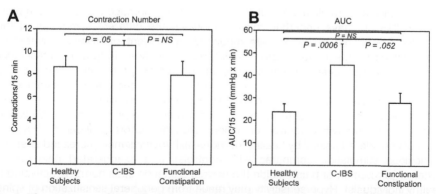

Fig. 1. The mean numbers (A) and areas under the pressure (AUC) values (B) of colon contractions less than 25 mm Hg in amplitude per 15 minutes of recording time are compared in healthy individuals, individuals with C-IBS, and individuals with functional constipation not meeting criteria for C-IBS. Numbers of colon contractions and AUC values were significantly greater in the C-IBS subset compared with healthy individuals. (*From* Hasler WL, Saad RJ, Rao SS, et al. Heightened colon motor activity measured by a wireless capsule in patients with constipation: relation to colon transit and IBS. Am J Physiol Gastrointest Liver Physiol 2009;297:G1111; with permission.)

contractions are found in some patients with IBS.[26] Delays in gastric emptying and gastric slow-wave dysrhythmias (tachygastria and bradygastria) and impaired slow-wave amplitude responses to meals are prevalent, especially in those with C-IBS and/or associated dyspepsia.[27,28] In addition, gastric-emptying impairments have been correlated with small bowel motility disruption in IBS.[27] Biliary tract abnormalities associated with IBS include impaired gallbladder emptying and sphincter of Oddi dysfunction with impaired sphincter relaxation in response to cholecystokinin stimulation. Outside the gastrointestinal tract, detrusor instability of the bladder and airway hyperreactivity to methacholine have been associated with IBS, suggesting the presence of a generalized dysfunction of smooth-muscle structures.

Possible Mediators of Motor Dysfunction

Several neurohumoral factors have been proposed to contribute to motor dysfunction in IBS. Serotonin (5-hydroxytryptamine [5-HT]) pathways play important roles in modulating gut motility, including elicitation of the peristaltic reflex. Platelet-depleted plasma 5-HT levels are increased in those with D-IBS, especially in men, and correlate positively with increased sigmoid colon contractility, but are decreased in C-IBS.[29] Likewise, the ratio of plasma 5-HT to 5-hydroxyindole acetic acid, a 5-HT metabolite, is increased in D-IBS, whereas small bowel mucosal 5-HT levels are reduced in C-IBS. As another measure of altered 5-HT metabolism, women with IBS have abnormal plasma kynurenine to tryptophan ratios, which relate to symptom severity.[30] Blood and tissue levels of other selected neuropeptides have been related to the presence of IBS. Patients with IBS show increased sigmoid colon and plasma cholecystokinin and vasoactive intestinal polypeptide levels and lower leptin levels. Neuropeptide Y levels in the plasma are lower in patients with D-IBS versus those with C-IBS; urinary levels of the melatonin metabolite 6-sulfatoxymelatonin are reduced in C-IBS, especially in men. Despite the observed associations, none of these neurohumoral factors has proved to be causative of any symptom profile in IBS.

ALTERED VISCERAL SENSORY ACTIVITY

As with motor abnormalities, alterations in visceral and somatic perception are prevalent in IBS but have uncertain roles in inducing the different symptoms of this disorder. Abdominal sensations are mediated by afferent pathways activated by stimuli acting on mechanoreceptors (which detect changes in tension), mesenteric nociceptors (which detect painful stimuli), and chemoreceptors (which sense osmolarity, temperature, and pH). Information from these receptors is transmitted by afferent pathways to the brain, where conscious perception occurs. Hypersensitivity may present as hyperalgesia (an increase in pain intensity reporting for a given painful stimulus compared with a control population), allodynia (reporting of pain from a stimulus not considered painful by healthy individuals), hypervigilance (increased attention to noxious stimulation compared with controls), and exaggerated pain referral patterns (perception of pain outside the normal anatomic sites normally activated in healthy individuals). Hypersensitivity may result from peripheral sensitization of spinal dorsal horn neurons or abnormal CNS processing of afferent information projecting from the gut.[31]

Visceral Sensory Dysfunction

Some patients with IBS experience normal physiologic events, not normally perceived by healthy individuals, as being uncomfortable or painful. Examples of this phenomenon include the observations that patients with IBS can sense different phases of the MMC, feel discomfort during passage of food residue from the ileum to the cecum, and experience pain during prolonged propagated contractions and discrete clustered contractions in the small intestine and HAPCs in the colon.[4,5,17,32]

Exaggerated perception is inducible by visceral stimulation in substantial percentages of patients with IBS. Most studies report that pain is experienced at lower volumes or pressures of rectal or ileal balloon inflation in patients with IBS than healthy controls, an effect not caused by altered visceral wall properties.[9,21,33–36] Some investigators report that hypersensitivity is specific for abrupt phasic distentions and that perception of a slow ramplike inflation is normal in IBS.[34] The degree of heightened sensation has been noted to be greater in women than men.[37] Increases in sensitivity to distention of more proximal gut regions also are observed in some patients with IBS, including the esophagus, stomach, and small bowel. Those with symptoms referable to multiple gut regions seem to have generalized hypersensitivity, whereas those with more localized symptoms seem to have heightened sensation in more restricted locations.[38] Hypersensitivity to ingestion of chili capsules, mucosal electrical and thermal stimulation, and intestinal lipid perfusion has been shown, suggesting that hyperalgesia is not specific for mechanoreceptor-activated pathways.[39] Evidence supporting a relation of visceral sensory abnormalities to symptom severity is conflicting, with some studies showing a positive correlation and others observing little or no association (**Fig. 2**).[24,34–36,40] Not all patients have a heightened perception of distention. Whereas individuals with D-IBS commonly have reduced thresholds for sensing luminal balloon inflation, some patients with C-IBS, hard stools, and no fecal urgency show reduced perceptual responses to distending stimuli.[21] A recent prospective study observed that only 20% of patients with IBS had increased sensation to luminal distention, whereas 16% showed reduced rectal sensation.[1] Patients with IBS also may show atypical pain referral patterns during gut distention, experiencing pain diffusely in the abdomen, back, shoulders, or chest.[34] One group has reported that 94% of patients with IBS show visceral sensory abnormalities when alterations in abdominal pain referral patterns are coupled with hypersensitive perception of rectal

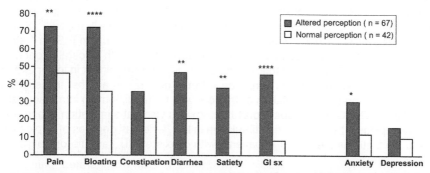

Fig. 2. Proportions of patients are shown who report at least moderate severity of individual and overall gastrointestinal symptoms (mean scores on Gastrointestinal Symptom Rating Scale domains ≥4) and clinically significant anxiety or depression (score on Hospital Anxiety and Depression Scale [HAD] anxiety or HAD depression ≥11) in those with altered versus normal rectal perception. More patients with hypersensitivity had overall symptoms of moderate or greater severity and reported moderate or greater abdominal pain, bloating, diarrhea, early satiety. Likewise, more patients with increased sensitivity reported significant anxiety. *P<.05; **P<.01; ****P<.0001. (*From* Posserud I, Syrous A, Lindstrom L, et al. Altered rectal perception in irritable bowel syndrome is associated with symptom severity. Gastroenterology 2007;133:1119; with permission.)

distention, but in light of more recent data to the contrary, this finding is not universally accepted as a biomarker for IBS.[34,41]

As with studies of motor dysfunction, abnormalities of sensory activity may be prominent under stimulated conditions. Colonic hypersensitivity is augmented by ingestion of cold water and high-fat nutrient meals, especially in D-IBS.[42] Repeated sigmoid colon distentions elicit prominent hyperalgesia as well as abnormal pain referral patterns in IBS, perhaps secondary to spinal dorsal horn neuronal sensitization.[43] Furthermore, repetitive inflations at levels less than those needed to elicit perception can lead to increased contractile activity in IBS. Rectal glycerol perfusion enhances sensitivity to distention.

Some investigators attribute exaggerated perception in IBS to psychological factors based on studies showing similar responses in patients with IBS and healthy controls when perceptual tests designed to minimize emotional influences were used.[41,44,45] Other investigations suggest that patients with IBS show a stronger tendency to report sensations as painful or negative during distention versus controls.[45,46] These findings have led some to propose that patients with IBS may show either peripheral hypersensitivity to distention or hypervigilance resulting from psychological dysfunction.[46] However, some studies comparing perception of true versus sham distentions in healthy controls and patients with IBS show no effect of psychological bias.[44]

Somatic Sensory Dysfunction

It remains controversial whether sensory dysfunction in IBS is restricted to the gut or is generalized to include hypersensitive responses in somatic structures. In some studies, responses to cutaneous electrical and thermal stimulation, including cold-water immersion, are similar in patients with IBS, healthy controls, and patients with organic disease.[35,47] Patients with IBS have shown reduced responsiveness to somatic pressure and electrical stimulation compared with patients with fibromyalgia.[47] Conversely, other investigations observed increased perception of calf and forearm heat pain in patients with IBS, impaired tolerance of cold-water stimulation in patients with functional disorders, and increased generalized somatic sensation in patients with IBS with coexisting fibromyalgia.[47–49] In addition, 3 subgroups were distinguished based on severity of somatic hypersensitivity in 1 report.[49] Several investigations have further characterized somatic sensory defects in IBS. In 1 study, hypersensitivity to thermal stimulation correlated positively with visceral hypersensitivity to distention.[48] Increased thermal sensitivity is more prominent in lower extremities sharing viscerosomatic convergence with the colon.[50] In another investigation, combining cold-pressor stimulation of the foot with rectal distention increased rectal perception in IBS. Other groups report that noxious visceral stimulation is perceived as more unpleasant than somatic stimulation in IBS, whereas degrees of unpleasantness to the 2 stimuli are similar in patients with coexistent IBS and fibromyalgia.[51]

Possible Mediators of Sensory Dysfunction

Several factors have shown associations with sensory dysfunction in IBS, suggestive of possible pathogenic roles in symptom induction. Local factors may contribute to hypersensitivity. Rectal sensitivity in patients with IBS is reduced by topical lidocaine administration, emphasizing the importance of sodium channels in this response.[52] Nerve-fiber sodium channels were decreased in rectal biopsy specimens from patients with hypersensitivity.[53] However, the observation that placebo jelly reduces perception of rectal distention more than distention without any topical treatment shows the importance of psychological factors as well. Mice with knockouts of the acid-sensing ion channel 3 (ASIC3) show impaired visceral sensitivity.[54] ASIC3 pathway defects have also been observed in animal models of IBS.

Neurohumoral abnormalities have been identified in patients with IBS and in animal models of visceral hypersensitivity. In D-IBS, heightened rectal sensation correlates with numbers of enterochromaffin cells in rectal biopsy specimens. In rats, intraperitoneal or intracerebroventricular $5-HT_{2B}$ antagonist treatment blunts visceral hypersensitivity.[55] Increases in substance-P immunoreactive nerve fibers have been identified in colon biopsies from patients with IBS.[56] Most unmyelinated C-fibers mediating perception of noxious gut stimuli express transient receptor potential vanilloid type 1 (TRPV1) receptors, which are activated by both capsaicin and cannabinoids. Involvement of TRPV1 receptors is reported in animal models of visceral hypersensitivity. Furthermore, studies of patients with IBS with rectal hypersensitivity show increases in TRPV1-expressing fibers in the colon.[56] Conversely, TRPV1 antagonists decrease colonic sensitivity to distention in rats given neonatal acetic acid perfusion and TRPV1 receptor knockout mice show analgesic responses to thermal stimulation.[57] In healthy humans, the cannabinoid receptor agonist dronabinol increases perception of painful colonic distention.[58] In animal models, cannabinoid CB_1 receptor antagonists increase rectal sensitivity to distention. Protease activated receptors (PARs) may participate in heightened visceral sensitivity in IBS. Supernatants from colonic biopsy specimens of patients with IBS sensitize cultured sensory neurons and induce hyperalgesia, an effect blocked by inhibitors of serine protease and not observed in sensory neurons not expressing PAR-2 receptors.[59] Intracolonic PAR-2 agonist perfusion initiates hypersensitivity to distention. In another study, a PAR-4 receptor agonist reduced responsiveness to colonic distention and blunted visceromotor responses to PAR-2 and TRPV4 agonists.[60] In other recent investigations, submucosal neuronal spike discharges elicited by supernatants from colonic biopsies of patients with IBS are inhibited by histamine antagonists, $5-HT_3$ antagonists, and protease inhibition (**Fig. 3**).[61] Visceral hypersensitivity in rats induced by maternal separation is associated with reduced glial excitatory amino acid transporter-1 and can be counteracted by spinal administration of riluzole, an agent that activates glutamate reuptake.[62] Inhibition of cystathione-β-synthase decreases the abdominal withdrawal reflex to colonic distention in rats. Expression of the $P_{2\times3}$ purinergic receptor protein is increased in some rat models of visceral hypersensitivity.[63] Visceromotor responses to mechanical distention are reduced in $P_{2\times3}$ +/− and −/− mice.[64] Visceral hypersensitivity can be reversed by antagonists of $P_{2\times1}$, $P_{2\times3}$, and $P_{2\times2/3}$ subtypes. The importance of any of these neurohumoral pathways in gut sensory dysfunction in IBS is undefined.

GUT SENSORIMOTOR DYSFUNCTION IN BLOATING AND DISTENTION

Evidence suggests that gut motor and sensory dysfunction as well as somatic factors participate in the sensation of bloating and the sign of visible distention in IBS. Bloating commonly is reported by patients with either D-IBS or C-IBS, but demonstrable distention detected by techniques such as impedance plethysmography is more prominent in those with C-IBS, who often have associated hard stools and delays in small intestinal or colonic transit.[65]

Insight into the pathogenesis of gas and bloating has been provided by studies involving intestinal gas perfusion. In healthy humans, jejunal delivery of physiologic gas mixtures mimicking venous gaseous concentrations produces steady-state flow with little distention and few symptoms. An older study using an argon washout method observed that total intestinal gas volumes in IBS are normal.[66] However,

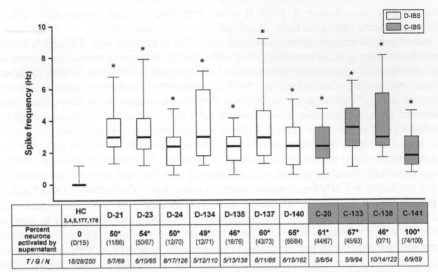

	HC 3,4,5,177,178	D-21	D-23	D-24	D-134	D-135	D-137	D-140	C-20	C-133	C-138	C-141
Percent neurons activated by supernatant	0 (0/15)	50* (11/66)	54* (50/67)	50* (12/70)	49* (12/71)	46* (18/76)	60* (43/73)	65* (56/84)	61* (44/67)	67* (45/93)	46* (0/71)	100* (74/100)
T / G / N	18/28/250	5/7/69	6/10/85	8/17/126	5/12/110	5/13/138	6/11/86	6/15/162	3/6/54	5/9/94	10/14/122	6/9/59

Fig. 3. Spike discharges in response to exposure to supernatants from patients with IBS are shown. Compared with healthy controls (HC), each of the IBS supernatants significantly increased spike discharge in 40% to 100% of the neurons per ganglion. This observation held for those with D-IBS (D-21, D-23, D-24, D-134, D-135, D-137, D-140) and C-IBS (C-20, C-133, C-138, C-141). Data for HC supernatants were pooled. Proportions of activated neurons are given as median percentage (25th and 75th percentiles). T/G/N, number of tissues/ganglia/neurons. *P<.05 compared with HC. (*From* Buhner S, Li Q, Vignali S, et al. Activation of human enteric neurons by supernatants of colonic biopsy specimens from patients with irritable bowel syndrome. Gastroenterology 2009;137:1429; with permission.)

abnormal retrograde gas reflux patterns were noted in some individuals, suggestive of transit defects. More recent jejunal gas perfusion studies observed pathologic gas retention in IBS associated with symptom development and increased abdominal girth.[67] Using radiolabeled xenon scintigraphy to localize sites of gas retention, patients with functional bloating show selective delays in gas transit in the small intestine.[68,69] This finding is supported by the observations that jejunal but not ileal gas perfusion produces gas retention, and duodenal lipid perfusion selectively delays gas transit in the small bowel in an exaggerated fashion in patients with IBS.[69] However, in a recent study, patients with IBS showed impaired gas clearance from the proximal colon during retrograde gas perfusion into the rectum, indicating participation of colonic motor defects as well.[70] Patients with IBS with objective distention also show increases in anal pressures and prolonged rectal balloon expulsion times, suggesting a role for anorectal outlet dysfunction as a contributor to gaseous symptoms in some cases.[71] However, others have observed rapid transit of solid-liquid meals in some patients with IBS with bloating, indicating heterogeneity in symptom pathogenesis.

The importance of perception is emphasized by observations from perfusion studies that, for similar degrees of gas retention, patients with bloating develop greater symptoms compared with healthy controls.[72] Furthermore, patients with bloating but no distention show heightened perception of gas perfusion, whereas those with bloating and distention show normal to reduced perceptual responses. Patients with IBS with bloating also show heightened sensation of rectal distention, whereas those with bloating plus distention show reduced perception, which indicates generalized gut hypersensitivity.[73]

Other contributors to bloating and distention in IBS include abnormal activities of the diaphragm and abdominal somatic musculature. In a computed tomography (CT) study in patients with bloating, severe distention episodes were associated with exaggerated diaphragmatic descent. Supporting a role for somatic muscle factors in IBS, patients with manometrically documented small intestinal dysmotility showed greater gas retention during jejunal gas perfusion than patients with IBS despite having similar symptoms and increases in abdominal girth.[74] Likewise using a CT method to quantify luminal gas, investigators observed increased gas retention with intestinal dysmotility associated with abdominal wall protrusion and cephalad diaphragmatic excursion, whereas those with functional bloating showed no increase in gas volume but showed protruded abdominal walls with caudad diaphragmatic movements (**Fig. 4**).[75] Recent rectal gas perfusion studies reported increases in perception in IBS and functional bloating, which were associated with changes in external and internal oblique muscle contraction, indicating an interaction of visceral and somatic musculature in production of gaseous symptomatology.[72]

AUTONOMIC NERVOUS SYSTEM DYSREGULATION

Disruption of normal autonomic nervous system activity has been observed in IBS and has been postulated to relate to the different subtypes of the disorder. In general, patients with D-IBS show abnormal sympathetic adrenergic activity, as measured by reduced fingertip blood flow responses, blood pressure responses to 35% carbon dioxide stress challenges, and skin conductance responses to repeated rectal distentions. Conversely, individuals with C-IBS show vagal parasympathetic dysfunction, measured by heart-rate variability profiles.[76–80] One group has specifically related heart-rate variability abnormalities in women to a pain-predominant pattern of illness, whereas others have observed exaggerated disturbances after meals or colonic distention.[80] In another study, autonomic dysfunction was greater in men with IBS compared with female patients.[81] Recent investigations observe persistence of autonomic defects even during sleep in IBS, suggesting that they are an intrinsic characteristic of the disease rather than a consequence of psychosocial influence.[77]

BRAIN-GUT INTERACTIONS

IBS may occur as a consequence of a primary alteration in gut sensorimotor function with modulation by CNS input or as a dominant CNS disturbance with centrally directed changes in gut sensorimotor function. Relative roles of peripheral versus central defects likely vary depending on symptom severity and between different symptom subsets. Perception of visceral stimulation is represented by several CNS regions. Localization and discrimination of perceptual characteristics of luminal pain occur in the primary (S1) and secondary (S2) somatosensory cerebral cortex. Emotional components of visceral perception of noxious stimuli are mediated by several CNS regions, including the insula, anterior cingulate cortex (ACC), and prefrontal cortex (PFC) (**Table 1**).[82,83] The ACC is postulated to participate in affective and cognitive components of luminal pain as well as initiating behavioral responses.[84,85] The insula integrates gut sensory, motor, and autonomic functions via interactions with the amygdala, hypothalamus, and brainstem.[83] Anticipation and hypervigilance may relate to activities of the dorsomedial and dorsolateral PFC and dorsal ACC, whereas pain inhibition may be controlled by the ventrolateral PFC.[86,87] Subcortical areas including the periaqueductal gray matter, hypothalamus,

Patient With Functional Bloating

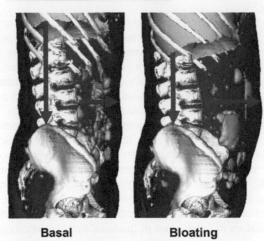

Basal   Bloating

Patient With Intestinal Dysmotility

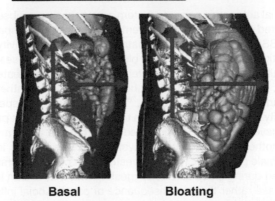

Basal   Bloating

Fig. 4. Abdominal imaging is shown from a patient with a functional disorder causing bloating and distention (*above*). In this individual, there is anterior abdominal wall protrusion and diaphragmatic descent during reports of bloating compared with basal conditions, which is associated with only a small increase (22 mL) in gas content. Abdominal imaging also is shown from a patient with manometrically proved intestinal dysmotility (*below*). In this case, there is a marked increment in gas content (3352 mL) during bloating, which is associated with anterior abdominal wall protrusion and diaphragmatic ascent. (*From* Accarino A, Perez F, Azpiroz F, et al. Abdominal distention results from caudo-ventral redistribution of contents. Gastroenterology 2009;136:1548, 1549; with permission.)

and thalamus also participate in visceral perception and regulate spinal transmission of painful luminal sensations.[83] Descending modulation of afferent input at the levels of the amygdala, brainstem, and spinal cord by the ACC has also been proposed.[88,89]

Brain Imaging Studies

Brain imaging methods such as positron emission tomography (PET) and functional MRI (fMRI) have been used to quantify regional cerebral blood flow as a measure of neuronal activation patterns in IBS. In an initial report, healthy individuals showed

Table 1
The primary connections and functions of human limbic structures in the brain

Limbic Structure	Primary Connection(s)	Functions	Responses to Stimulation	Results of Lesion
Hypothalamus	Autonomic nervous system (via hypothalamic-pituitary-endocrine axis); sensory structures in the brain	Govern CNS autonomic function; maintain homeostasis; generate coordinated and sophisticated emotional responses	Emotional responses, including anger, fear, curiosity, lethargy	Aberrant autonomic activity; emotional dysregulation
Amygdala	Thalamus; cortex	Process emotions; form emotional memories	Changes in emotion and autonomic function	Impairment in memory for emotionally charged events
ACC	PFC	Integrate visceral, attentional, and emotional information; regulate affect	Information processing; dispersal of pain inhibition signals	Profoundly impaired decision making
PFC	ACC	Represent goals; maintain vigilance to goal-directed behavior; process effect	Increased vigilance; affective processing	Tangential (ie, nongoal-directed) behavior

Data from Jones MP, Dilley JB, Drossman D, et al. Brain-gut connections in functional GI disorders: anatomic and physiologic relationships. Neurogastroenterol Motil 2006;18:91–103.

increased blood flow in the ACC during rectal distention, whereas patients with IBS showed reduced blood flow.[90] Conversely, sham distention elicited activation of the PFC in patients with IBS. Subsequent studies have yielded conflicting results, including exaggerated increases or decreases in activity in the anterior and medial cingulate cortex, increased activation in the posterior and middle dorsal cingulate cortex, increases in the PFC and thalamus, increases or decreases in insula and brain-stem activity, and reductions in activation of the amygdala, perigenual and temporal cortex, and striatum.[51,52,87,90–94] In 1 study, the degree of ACC activation correlated with symptom severity during luminal distention in healthy controls but not patients with IBS.[91] In another investigation, anticipation of distention reduced activity in the insula, supragenual ACC, amygdala, and brainstem.[94] Recent studies have also reported exaggerated activation of the S1 somatosensory cortex and then the thalamus and hypothalamus in response to graded distention in IBS.[95] In a comparison of different chronic functional pain syndromes, those with IBS were reported to show selective increases in ACC activation with luminal stimulation, whereas individuals with fibromyalgia showed similar activation patterns only with somatic stimuli.[51] Differences in brain activation have been related to gender and IBS subtype.[96] Repeated rectal distention over a 12-month period leads to normalization of heightened perception and reduced activation of the pregenual ACC and middle cingulate cortex but no changes in IBS symptom severity or subgenual ACC, insula, or thalamus activity.[84] These findings have been explained as reflecting excessive vigilance to sensory testing that improves over time. Although specific defects vary from study to study, results from PET and fMRI investigations taken as an aggregate suggest that patients with IBS show significant disruptions of CNS activity related to attention, arousal, emotional, and autonomic responses to gut stimulation.[87,91,97]

In addition to documenting functional abnormalities, recent CNS imaging studies have shown alterations in brain structure in IBS. In 1 investigation, IBS was associated with thinning of the right perigenual ACC, insula, and thalamus.[98] Another study observed associations of IBS with reduced gray matter density in the medial and ventrolateral PFC, posterior parietal cortex, ventral striatum, and thalamus and increased gray matter density in the pregenual ACC and orbitofrontal cortex.[99] Differences in the PFC and posterior parietal cortex persisted after accounting for coexistent anxiety and depression and were not dependent on bowel habit subtype. In a third investigation, patients with IBS showed increased hypothalamic gray matter and thinning in the ACC.[100] Pain catastrophizing correlated negatively with dorsolateral PFC thickness, whereas pain duration correlated positively with anterior insula thickness.

Other Methods to Assess Brain Function

Other methods to assess brain function have been used to characterize CNS activity in IBS. Evoked potential recordings in functional dyspepsia and IBS show shorter waveform latencies and increased waveform amplitudes, consistent with defects in visceral afferent pathways.[101] Further exaggerated decreases of evoked potential latencies are observed after ice-water ingestion in patients with IBS versus controls. Electroencephalographic waveforms including reduced α-power and increased β-power percentages are abnormal at rest, during psychological stress, or after neostigmine administration in patients with IBS.[102]

PSYCHOSOCIAL DISTRESS

Numerous studies confirm a high degree of psychosocial dysfunction in IBS. More recent investigations have attempted to characterize the patterns of psychological disturbance, ascribe a role for emotional factors in IBS symptom generation, and delineate mechanisms by which psychiatric disease disrupts gut sensorimotor and CNS function.

Epidemiology of Psychological Dysfunction

Psychiatric disturbances can be shown in most patients with IBS in tertiary practice.[103] Furthermore, psychosocial dysfunction is observed in patients with IBS managed in primary care and in individuals with IBS who do not seek care.[22,103,104] Rates of suicidal behavior are increased 2- to 4-fold in IBS.[105] Patients with IBS are more than twice as likely to be prescribed antidepressants, anxiolytics, antipsychotics, or sedatives in the first year after diagnosis.[106] Nevertheless, some studies report no increase in psychological abnormalities in patients with IBS who do not seek medical care for their gastrointestinal symptoms, whereas others report no increase in IBS symptoms in those with depression in remission.[107,108] Increased psychological distress has been observed in C-IBS versus D-IBS. Exposure to wartime early in life increased the risk of developing IBS in another investigation.[109]

No single psychiatric diagnosis predominates in IBS. Increases in patients with IBS compared with healthy controls have been reported for major depression, somatization disorder, generalized anxiety disorder, panic disorder, neuroticism, posttraumatic stress disorder, phobias, hypochondriasis, hostility, concealed aggression, and trait and suppressed anger.[110–112] Further associations of IBS with body preoccupation, interpersonal sensitivity, catastrophizing, ineffective coping, and impaired extroversion are reported.[9,110,113] The importance of somatization is emphasized by 1 study that observed that 43% of patients with IBS reported high degrees of somatic symptoms on a validated checklist versus 10% of controls.[114] Patients with IBS selectively recall gastrointestinal terminology with negative connotations, suggesting the presence of a cognitive-behavioral defect.[115] In addition to the increased prevalence of psychosocial dysfunction in patients with functional gastrointestinal disorders, symptoms of IBS are common in patients with depression, anxiety, or panic disorder.[108]

Psychiatric disturbances usually predate or occur concurrently with the onset of bowel symptoms, indicating that emotional illness is not a consequence of IBS. Recently, a matched cohort study observed that more patients with IBS than controls consulted specialists for care of depression in the 2 years before their IBS diagnosis.[116] Predictors of onset of IBS included high levels of illness behavior and anxiety in 1 study.[117]

Role of Stress

IBS shows a strong association with reports of psychological stress. Several studies have related IBS exacerbations with active, ongoing stressful events. Women with IBS show a correlation between current stress and daily symptoms. In another investigation, symptomatic flares were correlated with stress during the previous 2 days.[118] In a third study, data were consistent with a model in which effects of stress on gut symptomatology were most prominent 1 to 2 weeks after the stressful episode.[119] However, others have observed little relation of day-to-day stress variations with daily IBS symptom fluctuations. Severe emotional upheaval in the remote past is also frequently reported by patients with chronic IBS symptoms. Previous stressful life events, such as loss of a parent, marital difficulties, maladaptive family interactions, and career changes, are more common in patients with IBS than in healthy individuals or patients with organic disease.[110,111]

Sleep Disturbances

Sleep disturbances, such as repeated nocturnal awakening and arising in the morning feeling unrested, are reported by most patients with IBS. IBS patients had a longer latency to rapid eye movement sleep, increased duration of stage 3 and 4 sleep, and reduced duration of rapid eye movement sleep during psychological distress in a polysomnographic study.[120] In recent studies, IBS symptoms were greater in nurses who had rotating shifts than those who worked only during the day shift.[121] Sleep problems were predictive of IBS onset in 1 investigation.[117]

Physical and Sexual Abuse

IBS has been associated with histories of sexual and/or physical abuse.[112,122–124] Patients with IBS have a higher frequency of severe lifetime sexual trauma, severe childhood sexual abuse, and any lifetime sexual victimization than individuals with inflammatory bowel disease.[125] Forms of sexual abuse associated with IBS include verbal aggression, exhibitionism, sexual harassment, sexual touching, and rape. Women with IBS and a history of sexual abuse score higher on scales of self-blame and self-silencing.[126] Most studies examining associations of abuse with IBS have focused on patients followed in tertiary centers.[123,124] However, even in community populations, IBS-like symptoms are reported more often in those with previous abuse.[124]

Relation of Psychological Abnormalities to Motor/Sensory/CNS Function

Studies have attempted to relate circulating neurohumoral mediators to psychosocial factors in IBS; however, no definitive abnormalities have shown clear evidence as pathophysiologic contributors. Stress responsiveness of the gastrointestinal tract is postulated to be mediated by coordinated action of the hypothalamic-pituitary-adrenal (HPA) axis. Corticotropin-releasing hormone (CRH) administration modulates gut motor function and can evoke rectal hypersensitivity in the setting of repeated distentions.[127] However, HPA axis responsiveness shows no consistent pattern in IBS, with different studies observing heightened, reduced, or normal activity as measured by cortisol or adrenocorticotropic hormone levels in response to stressful stimulation, ischemic pain, lumbar puncture, or CRH administration.[128,129] In a recent study, early adverse life events were associated with increased cortisol levels (**Fig. 5**).[130] In another

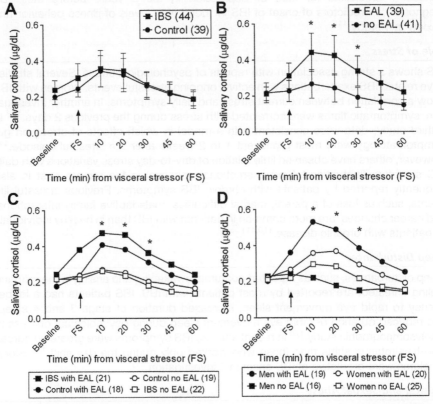

Fig. 5. Salivary cortisol responses to a visceral stressor (flexible sigmoidoscopy [FS]) are shown for (A) patients with IBS versus healthy controls, (B) subjects with and without early adverse life events (EALs), (C) subjects broken into groups by diagnosis and presence of EALs, and by (D) sex and EALs. In (B), the presence of EALs had a significant effect on the cortisol response (P<.05). In (C), EAL groups were significantly greater than IBS and controls without EALs. In (D), the effect of EALs on cortisol response was most pronounced among men. Where shown, error bars represent the 95% confidence interval around the mean. * Significant difference between the groups at that time point in post hoc analyses. (*From* Videlock EJ, Adeyemo M, Licudine A, et al. Childhood trauma is associated with hypothalamic-pituitary-adrenal axis responsiveness in irritable bowel syndrome. Gastroenterology 2009;137:1957; with permission.)

report, patients with C-IBS showed increased cortisol during sleep, whereas patients with D-IBS showed reduced levels.[131] In a third investigation, cortisol levels correlated with degrees of anxiety but not IBS symptom severity.[132]

Psychological dysfunction has shown a relation to sensorimotor and CNS abnormalities in some patients with IBS. Exaggerated colorectal motor activity is observed with stress and can be elicited by stressful interviews. More recent investigations report increases in colonic motor activity with stress and emotional triggers and changes in rectal tone when confronted with emotionally charged words.[133] Likewise, rectal hypersensitivity is increased by stress in IBS and has been associated with depression, anxiety, somatization, and neuroticism.[22,128] In a second investigation, anxiety and coping related to pain thresholds on rectal distention.[40] However, in another investigation, rectal sensation did not relate to psychological dysfunction.[22] Likewise, anxiety was not related to rectal hypersensitivity on multivariate analysis in a different study.[36] Patients with previous abuse have been reported to show normal, heightened, or reduced sensitivity to luminal distention.[122,134] Autonomic responses have shown correlations with anxiety and depression severity in D-IBS and with depression scores in patients with an alternating bowel pattern in different studies.[135] However, in another investigation, relations of IBS to sympathetic and parasympathetic activity in different symptom subtypes did not relate to the presence or absence of affective disease. In assessments of CNS activation patterns using PET and fMRI methods, acute stress has been reported to increase activation of the ACC and medial prefrontal cortex in patients with IBS.[136] Reduced supragenual ACC and increased middle and posterior cingulate cortex responses have been noted in patients with IBS with previous abuse.[93] Anxiety scores were associated with rectal distention-evoked activation of the ACC, whereas depression severity correlated with activation of the PFC and cerebellum.[92]

SUMMARY

Several abnormalities in gut sensorimotor profiles, autonomic nervous system activities, central pain processing, and psychosocial function have been identified in association with specific symptom profiles in different IBS subtypes. Their interactions with recently described immunologic and microbial disturbances in this condition are discussed in other articles in this issue. The importance of any one of these defects in an individual with IBS may be variable given the multifactorial nature of the disorder. Furthermore, most studies of peripheral or central dysfunction in IBS have focused on defects that are considered to be fixed and intrinsic properties of the nervous systems of affected patients. However, many patients with IBS show highly variable symptom patterns. In 1 large investigation, symptoms were experienced on only 7 days per month and 63% reported alternating bowel habits.[137] Other studies observe patient conversion from 1 bowel-habit subtype to the opposite pattern. Thus, conclusions derived from the impressive literature in this field must be tempered by the knowledge that any observed abnormalities of motor, sensory, or CNS function show plasticity, can be transitory in nature, and may not fully explain the symptomatic manifestations of IBS.

REFERENCES

1. Camilleri M, McKinzie S, Busciglio I, et al. Prospective study of motor, sensory, psychologic, and autonomic functions in patients with irritable bowel syndrome. Clin Gastroenterol Hepatol 2008;6:772–81.

2. Marciani L, Cox EF, Hoad CL, et al. Postprandial changes in small bowel water content in healthy subjects and patients with irritable bowel syndrome. Gastroenterology 2010;138:469–77.
3. Deiteren A, Camilleri M, Burton D, et al. Effect of meal ingestion on ileocolonic and colonic transit in health and irritable bowel syndrome. Dig Dis Sci 2010; 55:384–91.
4. Kellow JE, Phillips SF. Altered small bowel motility in irritable bowel syndrome is correlated with symptoms. Gastroenterology 1987;92:1885–93.
5. Kellow JE, Gill RC, Wingate DL. Prolonged ambulant recordings of small bowel motility demonstrate abnormalities in the irritable bowel syndrome. Gastroenterology 1990;98:1208–18.
6. Simren M, Castedal M, Stevland J, et al. Abnormal propagation pattern of duodenal pressure waves in the irritable bowel syndrome. Dig Dis Sci 2000; 45:2151–61.
7. Gorard DA, Libby GW, Farthing MJ. Ambulatory small intestinal motility in "diarrhea" predominant irritable bowel syndrome. Gut 1994;35:203–10.
8. Tornblom H, Lindberg G, Nyberg B, et al. Full-thickness biopsy of the jejunum reveals inflammation and enteric neuropathy in irritable bowel syndrome. Gastroenterology 2002;123:1972–9.
9. Whitehead WE, Engel BT, Schuster MM. Irritable bowel syndrome: physiological and psychological differences between diarrhea-predominant and constipation-predominant patients. Dig Dis Sci 1980;25:404–13.
10. Bazzocchi G, Ellis J, Villanueva-Meyer J, et al. Postprandial colonic transit and motor activity in chronic constipation. Gastroenterology 1990;98:686–93.
11. Sadik R, Stotzer PO, Simren M, et al. Gastrointestinal transit abnormalities are frequently detected in patients with unexplained GI symptoms at a tertiary centre. Neurogastroenterol Motil 2008;20:197–205.
12. Manabe N, Wong BS, Camilleri M, et al. Lower functional gastrointestinal disorders: evidence of abnormal colonic transit in a 287 patient cohort. Neurogastroenterol Motil 2010;22:293–e82.
13. Deiteren A, Camilleri M, Bharucha AE, et al. Performance characteristics of scintigraphic colon transit measurement in health and irritable bowel syndrome and relationship to bowel functions. Neurogastroenterol Motil 2010;22:415–23.
14. Snape WJ, Carlson GM, Matarazzo SA, et al. Colonic myoelectric activity in the irritable bowel syndrome. Gastroenterology 1976;70:326–30.
15. Latimer P, Sarna S, Campbell D, et al. Colonic motor and myoelectric activity: a comparative study of normal subjects, psychoneurotic patients, and patients with irritable bowel syndrome. Gastroenterology 1981;80:893–901.
16. Hasler WL, Saad RJ, Rao SS, et al. Heightened colon motor activity measured by a wireless capsule in patients with constipation: relation to colon transit and IBS. Am J Physiol Gastrointest Liver Physiol 2009;297:G1107–14.
17. Chey WY, Jin HO, Lee MH, et al. Colonic motility abnormality in patients with irritable bowel syndrome exhibiting abdominal pain and diarrhea. Am J Gastroenterol 2001;96:1499–506.
18. Clemens CH, Samsom M, Roelofs JM, et al. Association between pain episodes and high amplitude propagated pressure waves in patients with irritable bowel syndrome. Am J Gastroenterol 2003;98:1838–43.
19. Sullivan MA, Cohen S, Snape WJ. Colonic myoelectric activity in irritable-bowel syndrome. Effect of eating and anticholinergics. N Engl J Med 1978;298: 878–83.

20. Lembo T, Munakata J, Mertz H, et al. Evidence for the hypersensitivity of lumbar splanchnic afferents in irritable bowel syndrome. Gastroenterology 1994;107: 1686–96.
21. Prior A, Maxton DG, Whorwell PJ. Anorectal manometry in irritable bowel syndrome: differences between diarrhoea and constipation predominant subjects. Gut 1990;31:458–62.
22. van der Veek PP, van Rood YR, Masclee AA. Symptom severity but not psycho-pathology predicts visceral hypersensitivity in irritable bowel syndrome. Clin Gastroenterol Hepatol 2008;6:321–8.
23. Di Stefano M, Miceli E, Missanelli A, et al. Meal induced rectosigmoid tone modi-fication: a low caloric meal accurately separates functional and organic gastro-intestinal disease patients. Gut 2006;55:1409–14.
24. Kanazawa M, Palsson OS, Thiwan SI, et al. Contributions of pain sensitivity and colonic motility to IBS symptom severity and predominant bowel habits. Am J Gastroenterol 2008;103:2550–61.
25. Suttor VP, Prott GM, Hansen RD, et al. Evidence for pelvic floor dyssynergia in patients with irritable bowel syndrome. Dis Colon Rectum 2010;53:156–60.
26. Whorwell PJ, Clouter C, Smith CL. Oesophageal motility in the irritable bowel syndrome. Br Med J 1981;282:1101–2.
27. Evans PR, Bak YT, Shuter B, et al. Gastroparesis and small bowel dysmotility in irritable bowel syndrome. Dig Dis Sci 1997;42:2087–93.
28. van der Voort IR, Osmanoglou E, Seybold M, et al. Electrogastrography as a diagnostic tool for delayed gastric emptying in functional dyspepsia and Irri-table bowel syndrome. Neurogastroenterol Motil 2003;15:467–73.
29. Atkinson W, Lockhart S, Whorwell PJ, et al. Altered 5-hydroxytryptamine signaling in patients with constipation- and diarrhea-predominant irritable bowel syndrome. Gastroenterology 2006;130:34–43.
30. Fitzgerald P, Cassidy EM, Clarke G, et al. Tryptophan catabolism in females with irritable bowel syndrome: relationship to interferon-gamma, severity of symp-toms and psychiatric co-morbidity. Neurogastroenterol Motil 2008;20:1291–7.
31. Anand P, Aziz Q, Wilbert R, et al. Peripheral and central mechanisms of visceral sensitization in man. Neurogastroenterol Motil 2007;19:29–46.
32. Kellow JE, Eckersley CM, Jones MP. Enhanced perception of physiological intestinal motility in the irritable bowel syndrome. Gastroenterology 1991;101: 1621–7.
33. Ritchie J. Pain from the distention of the pelvic colon by inflating a balloon in the irritable colon syndrome. Gut 1973;14:125–32.
34. Mertz H, Naliboff B, Munakata J, et al. Altered rectal perception is a biological marker of patients with irritable bowel syndrome. Gastroenterology 1995;109: 40–52.
35. Whitehead WE, Holtkotter B, Enck P, et al. Tolerance for rectosigmoid distention in irritable bowel syndrome. Gastroenterology 1990;98:1187–92.
36. Posserud I, Syrous A, Lindstrom L, et al. Altered rectal perception in irritable bowel syndrome is associated with symptom severity. Gastroenterology 2007; 133:1113–23.
37. Chang L, Mayer EA, Labus JS, et al. Effect of sex on perception of rectosigmoid stimuli in irritable bowel syndrome. Am J Physiol Regul Integr Comp Physiol 2006;291:R277–84.
38. Bouin M, Lupien F, Riberdy M, et al. Intolerance to visceral distension in func-tional dyspepsia or irritable bowel syndrome: an organ specific defect or a pan intestinal dysregulation? Neurogastroenterol Motil 2004;16:311–4.

39. Gonlachanvit S, Mahayosnond A, Kullavanijaya P. Effects of chili on postprandial gastrointestinal symptoms in diarrhea predominant irritable bowel syndrome: evidence for capsaicin-sensitive visceral nociception hypersensitivity. Neurogastroenterol Motil 2009;21:23–32.

40. Sabate JM, Veyrac M, Mion F, et al. Relationship between rectal sensitivity, symptoms intensity and quality of life in patients with irritable bowel syndrome. Aliment Pharmacol Ther 2008;28:484–90.

41. Whitehead WE, Palsson OS. Is rectal pain sensitivity a biological marker for irritable bowel syndrome: psychological influences on pain perception. Gastroenterology 1998;115:1263–71.

42. Simren M, Abrahamsson H, Bjornsson ES. Lipid-induced colonic hypersensitivity in the irritable bowel syndrome: the role of bowel habit, sex, and psychologic factors. Clin Gastroenterol Hepatol 2007;5:201–8.

43. Munakata J, Naliboff B, Harraf F, et al. Repetitive sigmoid stimulation induces rectal hyperalgesia in patients with irritable bowel syndrome. Gastroenterology 1997;112:55–63.

44. Corsetti M, Ogliari C, Marino B, et al. Perceptual sensitivity and response bias during rectal distension in patients with irritable bowel syndrome. Neurogastroenterol Motil 2005;17:541–7.

45. Dorn SD, Palsson OS, Thiwan SI, et al. Increased colonic pain sensitivity in irritable bowel syndrome is the result of an increased tendency to report pain rather than increased neurosensory sensitivity. Gut 2007;56:1202–9.

46. Naliboff BD, Munakata J, Fullerton S, et al. Evidence for two distinct perceptual alterations in irritable bowel syndrome. Gut 1997;41:505–12.

47. Chang L, Mayer EA, Johnson T, et al. Differences in somatic perception in female patients with irritable bowel syndrome with and without fibromyalgia. Pain 2000;84:297–307.

48. Piche M, Arsenault M, Poitras P, et al. Widespread hypersensitivity is related to altered pain inhibition processes in irritable bowel syndrome. Pain 2010;148: 49–58.

49. Zhou Q, Fillingim RB, Riley JL, et al. Thermal hypersensitivity in a subset of irritable bowel syndrome patients. World J Gastroenterol 2009;15:3254–60.

50. Zhou Q, Fillingim RB, Riley JL, et al. Central and peripheral hypersensitivity in the irritable bowel syndrome. Pain 2010;148:454–61.

51. Chang L, Berman S, Mayer EA, et al. Brain responses to visceral and somatic stimuli in patients with irritable bowel syndrome with and without fibromyalgia. Am J Gastroenterol 2003;98:1354–61.

52. Verne GN, Robinson ME, Vase L, et al. Reversal of visceral and cutaneous hyperalgesia by local rectal anesthesia in irritable bowel syndrome (IBS) patients. Pain 2003;105:223–30.

53. Yiangou Y, Facer P, Chessel IP, et al. Voltage-gated ion channel Nav1.7 innervation in patients with idiopathic rectal hypersensitivity and paroxysmal extreme pain disorder (familial rectal pain). Neurosci Lett 2007;427:77–82.

54. Page AJ, Brierly SM, Martin CM, et al. Acid sensing channels 2 and 3 are required for inhibition of visceral nociceptors by benzamil. Pain 2007;133:150–60.

55. O'Mahony SM, Bulmer DC, Coelho AM, et al. 5-HT(2B) receptors modulate visceral hypersensitivity in a stress-sensitive animal model of brain-gut axis dysfunction. Neurogastroenterol Motil 2010;22:573–8.

56. Akbar A, Yiangou Y, Facer P, et al. Increased capsaicin receptor TRPV1-expressing sensory fibres in irritable bowel syndrome and their correlation with abdominal pain. Gut 2008;57:923–9.

57. Winston J, Shenoy M, Medley D, et al. The vanilloid receptor initiates and maintains colonic hypersensitivity induced by neonatal colon irritation in rats. Gastroenterology 2007;132:615–27.
58. Esfandyari T, Camilleri M, Ferber I, et al. Effects of a cannabinoid receptor agonist on colonic motor and sensory functions in humans: a randomized, placebo-controlled study. Am J Physiol Gastrointest Liver Physiol 2007;293:G137–45.
59. Cenac N, Andrews CN, Holzhausen M, et al. Role for protease activity in visceral pain in irritable bowel syndrome. J Clin Invest 2007;117:636–47.
60. Brandesi S. PAR4: a new role in the modulation of visceral nociception. Neurogastroenterol Motil 2009;21:1129–32.
61. Buhner S, Li Q, Vignali S, et al. Activation of human enteric neurons by supernatants of colonic biopsy specimens from patients with irritable bowel syndrome. Gastroenterology 2009;137:1425–34.
62. Gosselin RD, O'Connor RM, Tramullas M, et al. Riluzole normalizes early-life stress-induced visceral hypersensitivity in rats: role of spinal glutamate reuptake mechanisms. Gastroenterology 2010;138:2418–25.
63. Xu GY, Shenoy M, Winston JH, et al. P2x receptor-mediated visceral hyperalgesia in a rat model of chronic visceral hypersensitivity. Gut 2008;57:1230–7.
64. Shinoda M, Feng B, Gebhart GF. Peripheral and central P2x receptor contributions to colon mechanosensitivity and hypersensitivity in the mouse. Gastroenterology 2007;137:2096–104.
65. Houghton LA, Lea R, Agrawal A, et al. Relationship of abdominal bloating to distention in irritable bowel syndrome and effect of bowel habit. Gastroenterology 2006;131:1003–10.
66. Lasser RB, Bond JH, Levitt MD. The role of intestinal gas in functional abdominal pain. N Engl J Med 1975;293:524–6.
67. Serra J, Azpiroz F, Malagelada JR. Impaired transit and tolerance of intestinal gas in the irritable bowel syndrome. Gut 2001;48:14–9.
68. Salvioli B, Serra J, Azpiroz F, et al. Origin of gas retention and symptoms in patients with bloating. Gastroenterology 2005;128:574–9.
69. Salvioli B, Serra J, Azpiroz F, et al. Impaired small bowel gas propulsion in patients with bloating during intestinal lipid perfusion. Am J Gastroenterol 2006;101:1853–7.
70. Hernando-Harter AC, Serra J, Azpiroz F, et al. Colonic responses to gas loads in subgroups of patients with abdominal bloating. Am J Gastroenterol 2010;105:876–82.
71. Shim L, Prott G, Hansen RD, et al. Prolonged balloon expulsion is predictive of abdominal distension in bloating. Am J Gastroenterol 2010;105:883–7.
72. Tremolaterra F, Villoria A, Azpiroz F, et al. Impaired viscerosomatic reflexes and abdominal-wall dystony associated with bloating. Gastroenterology 2006;130:1062–8.
73. Agrawal A, Houghton LA, Lea R, et al. Bloating and distention in irritable bowel syndrome: the role of visceral sensation. Gastroenterology 2008;134:1882–9.
74. Serra J, Villoria A, Azpiroz F, et al. Impaired intestinal gas propulsion in manometrically proven dysmotility and in irritable bowel syndrome. Neurogastroenterol Motil 2010;22:401–6.
75. Accarino A, Perez F, Azpiroz F, et al. Abdominal distention results from caudoventral redistribution of contents. Gastroenterology 2009;136:1544–51.
76. Aggarwal A, Cutts TF, Abell TL, et al. Predominant symptoms in irritable bowel syndrome correlate with specific autonomic nervous system abnormalities. Gastroenterology 1994;106:945–50.

77. Thompson JJ, Elsenbruch S, Harnish MJ, et al. Autonomic functioning during REM sleep differentiates IBS symptom subgroups. Am J Gastroenterol 2002; 97:2865–71.

78. Elsenbruch S, Orr WC. Diarrhea- and constipation-predominant IBS patients differ in postprandial autonomic and cortisol responses. Am J Gastroenterol 2001;96:460–6.

79. Tanaka T, Manabe N, Hata J, et al. Characterization of autonomic dysfunction in patients with irritable bowel syndrome using fingertip blood flow. Neurogastroenterol Motil 2008;20:498–504.

80. Cain KC, Jarrett ME, Burr RL, et al. Heart rate variability is related to pain severity and predominant bowel pattern in women with irritable bowel syndrome. Neurogastroenterol Motil 2007;19:110–8.

81. Tillisch K, Mayer EA, Labus JS, et al. Sex specific alterations in autonomic function among patients with irritable bowel syndrome. Gut 2005;54:1396–401.

82. Aziz Q, Thompson DG, Ng VW, et al. Cortical processing of human somatic and visceral sensation. J Neurosci 2000;20:2657–63.

83. Derbyshire SW. A systematic review of neuroimaging data during visceral stimulation. Am J Gastroenterol 2003;98:12–20.

84. Naliboff BD, Mayer EA. Brain imaging in IBS: drawing the line between cognitive and non-cognitive processes. Gastroenterology 2006;130:267–70.

85. Yaguez L, Coen S, Gregory LJ, et al. Brain response to visceral aversive conditioning: a functional magnetic resonance imaging study. Gastroenterology 2005; 128:1819–29.

86. Sawamoto N, Honda M, Okada T, et al. Expectation of pain enhances responses to nonpainful somatosensory stimulation in the anterior cingulate cortex and parietal operculum/posterior insula: an event-related functional magnetic resonance imaging study. J Neurosci 2000;20:7438–45.

87. Mayer EA, Berman S, Suyenobu B, et al. Differences in brain responses to visceral pain between patients with irritable bowel syndrome and ulcerative colitis. Pain 2005;115:398–409.

88. Jones MP, Dilley JB, Drossman D, et al. Brain-gut connections in functional GI disorders: anatomic and physiologic relationships. Neurogastroenterol Motil 2006;18:91–103.

89. Dunckley P, Wise RG, Fairhurst M, et al. A comparison of visceral and somatic pain processing in the human brainstem using functional magnetic resonance imaging. J Neurosci 2005;25:7333–41.

90. Silverman DH, Munakata JA, Ennes H, et al. Regional cerebral activity in normal and pathological perception of visceral pain. Gastroenterology 1997;112:64–72.

91. Mertz H, Morgan V, Tanner G, et al. Regional cerebral activation in irritable bowel syndrome and control subjects with painful and nonpainful rectal distention. Gastroenterology 2000;118:842–8.

92. Elsenbruch S, Rosenberger C, Enck P, et al. Affective disturbances modulate the neural processing of visceral pain stimuli in irritable bowel syndrome: an fMRI study. Gut 2010;59:489–95.

93. Ringel Y, Drossman DA, Leserman JL, et al. Effect of abuse history on pain reports and brain responses to aversive visceral stimulation: an fMRI study. Gastroenterology 2008;134:396–404.

94. Berman SM, Naliboff BD, Suyenobu B, et al. Reduced brainstem inhibition during anticipated pelvic visceral pain correlates with enhanced brain response to the visceral stimulus in women with irritable bowel syndrome. J Neurosci 2008;28:349–59.

95. Kwan CL, Diamant NE, Pope G, et al. Abnormal forebrain activity in functional bowel disorder patients with chronic pain. Neurology 2005;65: 1268–77.
96. Naliboff BD, Berman S, Chang L, et al. Sex-related differences in IBS patients: central processing of visceral stimuli. Gastroenterology 2003;124: 1738–47.
97. Azpiroz F, Bouin M, Camilleri M, et al. Mechanisms of hypersensitivity in IBS and functional disorders. Neurogastroenterol Motil 2007;19(Suppl 1):62–88.
98. Davis KD, Pope G, Chen J, et al. Cortical thinning in IBS: implications for homeostatic, attention, and pain processing. Neurology 2008;70:153–4.
99. Seminowicz DA, Labus JS, Bueller JA, et al. Regional gray matter density changes in brains of patients with irritable bowel syndrome. Gastroenterology 2010;139:48–57.
100. Blankstein U, Chen J, Diamant NE, et al. Altered brain structure in irritable bowel syndrome: potential contributions of pre-existing and disease-driven factors. Gastroenterology 2010;138:1783–9.
101. Chan YK, Herkes GK, Badcock C, et al. Alterations in cerebral potentials evoked by rectal distension in irritable bowel syndrome. Am J Gastroenterol 2001;96: 2413–7.
102. Berman SM, Naliboff BD, Chang L, et al. Enhanced preattentive central nervous system reactivity in irritable bowel syndrome. Am J Gastroenterol 2002;97: 2791–7.
103. Whitehead WE, Palsson O, Jones KR. Systematic review of the comorbidity of irritable bowel syndrome with other disorders: what are the causes and implications? Gastroenterology 2002;122:1140–56.
104. Locke GR, Weaver AL, Melton LJ, et al. Psychosocial factors are linked to functional gastrointestinal disorders: a population based nested case-control study. Am J Gastroenterol 2004;99:350–7.
105. Spiegel B, Schoenfeld P, Naliboff B. Systematic review: the prevalence of suicidal behavior in patients with chronic abdominal pain and irritable bowel syndrome. Aliment Pharmacol Ther 2007;26:183–93.
106. Canavan JB, Bennett K, Feely J, et al. Significant psychological morbidity occurs in irritable bowel syndrome: a case-control study using a pharmacy reimbursement database. Aliment Pharmacol Ther 2009;29:440–9.
107. Drossman DA, McKee DC, Sandler RS, et al. Psychosocial factors in the irritable bowel syndrome: a multivariate study of patients and nonpatients with irritable bowel syndrome. Gastroenterology 1988;95:701–8.
108. Karling P, Danielsson A, Adolfsson R, et al. No difference in symptoms of irritable bowel syndrome between healthy subjects and patients with recurrent depression in remission. Neurogastroenterol Motil 2007;19:896–904.
109. Klooker TK, Braak B, Painter RC, et al. Exposure to severe wartime conditions in early life is associated with an increased risk of irritable bowel syndrome: a population-based cohort study. Am J Gastroenterol 2009;104:2250–6.
110. Creed F, Guthrie E. Psychological factors in the irritable bowel syndrome. Gut 1987;28:1307–18.
111. Whitehead WE, Crowell MD, Robinson JC, et al. Effects of stressful life events on bowel symptoms: subjects with irritable bowel syndrome compared with subjects without bowel dysfunction. Gut 1992;33:825–30.
112. Beesley H, Rhodes J, Salmon P. Anger and childhood sexual abuse are independently associated with irritable bowel syndrome. Br J Health Psychol 2010;15:389–99.

113. Heyman S, Maixner W, Whitehead WE, et al. Central processing of noxious somatic stimuli in patients with irritable bowel syndrome compared with healthy controls. Clin J Pain 2010;26:104–6.
114. Choung RS, Locke GR, Zinsmeister AR, et al. Psychosocial distress and somatic symptoms in community subjects with irritable bowel syndrome: a psychological component is the rule. Am J Gastroenterol 2009;104:1772–9.
115. Posserud I, Svedlund J, Wallin J, et al. Hypervigilance in irritable bowel syndrome compared with organic gastrointestinal disease. J Psychosom Res 2009;66:399–405.
116. Jones R, Latinovic R, Charlton J, et al. Physical and psychosocial co-morbidity in irritable bowel syndrome: a matched cohort study using the General Practice Research Database. Aliment Pharmacol Ther 2006;24:879–86.
117. Nicholl BI, Halder SL, MacFarlane GJ, et al. Psychosocial risk markers for new onset irritable bowel syndrome–results of a large prospective population-based study. Pain 2008;137:147–55.
118. Hislop IG. Psychological significance of the irritable colon syndrome. Gut 1971; 12:452–7.
119. Blanchard EB, Lackner JM, Jaccard J, et al. The role of stress in symptom exacerbation among IBS patients. J Psychosom Res 2008;64:119–28.
120. Heitkemper M, Charman AB, Shaver J, et al. Self-report and polysomnographic measures of sleep in women with irritable bowel syndrome. Nurs Res 1998;47: 270–7.
121. Nojkov B, Rubenstein JH, Chey WD, et al. The impact of rotating shift work on the prevalence of irritable bowel syndrome in women. Am J Gastroenterol 2010;105:842–7.
122. Drossman DA, Leserman J, Nachman G, et al. Sexual and physical abuse in women with functional or organic disorders. Ann Intern Med 1990;113:828–33.
123. Drossman DA, Talley NJ, Leserman J, et al. Sexual and physical abuse and gastrointestinal illness. Reviews and recommendations. Ann Intern Med 1995; 123:782–94.
124. Talley NJ, Fett SL, Zinsmeister AR, et al. Gastrointestinal tract symptoms and self-reported abuse: a population-based study. Gastroenterology 1994;107: 1040–9.
125. Drossman DA, Li Z, Leserman J, et al. Health status by gastrointestinal diagnosis and abuse history. Gastroenterology 1996;110:999–1007.
126. Ali A, Toner BB, Stickless N, et al. Emotional abuse, self-blame, and self-silencing in women with irritable bowel syndrome. Psychosom Med 2000;62:76–82.
127. Tache Y, Bonaz B. Corticotropin-releasing factor receptors and stress-related alterations of gut motor function. J Clin Invest 2007;117:33–40.
128. Posserud I, Agerforz P, Ekman R, et al. Altered visceral perceptual and neuroendocrine response in patients with irritable bowel syndrome during mental stress. Gut 2004;53:1102–8.
129. Dinan TG, Quigley EM, Ahmed SM, et al. Hypothalamic-pituitary-gut axis dysregulation in irritable bowel syndrome: plasma cytokines as a potential biomarker? Gastroenterology 2006;130:304–11.
130. Videlock EJ, Adeyemo M, Licudine A, et al. Childhood trauma is associated with hypothalamic-pituitary-adrenal axis responsiveness in irritable bowel syndrome. Gastroenterology 2009;137:1954–62.
131. Burr RL, Jarrett ME, Cain KC, et al. Catecholamine and cortisol levels during sleep in women with irritable bowel syndrome. Neurogastroenterol Motil 2009; 21:1148–e97.

132. Chang L, Sundaresh S, Elliott J, et al. Dysregulation of the hypothalamic-pituitary-adrenal (HPA) axis in irritable bowel syndrome. Neurogastroenterol Motil 2009;21:149–59.
133. Blomhoff S, Spetalen S, Jacobsen MB, et al. Rectal tone and brain information processing in irritable bowel syndrome. Dig Dis Sci 2000;45:1153–9.
134. Ringel Y, Whitehead WE, Toner BB, et al. Sexual and physical abuse are not associated with rectal hypersensitivity in patients with irritable bowel syndrome. Gut 2004;53:838–42.
135. Spetalen S, Sandvik L, Blomhoff S, et al. Autonomic function at rest and in response to emotional and rectal stimuli in women with irritable bowel syndrome. Dig Dis Sci 2008;53:1652–9.
136. Morgan V, Pickens D, Gautam S, et al. Amitriptyline reduces rectal pain related activation of the anterior cingulate cortex in patients with irritable bowel syndrome. Gut 2005;54:601–7.
137. Hungin AP, Whorwell PJ, Tack J, et al. The prevalence, patterns and impact of irritable bowel syndrome: an international survey of 40,000 subjects. Aliment Pharmacol Ther 2003;17:643–50.

The Role of Genetics in IBS

Yuri A. Saito, MD, MPH

KEYWORDS

- Irritable bowel syndrome • Genetics • Gene
- Complex genetic disease

As discussed in articles elsewhere in this issue, irritable bowel syndrome (IBS) is a chronic disorder characterized by abdominal pain or discomfort and diarrhea and/or constipation that can be associated with altered gastrointestinal motility and visceral sensation. The chronicity of IBS symptoms and the lack of a cure or effective treatments result in loss of work and school productivity and impaired personal and health-related quality of life.[1] Patients, their relatives, and friends frequently ask difficult questions, such as why they in particular developed IBS. Although diet, psychological factors, infection, and gut flora may attenuate IBS symptoms, there is no simple answer to this question. As other family members may concurrently have bowel disturbances, the role of genes in disease development—and the sense of personal destiny it invokes—is somewhat intuitive, easy to accept, but also difficult to refute with facts or objective findings arguing the contrary.

Great advances have been made in genetics in recent years. As the efficiency, ease, and cost of genotyping has decreased, our understanding of DNA sequence, structure, and function has improved dramatically. Previously, laboratory-based study of the human genome was often restricted to known genes and coding exon regions and study of a handful of genetic variants. Now, high-throughput technology allows genotyping of thousands to a million genetic markers across the genome, and sequencing of nearly the entire [coding] human genome is now possible. Furthermore, advances in data storage and analysis of these large quantities of data has led to the discovery of susceptibility loci for several diseases including, notably, Crohn's disease. These amazing scientific strides have led many to believe that "virtually every human ailment, except perhaps trauma, has some basis in our genes." (www.genome. gov). This premise has appealed to many IBS researchers, and several have commenced in trying to identify an IBS gene or set of genes.

Despite the acceptance by some that genes may cause—or at least contribute to the development of—IBS, careful examination of the body of literature is necessary

This work was supported by National Institutes of Health grant, DK76797.
The author has nothing to disclose.
Division of Gastroenterology and Hepatology, Mayo Clinic, 200 First Street SW, Rochester, MN 55905, USA
E-mail address: saito.yuri@mayo.edu

Gastroenterol Clin N Am 40 (2011) 45–67
doi:10.1016/j.gtc.2010.12.011
0889-8553/11/$ – see front matter © 2011 Elsevier Inc. All rights reserved.

gastro.theclinics.com

to determine whether there is sound basis for this theory, as gene discovery still requires considerable time, effort and, thus, financial resources. Alternative hypotheses, such as environmental exposures, certainly exist and cannot be ignored as important players in IBS. This article provides a summary of the studies around the competing hypotheses of "gene versus environment" or "nature versus nurture" in IBS. An overview of family studies, candidate gene studies, and alternative hypotheses for IBS are covered, to provide the reader an overview of the works conducted in this area.

IBS AS A COMPLEX GENETIC DISORDER

Classic Mendelian genetics diseases are typically caused by a few highly penetrant genetic defects on a single gene and are transmitted in a typical pattern through families. Mendelian diseases follow an autosomal dominant, recessive, codominant, or X-linked pattern of transmission through pedigrees. Recent genetic studies have focused less on Mendelian disorders and more on complex genetic diseases. A "complex genetic disease" is defined as a multifactorial genetic disorder resulting from multiple genetic variants on several genes (ie, polygenic) with contributions from environment and lifestyle. These genetic effects are modest in that the presence of a specific variant is rarely sufficient on its own to result in disease development. Complex genetic diseases are still heritable in that they tend to aggregate in families, but not in the same predictable fashion as classic Mendelian disorders.

Many common diseases of significant public health interest are thought to be complex disorders. Heart disease, hypertension, diabetes, obesity, autism, and mood disorders are a few of the diseases and disorders under study by geneticists and genetic epidemiologists. In gastroenterology, Crohn's disease is the best example of a complex genetic disorder with successful susceptibility loci identification. A combination of family-based linkage studies, candidate gene and fine-mapping studies, as well as genome-wide association studies have led to the identification of several genes—such as *NOD2, ATG16L1, IL23, IL12B, STAT3, NKX2-3*—found to be consistently associated with Crohn's disease.[2] These discoveries offer the promise that if gene discovery was possible in this complex gastrointestinal disorder, successful gene discovery is feasible in other multifactorial disorders and diseases including IBS.

Despite the discovery of several genetic loci involved in the development of Crohn's disease, it is clear that genes alone do not cause the disease and that environmental contributions, such as diet, smoking, early exposure to infectious organisms, and colonic microflora, are still important. A similar gene-environment paradigm could be proposed for IBS (**Fig. 1**) whereby a combination of genetic factors and environmental factors result in the alterations in gastrointestinal sensation and motor function that ultimately result in manifestation of symptoms. Genetic variation in genes that encode proteins that regulate gender-based biologic processes, control or modulate central or peripheral sensation and motility, or even regulate brain response to stress would be the obvious first candidates for IBS. These factors, interacting with environmental factors such as diet, infection, and early life trauma and stress, are likely responsible for the overall IBS phenotype. However, the specific combinations of genetic variants and environmental factors likely can in part explain the clinical heterogeneity of IBS. Hence, it is conceivable and likely that genes responsible for diarrhea are different to those responsible for constipation, and other genetic variants that predispose an individual to developing or sensing abdominal pain required for IBS are not generally present in the nonpainful functional disorders such as functional constipation and functional diarrhea. Exploring gene-environment interactions will be

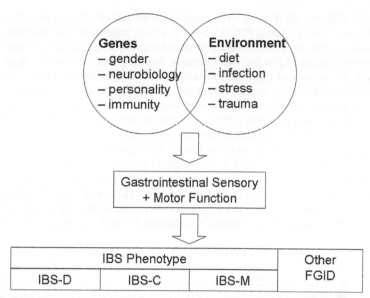

Fig. 1. Gene-environment paradigm in IBS development. A gene-environment paradigm supports the importance of both genes and environment in the development of IBS for both familial and sporadic IBS. Several combinations of individual genetic and environmental risk factors are possible, with each specific combination resulting in specific alterations in gastrointestinal motor and sensory function, and ultimately symptom presentation and the final clinical phenotype.

important if one postulates that IBS is a multifactorial, polygenic complex genetic disorder.

IBS AND HERITABILITY

Genetic diseases—complex or Mendelian—must run in families. Several studies of patients with IBS suggest that this disorder aggregates in families, and thus appears potentially heritable. Children with persistent recurrent abdominal pain who were found to report IBS-like symptoms as adults were almost threefold as likely to have at least one sibling with similar symptoms when compared with children-now-adults without IBS-like symptoms (40% vs 6%, $P<.05$).[3] Another study of IBS outpatients showed that one-third reported another family member with IBS, even in patients without a concurrent psychiatric diagnosis.[4] In another study, having a first-degree relative with IBS was one of the characteristics found to be predictive of IBS over other gastrointestinal disorders among outpatients consulting their general practitioner for chronic abdominal pain.[5]

The majority of original studies evaluating familial clustering of IBS has been based predominantly on patient reports of having another affected family member with IBS: proxy reporting. However, one study by the author's group has shown that accuracy of patient reporting on a specific relative's IBS status is poor.[6] As a consequence, a large family case-control study was performed, which collected bowel symptom and medical history data directly from cases, controls, and their first-degree relatives. This study of 477 cases, 1492 case-relatives, 297 controls, and 936 control-relatives found that 50% of case-families and 27% of control-families had at least one other relative with IBS (*P*<.05) (**Fig. 2**).[7] The magnitude of this effect was an odds ratio of 2.75 (95% confidence interval [CI]: 2.01–3.76). When looking at the absolute propor- tion of relatives affected, 25% of case-relatives reported having IBS compared with 12% of control-relatives (*P*<.05). Furthermore, the magnitude of familial aggregation did not vary by gender of the proband, with males and females being equally likely to have an affected relative or set of relatives. Although confidence intervals overlap- ped, there was a trend for the strength of aggregation to be greatest among probands with diarrhea, followed by constipation, and then mixed bowel habits. Prior intestinal infections, abuse, and depression or anxiety were more common among cases than controls, and among affected relatives than unaffected relatives. The overall preva- lence of these risk factors was 9% of affected relatives reporting a prior infection (vs 5% among controls), 35% reporting abuse (vs 25%), and 44% reporting depres- sion or anxiety (vs 22%). Thus, a family member of an individual with IBS is 2 to 3 times more likely to have IBS; familial clustering is present irrespective of predominant bowel pattern; and the known environmental risk factors for IBS are also common in IBS families.

Study of the pattern of IBS transmission through families has yielded additional interesting observations. A recent study of children with functional gastrointestinal disorders (FGIDs; but not IBS exclusively), their parents, and their child-aged siblings showed that all mothers, fathers, and siblings of cases were more likely to be affected with another FGID than matching control-relatives.[8] Mothers were the most likely to have an FGID (49.6% case-mothers vs 21.4% control-mothers, *P*<.05), followed by their child-aged siblings (26.4% vs 17.6%, not significant), then fathers (13.6% vs 9.3%, not significant). By contrast, a study of adult patients with IBS by the author's group showed that adult-aged case-siblings had the highest risk of concurrent IBS, followed by their adult-aged children, and then parents.[7] Although female relatives were more likely to be affected with IBS, both genders were still at risk for IBS compared with control-relatives. When formal segregation analysis was performed to determine whether the pattern of transmission of IBS through pedigrees is

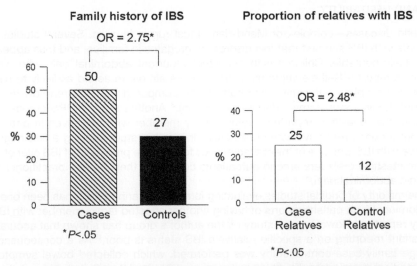

Fig. 2. Familial aggregation of IBS. Fifty percent of cases with IBS will have at least one other family member with IBS, but the overall proportion of first-degree relatives with IBS is 25%. Overall, case-relatives are 2 to 3 times as likely to have IBS than control-relatives.

consistent with Mendelian models (eg, autosomal dominant, recessive, X-linked, and so forth), IBS transmission was not consistent with the sporadic model, meaning IBS appeared consistently in families and in parents, arguing against random mutations causing IBS.[9] More importantly, there was general lack of convergence of the data with segregation analysis. This finding suggests that IBS does not result from a single, major locus, that there was incomplete penetrance, or that IBS could be the result of genetic and environmental factors. Overall findings indicate an underlying genetic basis for IBS.

Although IBS appears to run in families, the previously cited studies suggest that there may be individuals with "sporadic" or nonfamilial IBS as well as individuals with a familial form of IBS. This observation begs the question as to whether there are clinical characteristics suggesting a distinct mechanistic basis for the sporadic and familial forms of IBS. Genetic diseases may present at an earlier age or present with a more specific form of disease, as observed with hereditary colon cancer syndromes. The author's group found that cases with a stronger family history of IBS had more severe pain, had concurrent fibromyalgia, heartburn, and asthma, and reported symptoms of loose stools, urgency constipation, and pain compared with those with less of a family history of IBS ($P<.05$).[10] Age of onset was not predicted by family history of IBS, thus demonstrating that patients with a family history did not experience onset of IBS symptoms at a younger age than patients without a family history of IBS. Although at a univariate level of analysis, somatization level and personal or family history of psychiatric history or abuse were more common among individuals (probands and relatives) with IBS, these factors were not predictive of familial IBS with univariate or with multivariate analyses, suggesting that familial clustering was not related to psychological or psychiatric disease. Kanazawa and colleagues[11] has shown that among IBS patients reporting a parental history of bowel problems, these individuals exhibit higher levels of psychological distress. These studies suggest that familial forms of IBS are characterized by greater pain severity and greater comorbidity, including perhaps psychological distress.

Twin studies also support the concept that IBS may be a complex disorder with genetic as well as environmental contributors. To date, there have been at least 5 twin studies of IBS or functional bowel disorders, estimating that the genetic liability ranges between 1% and 20% with heritability estimates ranging between 0% and 57% (see **Fig. 2**).[12–16] In all but one study, the concordance rates for monozygotic twins (who are genetically identical) were higher than the concordance rates for dizygotic twins, suggesting an underlying genetic etiology. Nonetheless, Mohammed and colleagues[15] found that concordance rates for monozygotic and dizygotic twins were similar for IBS using a validated questionnaire and the Rome II diagnostic criteria to make the diagnosis of IBS, thus arguing that genes are not a major factor in IBS development, and certainly not a major gene with a strong effect. Studies with twins reared apart, which would permit greater discernment of the influence of different environments in genetically identical twins, are unfortunately lacking.

Heritability (h^2) is another statistical estimate to quantitate the relative genetic contribution to a trait, relative to its environmental contributors. Heritability is the amount or proportion of phenotypic variance of the disease of interest in the population that is inherited through genetic factors. The twin studies show that the heritability estimates range from 0% in the British Twin Study, 22% in the Minnesota Twin Study, 48% in the Norwegian Twin Study, to 57% in the Australian Twin study (**Fig. 3**). Using data collected from families and not twin pairs, when the IBS Rome criteria were converted into a quantitative trait based on number of Rome symptoms endorsed and severity, the heritability estimates for IBS ranged from 0.19 to 0.35 depending on the weighting

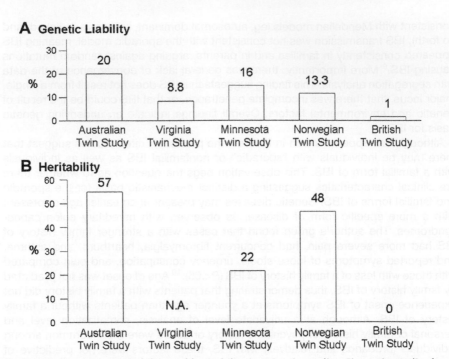

A Genetic Liability

Australian Twin Study: 20
Virginia Twin Study: 8.8
Minnesota Twin Study: 16
Norwegian Twin Study: 13.3
British Twin Study: 1

B Heritability

Australian Twin Study: 57
Virginia Twin Study: N.A.
Minnesota Twin Study: 22
Norwegian Twin Study: 48
British Twin Study: 0

Fig. 3. Estimated genetic liability and heritability in IBS twin studies. Five twin studies have evaluated the concordance of IBS between twin pairs. Genetic liability of IBS has been estimated to range between 1% and 20%, and heritability estimates in the best fit model ranged between 0% and 57% (*A, B*).

factors for each score. In summary, these studies suggest that the genetic contribution to IBS development is reasonably high and comparable to other diseases for which a genetic basis has been found.

ENVIRONMENTAL FACTORS AND FAMILIAL IBS

Despite the consistent observation that IBS clusters in families, this could still be explained by shared environmental contributors or, less likely, individual environmental exposures. Individual environmental contributors that are not likely to be shared among family members or across generations are not discussed in detail in this review. These exposures include early and later life experiences such as nasogastric tube placement at birth,[17] other painful stimuli experienced during infancy, maternal separation,[18] socioeconomic status,[19,20] military deployment,[21] and microflora.[22] These individual environmental factors are still potentially important to be included when gene-environment interactions may be required for disease development. This section discusses shared household exposures that could represent an alternative mechanism besides an underlying genetic basis for the familial aggregation observed in the families of patients with IBS. Environmental exposures that could have been shared between multiple family members include verbal abuse, physical abuse, sexual abuse, shared household stressors (eg, ill family member, unemployment, catastrophe), parenting style, and learned illness behavior.

Verbal, physical, and sexual abuse during childhood has been reported to be more common in patients with IBS than in matched controls in several studies. Up to 50% of patients with IBS may report a history of lifetime victimization.[6,23–26] The mechanism by which abuse is associated with, or possibly leads to development of IBS may be the result of psychological factors rather than a fundamental change in gastrointestinal motor and sensory function. Heitkempker and colleagues[27] have shown that among women with IBS, few differences were observed in characteristics in a comparison between those with and without an abuse history. Furthermore, when 4 groups of patients with and without IBS and with and without sexual abuse histories had rectal distension studies performed, although IBS again reported greater sensitivity to rectal distension, sexual abuse did not attenuate results.[28] Ringel and colleagues[29] have also recently shown that the presence or absence of abuse does not alter rectal sensation or lead to increased rectal pain sensation. By contrast, a population-based study found that although childhood abuse was associated with IBS, the abuse was no longer associated with IBS when neuroticism was accounted for and included in the analyses.[30] In the only family study examining the role of abuse, the author's group has shown that in family relatives, the association between abuse and IBS disappeared after inclusion of somatization in the multivariate model. This finding suggests that either somatization leads to overreporting of abuse or, perhaps more likely, abuse leads to somatization that ultimately results in IBS symptom development and reporting.[7] Furthermore, as the majority of patients with IBS report no history of abuse, abuse is clearly not required for the development of IBS. The familial clustering of IBS is unlikely to be explained by shared household exposure to an abuser, as the prevalence of abuse is the same among familial and nonfamilial, sporadic IBS.[10]

Besides household exposure to abuse, other shared stressors experienced in a family environment, particularly during childhood, could include adverse life events such as loss of a parent or close relative, significant illness in a household relative, singular or recurrent unemployment, and natural disasters. However, adverse childhood events appear very common—approximately 60% of 17,000 adults from a health maintenance organization reported one or more events during childhood, and no secular trends were observed across 4 birth cohorts.[31] Another study specifically comparing the role of early adverse life events among IBS patients and controls with respect to salivary cortisol measurements before and after a visceral stressor found that early adverse life events were present in nearly 50% of patients with IBS as well as their matched controls, and that IBS was equally common among individuals reporting adverse life events as compared with individuals reporting no early life events.[32] Although cortisol levels were higher among individuals reporting adverse childhood events than in those without early events, IBS patients did not have different salivary cortisol responses to stress than controls, and there was only a trend for an interaction between IBS patients who had reported life events and higher cortisol levels compared with controls ($P = .056$). Furthermore, although adverse life events appear to be common across time and thus possibly across generations, they are unlikely to be shared across multiple generations, making the hypothesis that they could contribute to familial clustering of IBS less viable.

Besides childhood or early adulthood exposures and stressors, others have suggested that the familial clustering of IBS may be a result of learned illness behavior modeled from parents. Whitehead and colleagues[33] surveyed a sample of the general population in metropolitan Cincinnati and found that individuals with IBS symptoms exhibited somatic behavior (eg, reporting more complaints, consulting physicians for minor complaints) but, importantly, reported being given gifts or special foods as children during illness—findings not found in those in acute diseases such as patients with peptic ulcer and the asymptomatic general population. Another study also confirmed that patients with IBS were more likely to miss school and have more doctor visits as children than individuals without IBS, suggesting that their parents paid greater attention to their illnesses, reinforcing chronic illness behaviors.[34] Levy and colleagues[35] conducted an interview study of mothers with IBS and their children, and compared them to mothers without IBS and their children. The study found that children of mothers with IBS have more gastrointestinal as well as nongastrointestinal symptoms, and have more school absences and physician visits. The investigators found that mother-IBS status was independent of maternal solicitousness (reinforcement of illness behavior) where parent-IBS status influenced children's perceptions of symptom severity but not their perception of the seriousness of gastrointestinal symptoms, whereas parental solicitousness appeared to influence the children's reporting of seriousness of symptoms but not severity. Ultimately, the study supported the role of learned illness behavior, although the investigators could not distinguish genetic and environmental contributors to gastrointestinal symptoms.

In summary, shared household environmental factors—whether abuse, other early adverse life events, or learned illness behavior from parental modeling—could explain a subset of cases with IBS, but the degree to which they contribute to familial clustering of IBS still remains to be fully elucidated.

GENETIC DISEASES THAT MIMIC IBS

One of the great challenges of studying the genetics of IBS is that there are several disorders with symptoms similar to IBS, and a group of these may also have an underlying genetic basis. These diseases include inflammatory bowel disease (eg, Crohn's disease, ulcerative colitis) and celiac sprue. These genetic traits may also coexist with IBS—lactose or fructose intolerance, for example—whose presence does not necessarily preclude an IBS diagnosis. As these disorders are not always ruled out before inclusion in family studies, there will always be some degree of uncertainty regarding the potential role of these disorders in the familial aggregation of IBS. Despite this concern of another genetic disorder mimicking IBS, the author's group found in more than 500 IBS cases that their IBS diagnoses endured over inflammatory conditions after extensive chart review as well as serologic testing for celiac sprue.[7] Celiac sprue was found in only 1% of IBS cases and in a comparable proportion of controls. When Villani and colleagues[36] screened loci associated with Crohn's disease and ulcerative colitis in their sample, IBD loci were not observed in the IBS group. Similarly, the prevalence of lactase nonpersistence was no different between IBS cases and controls (15% vs 14%),[37] suggesting that this autosomal recessive trait is unlikely to explain IBS, let alone explain the familial aggregation of IBS. Nonetheless, as a mimicker, testing for and adjustment for lactose intolerance, inflammatory bowel disease, and celiac disease may be necessary in gene studies of IBS.

In addition to gastrointestinal diseases, it may be important to account for the genetics of other nongastrointestinal disorders such as psychiatric diseases and traits in family studies of IBS, as psychiatric disorders are common in patients with IBS and select antidepressants can be used to treat IBS. Several studies have shown that there is a link between IBS and psychiatric illness, including in families. Sullivan and colleagues[38] reported that among outpatients receiving their first diagnosis of IBS, the prevalence of depression among blood relatives was higher than in controls (5.7% vs 1.8%, $P<.05$), at a level comparable with a group of individuals with major depression (5%). Although the proportion of relatives with depression was higher in IBS patients, the numbers were still quite low, but the investigators argue that self-report of family history is less reliable and likely represents an underestimate of the true prevalence of depression. Woodman and colleagues[39] conducted interviews of relatives of patients with IBS and patients who had undergone a laparoscopic cholecystectomy, and found that the relatives of IBS patients were more likely to report depressive disorders (33.3% vs 17.3%, $P = .05$) and anxiety disorders (41.7 vs 18.7, $P<.05$), but not somatoform (2.1% vs 1.8%, $P>.05$) or substance use disorders (18.8% vs 32.0%, $P>.05$). Whitehead and colleagues[40] performed a similar study interviewing probands with and without major depressive disorder (MDD) and found that IBS was more common in relatives of probands with MDD than in relatives of probands without MDD (16% vs 7%). In short, there has been a suggestion that IBS is part of a larger genetic psychiatric disorder. However, some could argue that because psychiatric comorbidity is related to health care seeking but is not a common feature in community IBS, it is unlikely that a broader psychiatric trait is the heritable component in IBS. The large family case-control study by the author's group did not find that a personal history of psychiatry disease, a family history of psychiatric disease, or a family history of alcohol abuse was predictive of familial IBS.[10] Moreover, as discussed in the next section, it was not observed that common genetic variants associated with mood disorders were associated with IBS in the absence of psychiatric disease.[41] Thus, although it is possible that there is a genetic variant responsible for a psychiatric trait linked to IBS, there is likely a separate genetic and biologic mechanism to explain the remaining symptoms of IBS.

CANDIDATE GENE AND PATHWAY STUDIES

To date, nearly 60 genes have been evaluated to determine whether specific genetic variants may be associated with IBS. The genes, the genetic markers, the findings, and references for these studies are summarized in **Table 1**. The genes studied lie in the following main pathways: serotonin, adrenergic, inflammation, intestinal barrier, and psychiatric. The genes studied were selected because of their proteins' putative role in gastrointestinal motor or sensory function or because of their potential role in resistance or response to microbial organisms. As gastrointestinal motility and sensation are abnormal in a subset of IBS patients, infection is a risk factor for IBS development, and antibiotic therapy can attenuate IBS symptoms, the genes encoding proteins and peptides related to gastrointestinal function pose an attractive target of study. Because the number of genetic markers and genes is too great to review in entirety, this section focuses primarily on genetic pathways and positive findings reported by investigators.

Serotonin has been well studied because of its presence in the intestinal tract and brain. More than 95% of the body's serotonin is located in intestinal enterochromaffin cells, but this neurotransmitter is best known for its effect on mood. Selective serotonin reuptake inhibitors (SSRIs) are one of the most effective antidepressant therapies available. Furthermore, serotonin receptor agonists and antagonists are known to accelerate and slow down gastrointestinal transit and have a positive impact on IBS symptoms.[42,43] The serotonin transporter linked polymorphic region (5-HTT LPR) is the best studied functional variant in the psychiatric and IBS field. Eleven candidate gene association studies and a meta-analysis have been published, largely demonstrating no link between this variable number tandem repeat (VNTR) polymorphism and IBS and its subtypes.[44] In contrast to the psychiatric literature in which several studies suggest gene-environment interactions between this variant and abuse or other stressors, no similar interaction was seen between this variant and environmental factors such as abuse, parental psychiatric disease, and gastrointestinal infection.[45]

Table 1
List of candidate genes tested in IBS patients

Gene	SNP rs ID #	Variant	Associated with IBS?	References
Serotonin pathway genes				
SLC6A4	rs4795541	5-HTT LPR (44 bp ins/del)	No; LS, LL α IBS-C	36,44,50,64
	—	STin2 VNTR	No	73–75
	rs25531	—	G allele	75
	rs3813034	G>T	No	50
HTR2A	rs6313	102T>C	No	50,76
	rs6311	−1438G>A	No	50,76
	rs6314	H452Y	No	50
HTR3A	—	−42C>T	CT α IBS-D	46
	—	−25C>T	No	46
	—	*70C>T	No	46
	—	*503C>T	No	46
HTR3B	—	386A>C	AC/CC	48
HTR3C	—	489C>A	CC α IBS-D	77
HTR3E	rs62625044	*76G>A	GA α IBS-D	46
	—	*115T>G	No	46
	—	*138C>T	No	46
	—	−189A>G	No	46
TPH1	rs1800532	218A>C	No	50
	rs1799913	779A>C	No	50
TPH2	rs11178997	−473T>A	No	50
	rs4570625	−703G>T	No	50
	rs4565946	90A>G	No	50
Inflammatory/Immune pathway genes				
IL10	rs1800896	−1082G>A	A α IBS; No; G α IBS; GA α IBS	36,50–52,78
	—	−819C>T	No	52
	rs1800872	−592A>C	No	50
TNFα	—	−308G>A	GA α IBS; No; No	52,79,80
	—	−238G>A	G α IBS	79
TGFβ1	rs1982073	+869T>C	No	51
	rs1800469	−509C>T	No	50
NOD2	rs2066847	Leu1007insC	No	50
	rs2066844	R702W	No	50
	rs2066845	G908R	No	50
	rs2076756	—	No	50
NOD1	rs6958571	ND1+32656*1	No	50
CARD8	rs2043	Cys10Stop	No	50
TLR4	rs4986790	D299G	No	50
TLR5	rs5744168	1174C>T	No	50
TLR9+	rs5743836	−1237T>C	T α PI-IBS	50
	rs352139	2848G>A	A α PI-IBS	50
CD14	rs2569190	−159T>C	No	50
NFKB1	rs28362491	−94delATTG	No	50
ATG16L1	rs2241880	T300A	No	50
PTGER4	rs4495224	—	No	50
	rs6313763	—	No	50
	rs9292777	—	No	50
IRGM	rs4958847	—	No	50
	rs13361189	—	No	50
NKX2-3	rs10883365	—	No	50
	rs7078219	—	No	50

(continued on next page)

Table 1
(continued)

Gene	SNP rs ID #	Variant	Associated with IBS?	References
PTPN2	rs2542151	—	No	[50]
	rs2847297	—	No	[50]
IFNA	—	874T>A	No	[80]
TNF	rs1800629	−308G>A	No	[50]
	rs1799724	−857C>T	No	[50]
	rs1800630	−863C>A	No	[50]
	rs1799964	−1031T>C	No	[50]
IL1A	—	−889T>C	No	[79]
IL1B	rs1143627	−31C>T	No	[50]
	rs1143634	F105F	No	[50]
	rs16944	−511C>T	No	[50,79]
	—	+3962C>T	No	[79]
IL1R	—	Pst-I 1970C>T	C α IBS	[79]
IL1RA	—	Mspa-I 11100T>C	No	[79]
IL4	rs2243250	−590C>T	No; C α IBS	[50,78]
	—	−33T	T α IBS	[78]
IL4R	rs1801275	Q576R	No	[50]
	rs1805015	S503P	No	[50]
IL6	rs1800795[+]	−174G>C	C α PI-IBS; G α IBS	[50,79,80]
	—	nt565	No	[79]
	—	−1082A>G	No	[80]
	—	−819T>C	No	[80]
	—	−592A>C	No	[80]
IL6R	rs4537545	—	No	[50]
	rs8192284/ rs2228145	D358A	No	[50]
IL7R	rs6897932	T244I	No	[50]
IL8	rs4073	−251T>A	No	[50]
IL12B	rs10045431	—	No	[50]
	rs6887695	—	No	[50]
IL13	rs20541	R130Q	No	[50]
	rs1800925	−1112C>T	No	[50]
IL23R	rs11209026	R381Q	No	[50]
(3p21)	rs9858542	—	No	[50]
(10q21.1)	rs224136	—	No	[50]
	rs224135	—	No	[50]
(5q31)	rs2188962	—	No	[50]
Intestinal barrier genes				
SLC22A4	rs1050152	1672C>T	No	[50]
SLC22A5	rs2631367	−207G>C	No	[50]
CDH1	rs16260	−160C>A	A α PI-IBS	[50]
	rs5030625	−347G>A	No	[50]
ICAM1	rs5498	K469E	No	[50]
	rs1799969	G241R	No	[50]
DLG5	rs1248696	R30Q	No	[50]
MYO9B	rs1545620	S1011A	No	[50]
ABCB1	rs1045642	3435C>T	No	[50]
	rs3789243	—	No	[50]
NR1I2	rs3814055	−25385C>T	No	[50]
	rs6785049	7635A>G	No	[50]
LTF	rs7645243	Leu632Leu	No	[50]

(continued on next page)

Table 1
(continued)

Gene	SNP rs ID #	Variant	Associated with IBS?	References
BPI	rs4358188	E216K	No	50
Adrenergic pathway genes				
NET	—	237G>C	No	81
ADRA2A	rs1800035	753C>G	No	50,64,81
	rs1800544	−1291C>G	G α IBS-C; CG/GG α IBS-D; No	50,81,82
ADRA2C	—	Del 332–335	IBS-C	81
Psychiatric genes				
FKBP5	rs3800373	—	No	41
	rs1360780	—	No	41
	rs9470080	—	No	41
COMT	rs4680	Val158Met	Met α IBS-C	41
NPY	rs16147	—	No	41
BDNF	rs6265	Val166Met	Met α psychiatric IBS	41
ANKK1	rs1800497	—	No	41
DRD2	rs12364283	Ser311Cys	No	41
OPRM1	rs1799971	118A>G	G α IBS-M, IBS-D females	41
Other tested genes				
CCK	rs1800857	779T>C	No	50
CCK1R	—	Intron1 779T>C	C α IBS-C	83
	—	Exon1 G>A	No	83
	—	266G>C	No	84
	—	8641G>A	No	84
	—	984T>C	No	84
CNR1	—	AAT repeats	Yes	85
FAAH	rs324420	385C>A	A α IBS-D, IBS-M. No	41,65
GNβ3	rs5443	825C>T	No, but possible interaction with gastrointestinal infection	45,50,64,86–88
NPSR1	rs2609234	—	No	66
	rs714588	—	No	66
	rs1963499	—	No	66
	rs2168890	—	No	66
	rs2530547	—	No	66
	rs887020	—	No	66
	rs1379928	—	No	66
	rs323917	—	No	66
	rs323922	—	No	66
	rs324377	—	No	66
	Hopo546333	—	No	66
	rs324396	—	No	66
	rs10278663	—	No	66
	rs740347	—	No	66
	rs324981	Ile107Asn	No	66
	rs727162	Arg241Ser	No	66
	rs6972158	Arg344Gln	No	66
SCN5A	—	G298S	IBS-D	89

Abbreviations: 5-HTT LPR, serotonin transporter linked polymorphic region; IBS-C, constipation-predominant IBS; IBS-D, diarrhea-predominant IBS; PI-IBS, postinfectious IBS; SNP, single nucleotide polymorphism; VNTR, variable number tandem repeat.

In addition to studies of other genetic variants on the serotonin transporter gene (*SLC6A4*), several studies have examined functional single nucleotide polymorphisms (SNPs) on the genes encoding serotonin receptors. These genes that encode various receptor subtypes include *HTR2A*, *HTR3A*, *HTR3B*, *HTR3C*, and *HTR3E*. Three studies had positive findings. One study found that the *HTR3A* −42C>T C/T genotype was more common in diarrhea-predominant IBS (IBS-D) patients.[46] Unfortunately, this finding was not replicated in a second cohort. By contrast, the *76G>A SNP on the *HTR3E* gene was found to be associated with IBS-D in 2 separate cohorts.[46] This finding is intriguing because the 5-HT$_{3E}$ receptor is expressed in colon, small intestine, and stomach, and in vitro studies show that there is increased expression of 5-HT$_{3E}$ subunits and thus may have direct effects on the function of 5-HT$_3$ receptors.[47] Fukudo and colleagues[48] studied the 386A>C polymorphism on the *HTR3B* gene and found that regions of brain activation differed between AA subjects and AC and CC subjects. The author's group has recently performed a comprehensive study of more than 20 serotonin-related genes in 968 cases and controls, and have observed the following associations: (1) 27 SNP associations on 9 genes with IBS with several associations on *TDO2*, *HTR2A*, and *HTR7*; (2) 32 SNPs on 15 genes with constipation-predominant IBS (IBS-C) with multiple associations on *HTR4* and *HTR7*; (3) 26 SNPs on 7 genes with IBS-D with multiple associations on *HTR2A*; and (4) 32 associations on 9 genes with multiple associations on *TPH2*, *DDC*, *TDO2*, *HTR1E*, *HTR2A*, and *HTR7*.[49] Thus, there are several lines of evidence to suggest that genes involved with serotonin processing are important in the pathophysiology of IBS.

Genes encoding intestinal barrier proteins have also been studied because of a subgroup of IBS patients whose symptoms began after an acute gastroenteritis, known as postinfectious IBS (PI-IBS). Villani and colleagues[50] conducted an extensive study using the Walkerton Health Study (WHS), a population cohort created after contamination of a municipal water supply in Walkerton, Canada, that resulted in a large outbreak of acute *Escherichia coli* 0157:H7 and *Campylobacter jejuni* gastroenteritis, with more than 2300 individuals developing acute gastroenteritis. This cohort has undergone clinical assessments as well as intensive surveys to define past and current health, and has been followed longitudinally to provide a unique resource to better understand the epidemiologic features of PI-IBS. In this study, the investigators selected 79 functional variants in 51 candidate genes that encoded proteins involved in intestinal epithelial barrier function, innate immune response, or the serotonin pathways, as well as other genes postulated by others to be potentially associated with IBS, and tested these variants in 228 cases with PI-IBS and 581 controls. Four of the SNPs were associated with PI-IBS. Two variants were on the *TLR9* gene encoding the toll-like receptor 9; one was on *CDH1* gene encoding the tight junction protein, cadherin; and one variant was on *IL6*, which encodes the cytokine, interleukin-6. Fine mapping was then performed with selection of additional SNPs in these 3 genomic regions including functional SNPs associated with inflammatory conditions, nonsynonymous SNPs reported in dbSNP with minor allele frequencies greater than 1%, SNPs disrupting transcription-factor, microRNA, or enhancer binding sites, SNPs located in regulator regions, and tagging SNPs to cover the remaining regions of the 3 genes (defined as 10 kb upstream and 10 kb downstream of coding sequence). When multiple logistic regression to identify risk factors for PI-IBS was performed again, now including the 3 candidate polymorphisms from *TLR9*, *IL6*, and *CDHI*, the original risk factors (younger age, female gender, and so forth) as well as these 3 genetic variants were found to be independent risk factors for development of PI-IBS. These findings appear to be specific to PI-IBS, because when the genetic variants were retested in a separate cohort of non–PI-IBS cases and controls, the results were not reproduced.[36]

In addition to the genes cited, other genes in the inflammation pathway have been studied because of reports of cytokine abnormalities in patients with IBS. *IL10* is the gene that has been studied by 3 groups. Gonsalkorale and colleagues[51] tested one SNP, -1082G>A, and found that IBS patients were less likely to have the high producer genotype. Van der Veek and colleagues[52] subsequently observed no association between the same SNP and IBS, as well as no association between the -819C>T SNP and IBS. Villani and colleagues[36] noted an association between 2 SNPs on *IL10* with noninfectious IBS (-592A>C, -1082G>A). With further fine mapping, 16 SNPs on the *IL10* gene were genotyped and 5 additional SNPs were found to be associated with noninfectious IBS. Three of the 5 new associations could be explained by linkage disequilibrium with the 2 original variants, but 2 variants were still associated with noninfectious IBS, suggesting that genetic variation in the *IL10* promoter region may lead to IBS susceptibility. Nonetheless, the inconsistency in findings between study populations, particularly over the -1082G>A polymorphism, suggests that additional confirmatory work on the *IL10* gene and cytokine is needed.

Because depression, anxiety, and somatoform disorders have been reported to occur in up to 94% of IBS patients,[53] the author's group was interested in evaluating the relationship between functional SNPs that have been consistently associated with psychiatric disorders and clinical traits such as mood disorders and pain sensitivity. To this end, 10 SNPs on 8 genes (*FKBP5, COMT, NPY, BDNF, ANKK1, DRD2, OPRM1, FAAH*) were evaluated.[41] None of the 10 tested SNPs were observed to be associated with IBS overall. However, the *COMT* Val158Met variant was associated with IBS-C (odds ratio [OR] = 1.81, 95% CI: 1.01–3.25), the *OPRM1* 118A>G variant was associated with mixed IBS (IBS-M) (OR = 1.57, 95% CI: 1.06–2.30) and IBS-D in females (OR = 1.69, 95% CI: 1.00–2.85), and the *BDNF* Val166Met SNP was associated in IBS individuals with a psychiatric disorder. These findings are of interest because the *COMT* variant has been linked to anxiety, obsessive-compulsive disorder, panic disorder, and cognitive performance,[54–56] while the *OPRM1* variant has been linked to pain sensitivity, opioid dependence, and social sensitivity.[57,58] The *BDNF* variant has also been linked to emotional reactivity and post-traumatic stress disorder, mood disorders, and schizophrenia.[59–61]

In conclusion, genes *HTR2A, HTR3E, IL10, IL6,* and other genes are intriguing potential candidate genes for IBS (**Fig. 4**). Furthermore, distinct genes—*IL6, CDH1,* and *TLR9*—may represent susceptibility loci for PI-IBS, with genetic studies suggesting that there is a different genetic basis for sporadic, noninfectious IBS and PI-IBS. However, it is clear that the role of these genetic variants in IBS development still bears further replication in other patient cohorts, as well as confirmation through additional clinical and laboratory testing.

ENDOPHENOTYPES IN IBS

Clinical disease can be the result of an aberrant single physiologic pathway, but can also be the result of multiple abnormalities in several biologic pathways. In the latter case, understanding and discovering the individual pathophysiological mechanisms that result in disease presentation can be difficult, and can be even more difficult if the disease has heterogeneous clinical features that vary from individual to individual. The term "endophenotype" originated in the psychiatric literature with the idea that an objective, measurable, and ideally reproducible phenotype of a more abstract or complex clinical phenotype would be more closely related to an underlying biologic

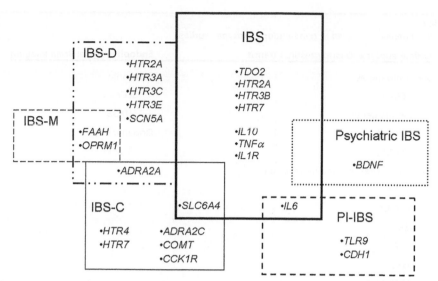

Fig. 4. Summary of positive gene associations, by IBS type and subtype. Positive gene associations shown in **Table 1** are summarized by IBS phenotype. Some genetic associations are unique to specific IBS types and subtypes, whereas others are shown to overlap between IBS subtypes.

process. Use of endophenotypes in research implies that the complex biologic processes causing disease are more easily discoverable if study of the disease can be parsed out into individual, smaller components. Endophenotypes may be a biomarker, or may be referred to as an *intermediate phenotype* or subclinical trait. In genetics research, endophenotypes should generally have the following characteristics: be associated with illness in the general population, be heritable, cosegregate with illness in families, manifest in an individual irrespective of whether the disease is active or inactive, and be found in affected and unaffected family members of an individual with disease at a higher rate than in the general population.[62] Because of the lack of objective findings and the clinical heterogeneity of functional gastrointestinal disorders such as IBS, use of an endophenotype strategy in gene discovery for IBS has appeal. Although none have yet been validated as endophenotypes using the Gottesman criteria, at least 2 testing modalities have been proposed to be potential endophenotypes for IBS: gastrointestinal transit, and brain imaging with visceral stimulation (**Box 1.**)

Gastrointestinal transit as an intermediate phenotype has been studied extensively by Camilleri and colleagues.[63] This group first postulated that because adrenergic and serotonergic mechanisms modulate gastrointestinal motility, an exploratory study was performed examining these 4 functional variants—*ADRA2A* −1291C>G, *ADRC2A* Del 332–325, *GNβ3* 825C>T, and 5-HTT LPR—in 251 patients with FGIDs and healthy volunteers. No direct correlation was seen between these 4 genotypes and upper and lower gastrointestinal emptying and transit time, but when interactions between phenotype (eg, IBS subtype) and genotype were evaluated, several specific interactions were observed. The *GNβ3* CC genotype appeared to be predictive of faster gastric emptying among IBS-D patients, the *ADRA2A* CC genotype was predictive of faster gastric emptying among IBS-M patients, and the *ADRA2C* heterozygous genotype was associated with slower gastric emptying among IBS-M patients but

Box 1
List of genes evaluated in gene-endophenotype studies

Endophenotype: Gastrointestinal Transit	**Endophenotype: Brain Imaging**
Serotonin genes	Serotonin
SLC6A4	*SLC6A4*
Adrenergic genes	*HTR3B*
ADRA2A	Dopamine
ADRA2C	*COMT*
Bile acid processing and metabolism	
NROB2	
SC10A2	
KLB	
FGFR4	
OSTα	
OSTβ	
CYP7A1	
Cannabinoid genes	
FAAH	
Cholecystokinin	
CCK	
CCKAR	
CCKBR	
Neuropeptide S	
NPSR1	
Other	
GNβ3	

faster gastric emptying among IBS-C patients. In a subsequent study, in addition to reporting associations with IBS phenotypes (also summarized in **Table 1**), this group[64] studied the role of the same 4 genetic markers and rectal compliance and pain sensation, and found an association between 5-HTT LPR LS/SS and increased pain sensation and rectal compliance. Besides these genetic markers, these investigators[65] evaluated the role of *FAAH* 385C>A in a group of 482 individuals with FGIDs (predominantly IBS patients) with the underlying hypothesis that because cannabinoid receptors are located on brain stem, gastric, and colonic neurons, functional variants that affect endocannabinoid metabolism could affect gastrointestinal motility and/or sensation, and therefore potentially explain IBS-type symptoms. It was found that the A allele was associated with IBS-D and IBS-M ($P<.05$) as well as accelerated transit in patients with IBS-D. In another study, Camilleri and colleagues[66] proposed that 20 SNPs on the *NPSR1* gene, which encodes a receptor for neuropeptide S that is localized in gut enteroendocrine cells, could potentially play a role in modulating gastrointestinal motor function, and found that 4 SNPs were associated with colon transit time, with significance that persisted after false detection rate correction for multiple tests.

These studies suggest that the genetic mechanisms for gastrointestinal transit may be specific to IBS subtype. In addition to the previous studies evaluating a mixed group of IBS patients with subanalysis of IBS subtypes, other studies have looked at isolated subgroups. One study of IBS-C patients and 7 variants in genes encoding cholecystokinin (CCK), CCK_A receptors (CCKAR), and CCK_B receptors (CCKBR) found that the intronic 779C>T polymorphism appeared to be associated with delayed gastric emptying in IBS-C patients, but was not associated with small intestinal or colonic transit.[67] A more recent study evaluated variations in genes controlling bile acid absorption, processing, and metabolism with colon transit in a clinical trial evaluating the effects of sodium chenodeoxycholate (CDC) on colon transit and symptoms in patients with IBS-C.[68] Sixteen nonsynonymous SNPs on 7 genes (NROB2, SC10A2, KLB, FGFR4, OSTα, OSTβ, and CYP7A1) were genotyped and analyzed to determine whether they predicted colon transit time in 36 patients with IBS-C. One SNP on the FGFR4 gene was found to be associated with filling of the ascending colon ($P = .015$) and borderline associations between a SNP on the CYP7A1 gene and colon transit ($P = .08$) were seen as well. The same group has also reported an association between rs17618244 on the KLB gene and colon transit time in healthy volunteers as well as those with all IBS subtypes.[69]

Fewer studies have been published regarding the role that genetic variants play in modulating brain activation and processing of visceral stimuli. The only article published as a full manuscript is a study from Fukudo and colleagues[70] evaluating the role of the 5-HTT LPR polymorphism in brain processing of rectal stimuli by rectal barostat. The investigators postulated that because serotonin neurons in the brain are important in mood as well as anxiety-related behaviors, 5-HTT LPR could potentially predict activation of prefrontal-limbic circuits. Specifically, they hypothesized that the s allele (resulting in lower transcription of the serotonin transporter, leading to greater synaptic quantities of serotonin) could lead to greater activation of the anterior cingulate cortex (ACC) and amygdala. The investigators found that individuals (not IBS patients) with the s/s genotype were more likely to activate left ACC, right parahippocampal gyrus, and left orbitofrontal cortex (OFC) on positron emission tomography (PET) imaging than those bearing the l allele. Because these regions are important in central emotional processing, these findings suggest that this variant may also be relevant in brain activation after colorectal distension in patients with IBS. Labus and colleagues[71] reported similar findings that the s/s genotype appears to result in altered activation of brain regions regulating emotional arousal. In contrast to l carriers who exhibited the expected negative connectivity between the sACC and the amygdala, s/s carriers lacked the feedback inhibition of the amygdala, which they postulated could result in magnified perception of visceral sensation and thus represent a "vulnerability factor" for IBS. The findings from these 2 studies suggest the 5-HTT LPR, although not a risk factor for the clinical IBS phenotype, could represent a susceptibility factor for components of IBS such as central processing of visceral events.

In addition to studies of the much-studied 5-HTT LPR variant, 2 additional variants have been studied in the context of brain processing. Fukudo and colleagues[48] subsequently genotyped the rs1176744 polymorphism on the gene encoding the 5-HT_{3B} receptor subunit (HTR3B) using similar methodology to the previous study, and found that those with the AC or CC genotype demonstrated more activation of the right amygdala, left insula, and left OFC—regions controlling negative emotion—than AA subjects. Truong and colleagues[72] used a different strategy to evaluate amygdala-based responses by measuring acoustic startle response by threats (fear potentiation [FP] and prepulse inhibition [PPI]) in relation to the COMT gene, which encodes the catechol O-methyltransferase enzyme, an important regulator of synaptic dopamine levels. This group found that there was an interaction between genotype, diagnosis (IBS, fibromyalgia, controls) and threat condition whereby Met carriers in patients showed enhanced FP when faced with imminent threat. The investigators speculate that reduced synaptic dopamine in these individuals impairs down-regulation of amygdala-based startle responses that may lead to hypervigilance to symptoms.

THE FUTURE OF GENETIC STUDIES IN IBS

Genetics is rapidly evolving, with technological advances making it increasingly possible to identify common and rare variants on genomic DNA. Current approaches to gene discovery range considerably from the established candidate gene association studies, to the newer genome-wide association studies (GWAS), to newest techniques that involve deep sequencing to identify less common variants. Although the candidate genes have been studied in IBS, the newer methods have not yet been applied to the study of IBS for several reasons and limitations. Ultimately, the greatest constraint on IBS gene discovery is the IBS phenotype. IBS is a heterogeneous, unstable disorder, without a well-defined molecular pathway or established biomarkers, whose development is clearly multifactorial. Twin studies suggest that there are genes of modest effect that in part explain IBS, but environmental exposures are clearly important in determining the clinical manifestations of IBS. The importance of these environmental factors—such as early or childhood trauma or stress—cannot be ignored, as they may be crucial components to IBS vulnerability.

Although twin studies suggest a modest contribution of genetics to IBS and other functional disorders, such studies are limited by the same concerns regarding heterogeneous or even vague disease definitions. Although there does not appear to be a single or dominant Mendelian gene causing IBS, the fact that IBS clusters in families and through multiple generations suggests that there is likely a heritable component to IBS. Nonetheless, future genetic studies will need to study well-characterized, homogeneous groups or subgroups of IBS patients. Based on the candidate gene studies, it appears that there may be a different molecular basis for constipation versus diarrhea, sporadic IBS versus PI-IBS, and perhaps even for anxiety-associated IBS versus nonanxiety-associated IBS. In addition to studying IBS clinical phenotypes, validated endophenotypes—whether gastrointestinal transit, brain imaging, or another modality such as visceral sensation measures—will provide a complementary approach for successful gene identification. Because environment clearly affects IBS development and symptom manifestation, these gene-environment interactions should be included in analyses of future genetic studies of IBS. Similarly, studies of epigenetics—environment-induced DNA methylation or histone modification that are heritable but do not result in DNA sequence changes—have not formally been performed but perhaps should be evaluated in future IBS genetic studies. Although genetic studies of IBS need not be family-based and can certainly be performed using information collected from unrelated cases and controls, families represent a unique opportunity to discern the genetic and environmental contributors to the development of IBS. Much work still remains to be done in IBS genetics, presenting an exciting opportunity to make great strides in our understanding of the underlying mechanisms of IBS.

REFERENCES

1. El-Serag HB, Olden K, Bjorkman D. Health-related quality of life among persons with irritable bowel syndrome: a systematic review. Aliment Pharmacol Ther 2002; 16(6):1171–85.

2. Cho JH. The genetics and immunopathogenesis of inflammatory bowel disease. Nat Rev Immunol 2008;8(6):458–66.

3. Pace F, Zuin G, Di Giacomo S, et al. Family history of irritable bowel syndrome is the major determinant of persistent abdominal complaints in young adults with a history of pediatric recurrent abdominal pain. World J Gastroenterol 2006; 12(24):3874–7.

4. Whorwell PJ, McCallum M, Creed FH, et al. Non-colonic features of irritable bowel syndrome. Gut 1986;27(1):37–40.

5. Bellentani S, Baldoni P, Petrella S, et al. A simple score for the identification of patients at high risk of organic diseases of the colon in the family doctor consulting room. The Local IBS Study Group. Fam Pract 1990;7(4):307–12.

6. Saito YA, Zimmerman JM, Harmsen WS, et al. Irritable bowel syndrome aggregates strongly in families: a family-based case-control study. Neurogastroenterol Motil 2008;20:790–7.

7. Saito YA, Petersen GM, Larson JJ, et al. Familial aggregation of irritable bowel syndrome: a family case-control study. Am J Gastroenterol 2010;105(4):833–41.

8. Buonavolonta R, Coccorullo P, Turco R, et al. Familial aggregation in children affected by functional gastrointestinal disorders. J Pediatr Gastroenterol Nutr 2010;50(5):500–5.

9. Saito-Loftus Y, Larson J, Atkinson E, et al. Irritable bowel syndrome (IBS) is not a major gene, Mendelian disorder. Am J Gastroenterol 2008;103(Suppl S):S472.

10. Saito Y, Zimmerman J, Almazar-Elder A, et al. Clinical characteristics of familial irritable bowel syndrome (IBS) differ from sporadic IBS. Gastroenterology 2008; 134(4 Suppl 1):A-30.

11. Kanazawa M, Endo Y, Whitehead WE, et al. Patients and nonconsulters with irritable bowel syndrome reporting a parental history of bowel problems have more impaired psychological distress. Dig Dis Sci 2004;49(6):1046–53.

12. Morris-Yates A, Talley NJ, Boyce PM, et al. Evidence of a genetic contribution to functional bowel disorder. Am J Gastroenterol 1998;93(8):1311–7.

13. Levy RL, Jones KR, Whitehead WE, et al. Irritable bowel syndrome in twins: heredity and social learning both contribute to etiology. Gastroenterology 2001; 121(4):799–804.

14. Lembo A, Zaman M, Jones M, et al. Influence of genetics on irritable bowel syndrome, gastro-oesophageal reflux and dyspepsia: a twin study. Aliment Pharmacol Ther 2007;25(11):1343–50.

15. Mohammed I, Cherkas LF, Riley SA, et al. Genetic influences in irritable bowel syndrome: a twin study. Am J Gastroenterol 2005;100(6):1340–4.

16. Svedberg P, Johansson S, Wallander MA, et al. Extra-intestinal manifestations associated with irritable bowel syndrome: a twin study. Aliment Pharmacol Ther 2002;16(5):975–83.

17. Anand K, Runeson B, Jacobson B. Gastric suction at birth associated with long-term risk for functional intestinal disorders in later life. J Pediatr 2004;144(4): 449–54.

18. Barreau F, Ferrier L, Fioramonti J, et al. New insights in the etiology and pathophysiology of irritable bowel syndrome: contribution of neonatal stress models. Pediatr Res 2007;62(3):240–5.

19. Howell S, Talley N, Quine S, et al. The irritable bowel syndrome has origins in the childhood socioeconomic environment. Am J Gastroenterol 2004;99(8): 1572–8.

20. Mendall M, Kumar D. Antibiotic use, childhood affluence and irritable bowel syndrome (IBS). Eur J Gastroenterol Hepatol 1998;10(1):59–62.

21. Gray GC, Reed RJ, Kaiser KS, et al. Self-reported symptoms and medical conditions among 11,868 Gulf War-era veterans: the Seabee Health Study. Am J Epidemiol 2002;155(11):1033–44.
22. Gasbarrini A, Lauritano EC, Garcovich M, et al. New insights into the pathophysiology of IBS: intestinal microflora, gas production and gut motility. Eur Rev Med Pharmacol Sci 2008;12(Suppl 1):111–7.
23. Drossman DA. Irritable bowel syndrome and sexual/physical abuse history. Eur J Gastroenterol Hepatol 1997;9(4):327–30.
24. Walker EA, Katon WJ, Roy-Byrne PP, et al. Histories of sexual victimization in patients with irritable bowel syndrome or inflammatory bowel disease. Am J Psychiatry 1993;150(10):1502–6.
25. Talley NJ, Fett SL, Zinsmeister AR, et al. Gastrointestinal tract symptoms and self-reported abuse: a population-based study. Gastroenterology 1994;107(4): 1040–9.
26. Talley NJ, Fett SL, Zinsmeister AR. Self-reported abuse and gastrointestinal disease in outpatients: association with irritable bowel-type symptoms. Am J Gastroenterol 1995;90(3):366–71.
27. Heitkemper M, Jarrett M, Taylor P, et al. Effect of sexual and physical abuse on symptom experiences in women with irritable bowel syndrome. Nurs Res 2001; 50(1):15–23.
28. Whitehead WE, Crowell MD, Davidoff AL, et al. Pain from rectal distension in women with irritable bowel syndrome: relationship to sexual abuse. Dig Dis Sci 1997;42(4):796–804.
29. Ringel Y, Whitehead WE, Toner BB, et al. Sexual and physical abuse are not associated with rectal hypersensitivity in patients with irritable bowel syndrome. Gut 2004;53(6):838–42.
30. Talley NJ, Boyce PM, Jones M. Is the association between irritable bowel syndrome and abuse explained by neuroticism? A population based study. Gut 1998;42(1):47–53.
31. Dube SR, Felitti VJ, Dong M, et al. The impact of adverse childhood experiences on health problems: evidence from four birth cohorts dating back to 1900. Prev Med 2003;37(3):268–77.
32. Videlock EJ, Adeyemo M, Licudine A, et al. Childhood trauma is associated with hypothalamic-pituitary-adrenal axis responsiveness in irritable bowel syndrome. Gastroenterology 2009;137(6):1954–62.
33. Whitehead W, Winget C, Fedoravicius A, et al. Learned illness behavior in patients with irritable bowel syndrome and peptic ulcer. Dig Dis Sci 1982;27(3): 202–8.
34. Lowman B, Drossman D, Cramer E, et al. Recollection of childhood events in adults with irritable bowel syndrome. J Clin Gastroenterol 1987;9(3):324–30.
35. Levy R, Whitehead W, Walker L, et al. Increased somatic complaints and health-care utilization in children: effects of parent IBS status and parent response to gastrointestinal symptoms. Am J Gastroenterol 2004;99(12):2442–51.
36. Villani A, Saito Y, Lemire M, et al. Validation of genetic risk factors for post-infectious irritable bowel syndrome (IBS) in patients with sporadic IBS. Gastroenterology 2009;136(5 Suppl 1):289.
37. Chang J, Locke G, Talley N, et al. Comparison of lactase variant MCM6-13910C>T testing and self-report of dairy sensitivity in patients with irritable bowel syndrome. Am J Gastroenterol 2010;105(Suppl 1):S499.
38. Sullivan G, Jenkins PL, Blewett AE. Irritable bowel syndrome and family history of psychiatric disorder: a preliminary study. Gen Hosp Psychiatry 1995;17(1):43–6.

39. Woodman CL, Breen K, Noyes R Jr, et al. The relationship between irritable bowel syndrome and psychiatric illness. A family study. Psychosomatics 1998;39(1): 45–54.

40. Whitehead WE, Bosmajian L, Zonderman AB, et al. Symptoms of psychologic distress associated with irritable bowel syndrome. Comparison of community and medical clinic samples. Gastroenterology 1988;95(3):709–14.

41. Saito Y, Larson J, Atkinson E, et al. A candidate gene association study of functional "psychiatric" polymorphisms in irritable bowel syndrome. Gastroenterology 2010;138(5 Suppl 1):348.

42. Ford AC, Brandt LJ, Young C, et al. Efficacy of 5-HT$_3$ antagonists and 5-HT$_4$ agonists in irritable bowel syndrome: systematic review and meta-analysis. Am J Gastroenterol 2009;104:1831–43.

43. Tack J, Muller-Lissner S, Bytzer P, et al. A randomised controlled trial assessing the efficacy and safety of repeated tegaserod therapy in women with irritable bowel syndrome with constipation. Gut 2005;54(12):1707–13.

44. Van Kerkhoven LA, Laheij RJ, Jansen JB. Meta-analysis: a functional polymorphism in the gene encoding for activity of the serotonin transporter protein is not associated with the irritable bowel syndrome. Aliment Pharmacol Ther 2007;26(7):979–86.

45. Saito Y, Larson J, Atkinson E, et al. The role of 5-HTT LPR and GNbeta3 825C>T polymorphisms and gene environment interactions in irritable bowel syndrome. Gastroenterology 2009;136(5 Suppl 1):289.

46. Kapeller J, Houghton L, Monnikes H, et al. First evidence for an association of functional variant in the microRNA-510 target site of the serotonin receptor-type 3E gene with diarrhea predominant irritable bowel syndrome. Hum Mol Genet 2008;17(19):2967–77.

47. Niesler B, Frank B, Kapeller J, et al. Cloning, physical mapping and expression analysis of the human 5-HT3 serotonin receptor-like genes HTR3C, HTR3D and HTR3E. Gene 2003;310:101–11.

48. Fukudo S, Ozaki N, Watanabe S, et al. Impact of serotonin-3 receptor gene polymorphism on brain activation by rectal distention in human. Gastroenterology 2009;136(5 Suppl 1):A-170.

49. Saito Y, Larson J, Atkinson E, et al. A serotonin-pathway candidate gene association study of irritable bowel syndrome (IBS). Gastrenterology 2010;138(5 Suppl 1):348.

50. Villani A-C, Lemire M, Thabane M, et al. Genetic risk factors for post-infectious irritable bowel syndrome following a waterborne outbreak of gastroenteritis. Gastroenterology 2010;138(4):1502–13.

51. Gonsalkorale WM, Perrey C, Pravica V, et al. Interleukin 10 genotypes in irritable bowel syndrome: evidence for an inflammatory component? Gut 2003;52(1): 91–3.

52. van der Veek PP, van den Berg M, de Kroon YE, et al. Role of tumor necrosis factor-alpha and interleukin-10 gene polymorphisms in irritable bowel syndrome. Am J Gastroenterol 2005;100(11):2510–6.

53. Whitehead WE, Palsson O, Jones KR. Systematic review of the comorbidity of irritable bowel syndrome with other disorders: what are the causes and implications? Gastroenterology 2002;122(4):1140–56.

54. Dickinson D, Elvevag B. Genes, cognition and brain through a COMT lens. Neuroscience 2009;164(1):72–87.

55. Domschke K, Deckert J, O'Donovan MC, et al. Meta-analysis of COMT val158met in panic disorder: ethnic heterogeneity and gender specificity. Am J Med Genet B Neuropsychiatr Genet 2007;144B(5):667–73.

56. Hosak L. Role of the COMT gene Val158Met polymorphism in mental disorders: a review. Eur Psychiatry 2007;22(5):276–81.
57. Way BM, Lieberman MD. Is there a genetic contribution to cultural differences? Collectivism, individualism and genetic markers of social sensitivity. Soc Cogn Affect Neurosci 2010;5(2–3):203–11.
58. Tan EC, Lim EC, Teo YY, et al. Ethnicity and OPRM variant independently predict pain perception and patient-controlled analgesia usage for post-operative pain. Mol Pain 2009;5:32.
59. Frielingsdorf H, Bath KG, Soliman F, et al. Variant brain-derived neurotrophic factor Val66Met endophenotypes: implications for posttraumatic stress disorder. Ann N Y Acad Sci 2010;1208:150–7.
60. Cirulli F, Berry A, Bonsignore LT, et al. Early life influences on emotional reactivity: evidence that social enrichment has greater effects than handling on anxiety-like behaviors, neuroendocrine responses to stress and central BDNF levels. Neurosci Biobehav Rev 2010;34(6):808–20.
61. Fan J, Sklar P. Genetics of bipolar disorder: focus on BDNF Val66Met polymorphism. Novartis Found Symp 2008;289:60–72 [discussion: 72–3, 87–93].
62. Gottesman II, Gould TD. The endophenotype concept in psychiatry: etymology and strategic intentions. Am J Psychiatry 2003;160(4):636–45.
63. Grudell AB, Camilleri M, Carlson P, et al. An exploratory study of the association of adrenergic and serotonergic genotype and gastrointestinal motor functions. Neurogastroenterol Motil 2008;20(3):213–9.
64. Camilleri M, Busciglio I, Carlson P, et al. Candidate genes and sensory functions in health and irritable bowel syndrome. Am J Physiol Gastrointest Liver Physiol 2008;295(2):G219–25.
65. Camilleri M, Carlson P, McKinzie S, et al. Genetic variation in endocannabinoid metabolism, gastrointestinal motility, and sensation. Am J Physiol Gastrointest Liver Physiol 2008;294(1):G13–9.
66. Camilleri M, Carlson P, Zinsmeister AR, et al. Neuropeptide S receptor induces neuropeptide expression and associates with intermediate phenotypes of functional gastrointestinal disorders. Gastroenterology 2010;138(1):98–107, e104.
67. Cremonini F, Camilleri M, McKinzie S, et al. Effect of CCK-1 antagonist, dexloxiglumide, in female patients with irritable bowel syndrome: a pharmacodynamic and pharmacogenomic study. Am J Gastroenterol 2005;100(3):652–63.
68. Rao AS, Wong BS, Camilleri M, et al. Chenodeoxycholate in females with irritable bowel syndrome-constipation: a pharmacodynamic and pharmacogenetic analysis. Gastroenterology 2010;139(5):1549–58, 1558 e1541.
69. Wong B, Camilleri M, Carlson P, et al. Klotho-beta gene polymorphism is associated with colonic transit in health and lower functional gastrointestinal disorders. Gastroenterology 2010;138(5 Suppl 1):S-624.
70. Fukudo S, Kanazawa M, Mizuno T, et al. Impact of serotonin transporter gene polymorphism on brain activation by colorectal distention. Neuroimage 2009; 47(3):946–51.
71. Labus JS, Mayer EA, Hamaguchi T, et al. 5-HTTLPR gene polymorphism modulates activity and connectivity within an emotional arousal network of healthy control subjects during visceral pain. Gastroenterology 2008;134(4 Suppl 1): A121.
72. Truong T, Kilpatrick L, Naliboff B, et al. COMT genetic polymorphism is associated with alterations in attentional processing in patients with IBS and other functional pain syndromes. Gastrenterology 2009;136(Suppl 1):A-74.

73. Pata C, Erdal ME, Derici E, et al. Serotonin transporter gene polymorphism in irritable bowel syndrome. Am J Gastroenterol 2002;97(7):1780–4.

74. Niesler B, Kapeller J, Fell C, et al. 5-HTTLPR and STin2 polymorphisms in the serotonin transporter gene and irritable bowel syndrome: effect of bowel habit and sex. Eur J Gastroenterol Hepatol 2010;22(7):856–61.

75. Kohen R, Jarrett M, Cain K, et al. The serotonin transporter polymorphism rs25531 is associated with irritable bowel syndrome. Dig Dis Sci 2009;54(12): 2663–70.

76. Pata C, Erdal E, Yazc K, et al. Association of the -1438 G/A and 102 T/C polymorphism of the 5-HT2A receptor gene with irritable bowel syndrome 5-HT2A gene polymorphism in irritable bowel syndrome. J Clin Gastroenterol 2004;38(7): 561–6.

77. Kapeller J, Houghton L, Walstab J, et al. A coding variant in the serotonin receptor 3C subunit is associated with diarrhea-predominant irritable bowel syndrome. Gastroenterology 2009;136(5 Suppl 1):A-155–6.

78. Barkhordari E, Rezaei N, Mahmoudi M, et al. T-helper 1, T-helper 2, and T-regulatory cytokines gene polymorphisms in irritable bowel syndrome. Inflammation 2010;33(5):281–6.

79. Barkhordari E, Rezaei N, Ansaripour B, et al. Proinflammatory cytokine gene polymorphisms in irritable bowel syndrome. J Clin Immunol 2010;30(1):74–9.

80. Santhosh S, Dutta A, Samuel P, et al. Cytokine gene polymorphisms in irritable bowel syndrome in Indian population—a pilot case control study. Trop Gastroenterol 2010;31(1):30–3.

81. Kim HJ, Camilleri M, Carlson PJ, et al. Association of distinct alpha(2) adrenoceptor and serotonin transporter polymorphisms with constipation and somatic symptoms in functional gastrointestinal disorders. Gut 2004;53(6):829–37.

82. Sikander A, Rana SV, Sharma SK, et al. Association of alpha 2A adrenergic receptor gene (ADRα2A) polymorphism with irritable bowel syndrome, microscopic and ulcerative colitis. Clin Chim Acta 2010;411(1–2):59–63.

83. Park S, Rew J, Lee S, et al. Association of CCK(1) receptor gene polymorphisms and irritable bowel syndrome in Korean. J Neurogastroenterol Motil 2010;16(1): 71–6.

84. Colucci R, Ghisu N, Bellini M, et al. Analysis of cholecystokinin type 1 receptor gene polymorphisms in patients with irritable bowel syndrome. Gastroenterology 2009;136(5 Suppl 1):A-225.

85. Park J, Choi M, Cho Y, et al. Cannabinoid receptor 1 gene polymorphism and irritable bowel syndrome in the Korean population: a hypothesis-generating study. J Clin Gastroenterol 2011;45(1):45–9.

86. Holtmann G, Siffert W, Haag S, et al. G-protein beta 3 subunit 825 CC genotype is associated with unexplained (functional) dyspepsia. Gastroenterology 2004; 126(4):971–9.

87. Andresen V, Camilleri M, Kim HJ, et al. Is there an association between GNbeta3-C825T genotype and lower functional gastrointestinal disorders? Gastroenterology 2006;130(7):1985–94.

88. Saito YA, Locke GR 3rd, Zimmerman JM, et al. A genetic association study of 5-HTT LPR and GNbeta3 C825T polymorphisms with irritable bowel syndrome. Neurogastroenterol Motil 2007;19(6):465–70.

89. Saito YA, Strege PR, Tester DJ, et al. Sodium channel mutation in irritable bowel syndrome: evidence for an ion channelopathy. Am J Physiol Gastrointest Liver Physiol 2009;296(2):G211–8.

Inflammation and Microflora

Mark Pimentel, MD, FRCP(C)*, Christopher Chang, MD, PhD

KEYWORDS

- Irritable bowel syndrome • Inflammation • Microflora
- Methanogenic flora

Irritable bowel syndrome (IBS) is a chronic bowel condition characterized by abdominal pain, altered bowel function, and bloating. It is in fact the most common gastrointestinal condition, affecting 10% to 20% of adults in developed countries[1,2] and accounting for 50% of all gastrointestinal office visits.[2] Due to the high prevalence, the health care costs related to IBS are estimated to exceed $30 billion per year.[3] Moreover, this condition has serious implications for quality of life, which have been likened to diabetes or heart disease, in young adults who should otherwise be productive and healthy.[4] However, despite the seriousness of IBS as a health care issue, the underlying causes remain largely unknown.

Although the etiology of IBS has remained unclear, many hypotheses have emerged, based on associations between IBS and stressful life events in the past[5] as well as altered gut sensations.[6] The association between stress, psychological trauma, and findings of lower thresholds for rectal balloon sensation in IBS[7] led to the concept of the brain-gut dysregulation as a hypothesis in IBS.[8] The brain-gut concept has continued to be a fertile area of work in IBS but unfortunately, it is difficult to prove a cause-and-effect relationship between life events and IBS. In fact, the United States householder study suggested that in the community, psychological problems are not more common in subjects with IBS.[9]

The human intestinal tract is composed of more than 500 different species of bacteria that usually function in symbiosis with the host. Although the composition and number of bacteria in the gut depends on many factors,[10–12] by adulthood, if not earlier, most humans reach an established balance of type and numbers of bacteria that is unique to a given individual, much like a fingerprint. Over the last few years, growing evidence has supported a new hypothesis for IBS based on alterations in intestinal bacterial composition. Several nonmutually exclusive mechanisms may explain how altered gut flora can lead to IBS. First, gut microbes interact with the gut mucosal immune system through innate and adaptive mechanisms. Second,

---

GI Motility Program, Cedars-Sinai Medical Center, 8730 Alden Drive, Suite 225E, Los Angeles, CA 90048, USA
* Corresponding author.
E-mail address: pimentelm@cshs.org

Gastroenterol Clin N Am 40 (2011) 69–85
doi:10.1016/j.gtc.2010.12.010
0889-8553/11/$ – see front matter © 2011 Elsevier Inc. All rights reserved.

altered flora can lead to changes in the intestinal epithelial barrier. Third, neuroimmune and pain modulation pathways may be influenced by the flora.[13,14] Fourth, changing flora can increase food fermentation and subsequent intestinal gas production. Finally, bile acid malabsorption can result from expansion of gut flora into the small bowel.[15] For any or all of these reasons, gut flora can produce IBS-like symptoms.

Further epidemiologic and clinical data support this new bacterial concept of IBS. First, there has been growing data linking the development of IBS to an initial episode of acute gastroenteritis[16,17]; this is now termed postinfectious IBS (PI-IBS). The second area of interest in IBS related to gut microbes is the concept that IBS patients have alterations in the balance of fecal flora. It is on this basis that probiotic studies in IBS began to be conducted. The final and most promising area is that of alterations in small intestinal flora. Relevant studies suggest that IBS subjects have excessive coliform bacteria in their small intestine (otherwise known as SIBO). The link to SIBO has led to clinical trials of antibiotics in IBS. In this article the authors review the evidence for a bacterial concept in IBS, and by the end begin to formulate a hypothesis of how these bacterial systems could integrate in a new pathophysiologic mechanism in the development of IBS. In addition, there have been data to suggest an interaction between this gut flora and inflammation in the context of IBS, and this is also be presented.

GUT MICROBES AND IBS
Altered Intestinal Flora Composition and IBS

The effect of gut microflora on gastrointestinal physiology has been most clearly demonstrated in animal experiments under controlled conditions not feasible in human studies. For example, germ-free rats had delayed gastric emptying and intestinal transit, and a prolonged interdigestive migrating motor complex (MMC) as compared with rats with conventional flora.[18–21] Moreover, introduction of normal gut flora to these germ-free rats normalized their motility.[21,22] Of interest, when germ-free rats were mono-associated with either *Lactobacillus acidophilus* or *Bifidobacterium bifidum*, their small intestine transit accelerated and their MMC frequency increased.[22] Hooper and Gordon[23] profiled gene expression patterns in germ-free mice, and showed reduction of several enteric neuron and intestinal smooth muscle genes. Subsequent mono-association with *Bacteroides thetaiotaomicron*, a highly adapted and abundant commensal of the human and murine colon, restored the normal expression pattern. These experiments, which involve profound changes in the gut flora of rodents, imply a critical role of the resident flora in establishing and maintaining normal intestinal function, and suggest that changes in the gut microflora can lead to significant alterations in gastrointestinal function.

Changes in gut flora of patients with gastrointestinal disorders, including IBS, have been sought for decades. Efforts have been hampered by (1) disease heterogeneity and multifactorial pathophysiology; (2) studies not controlling for diet and medication use that can influence flora composition; (3) potential fluctuations in stability of gut flora and topographic/geographic variability, both in "normal" and affected subjects; and (4) inherent limitations in methodologies to assess gut flora composition. The last challenge in this area will be overcome by evolving technology.

Although culture of the bowel flora has been the mainstay of evaluating intestinal bacterial composition, the majority of intestinal flora are nonculturable, based on fastidious requirements and limited understanding of the vast expanse of human colonizers. DNA-based strategies such as high-throughput pyro-sequencing are considered more sensitive and accurate, but are still costly and technology intensive.

Despite these limitations, culture studies have consistently demonstrated a paucity of *Lactobacillus*[24] and *Bifidobacterium*[25,26] species in the feces of IBS patients compared with controls (**Table 1**), with the exception of Tana and colleagues[27] who noted increased *Lactobacillus*. Although the influence of *Lactobacillus*, *Bifidobacterium*, and other so-called beneficial bacteria have been studied extensively based on their effects on the epithelium, host immune response, and other factors, this is beyond the scope of this article. However, one finding is notable. Balb/c mice infected with a probiotic *L acidophilus* strain had elevated expression of several intestinal pain receptors that led to decreased visceral sensitivity.[28]

While these results sparked the use of these specific probiotics in IBS, there were inherent problems with this initial research. The results are difficult to interpret because of the failure of these studies to control for diet. A common finding in the literature related to IBS is the association between IBS and lactose intolerance.[29] The reason for this remains unclear, yet it is recognized that more than 60% of IBS sufferers have dairy intolerance on this basis.[30] Because dairy products are the prebiotic for *Lactobacillus* and *Bifidobacterium* species, not accounting for diet, leaves the finding of reduced counts of these organisms possibly secondary to intrinsic diet issues in IBS subjects. The ideal study of this topic would be to put IBS and controls on an identical diet for 2 weeks followed by stool evaluation. This lack of control may explain the overall failure of *Lactobacillus*-based treatment in IBS, as discussed later.

Table 1
Studies demonstrating altered intestinal flora in IBS subjects

IBS Subjects, #	Methodology	Findings in IBS Subjects	Citation
Unsubtyped, n = 25	Culture	Decreased Bifidobacteria and increased Enterobacteriaceae	Si et al,[25] 2004
IBS-D, n = 12 IBS-C, n = 9 IBS-M, n = 5	Culture PCR-DDGE	Increased coliforms and aerobic bacteria/total bacteria Increased *Clostridium* and decreased *Eubacterium*	Matto et al,[98] 2005
IBS-D, n = 12 IBS-C, n = 9 IBS-M, n = 6	Q-RTPCR	Decreased *Lactobacillus* in IBS-D, increased *Veillonella* in IBS-C	Malinen et al,[24] 2005
IBS-D, n = 7 IBS-C, n = 6 IBS-M, n = 3	PCR-DDGE RTPCR-DDGE	Decreased *Clostridium coccoides-Eubacterium rectale* in IBS-C	Maukonen et al,[99] 2006
IBS-D, n = 10 IBS-C, n = 8 IBS-M, n = 6	Q-RTPCR (nucleic acid fractionation)	Decreased *Collinsella*, *Clostridium,* and *Coprococcus*	Kassinen et al,[31] 2007
IBS-D, n = 14 IBS-C, n = 11 IBS-M, n = 16	FISH	Decreased *Bifidobacterium*	Kerckhoffs et al,[26] 2009
IBS-D, n = 8 IBS-C, n = 11 IBS-M, n = 7	Culture Q-RTPCR	Increased *Lactobacillus* Increased *Veillonella*	Tana et al,[27] 2010

Abbreviations: DDGE, denaturing gradient gel electrophoresis; FISH, fluorescent in situ hybridization; IBS-C, constipation predominant IBS; IBS-D, diarrhea predominant IBS; IBS-M, mixed IBS; PCR, polymerase chain reaction; Q-RTPCR, quantitative real-time PCR.

Recently, more sophisticated techniques have been used to examine subjects with IBS and their fecal content. In a recent study, molecular techniques were used to determine shifts in flora between IBS and controls.[31] In addition to finding differences categorically, subjects with constipation predominant IBS (C-IBS) also appeared to have unique differences in contrast to diarrhea predominant IBS (D-IBS). Specifically, a lack of *Lactobacillus* and *Collinsella* species were seen in IBS. Of note, C-IBS subjects had an abundance of *Ruminococcus*. In D-IBS, a decrease in *Bifidobacterium* was seen. Even in this sophisticated study, however, diet was not controlled, making interpretation an ongoing issue.

Though not specifically a chronic change in intestinal microflora, acute changes may have an impact on IBS and its development. This process involves the association between IBS and acute gastroenteritis. While this is discussed in detail in this article, animal models used to study PI-IBS further suggest a link between altered gut microflora and IBS. The most characterized postinfectious model of IBS used the organism *Trichinella spiralis*. This parasitic mouse infection model was found to produce reduced gut motility and increased visceral sensitivity to colorectal distention,[32] and has been likened to IBS. However, the stool flora have not been characterized in this model.

Small Intestinal Bacterial Overgrowth and IBS

SIBO is a situation whereby coliform bacterial counts in the small bowel become excessive. Symptoms of SIBO are similar to IBS. In the last decade, growing data have linked SIBO and IBS. Whereas the initial criticism of the work was a consequence of inaccuracies of breath testing as a means of diagnosing SIBO, recent work has begun to confirm the results of breath testing in IBS, supported by small bowel culture.

As early as 2000, work began to emerge suggesting that subjects with IBS have bacterial overgrowth, based on the lactulose breath test.[33] In this initial study, SIBO was suspect in 76% of IBS subjects and although based on a prospective database, appeared to improve after antibiotic therapy using an open-label approach. In the first follow-up study to this work, a higher rate of positive lactulose breath test results (up to 84%) were identifed.[33,34] This rate was noted to be far greater than in healthy control subjects. After this work was published there was a high degree of skepticism, due to the complexities of the breath-testing techniques. Now 10 years later, meta-analyses have been conducted that support the breath test findings in IBS compared with controls. In the first of 2 meta-analyses, Ford and colleagues[35] demonstrated that IBS subjects appear to have a higher prevalence of abnormal breath test results in IBS, but only using the most conservative interpretation of the test compared with controls. The second meta-analysis used a different approach based on simply combining the results of studies using breath testing in IBS versus controls in general.[36] This study demonstrated that IBS patients have a greater likelihood of a positive test compared with controls. When only the best studies were used (age- and sex-matched studies), the odds ratio of a positive test in IBS was 9.64 (confidence interval = 4.26–21.82) compared with controls.[36]

Further validation of the SIBO concept in IBS is based on culture and antibiotic trials. In the largest published study of small bowel culture in IBS, aspirates of jejunal fluid in IBS were found to harbor a greater number of coliform bacteria compared with healthy controls (using >5000 coliforms/mL) ($P<.001$).[37] Studies of antibiotic response also support SIBO in IBS (**Table 2**). Controlled trials in IBS[34,38,39] Pimentel and colleagues,[40] and functional bloating[41] demonstrate successful treatment of IBS with antibiotics based on this excessive flora. Using breath testing as an outcome measure, antibiotic therapy led to improvement of SIBO,[34,41] with a 75% improvement in IBS symptoms observed if normalization of the breath test is seen with antibiotics.[34]

Table 2
Controlled studies demonstrating benefit of antibiotics in IBS

Citation	# of Subjects	Diagnostic Criteria	Antibiotic Used	Length (days)	Primary Outcome Measure	Placebo	Antibiotic
Pimentel et al[34]	111	Rome I	Neomycin 500 mg twice daily	10	Symptom composite	11	35%
Sharara et al[41]	124 (70 IBS)	Rome II	Rifaximin 400 mg twice daily	10	Global symptoms	23	41
Pimentel et al[77]	87	Rome I	Rifaximin 400 mg 3 times a day	10	Global symptoms	21	36
Lembo et al[78]	388	Rome II	Rifaximin 550 mg twice daily	14	Adequate relief of IBS	44	52
Pimentel et al[40]	1260	Rome II[a]	Rifaximin 550 mg 3 times a day	14	Adequate relief of IBS	31.7	40.7

[a] Nonconstipated IBS.

Another controlled trial demonstrated improvement in IBS symptoms that were sustained for a full 10 weeks of follow-up after cessation of antibiotics.[38] Taken together, these findings strongly support a role for the gut microbiome and perhaps SIBO in the pathophysiology of symptoms in a subset of IBS sufferers.

Evidence suggests that SIBO in IBS may be caused by a deficiency in phase III of interdigestive motor activity. During the fasting state, the small bowel cycles through 3 phases of activity, phases I to III.[42] Phase III is a high-amplitude multiphasic motor event, and an absence or reduced frequency of these contractions is known to induce SIBO.[43,44] The authors recently demonstrated that IBS patients with SIBO have significantly reduced phase III frequency, suggesting that attenuated gut motility may underlie the development of SIBO in IBS.[44] Although the physiologic basis for this reduced phase III frequency remains unknown, the interstitial cells of Cajal (ICC) are known to be required for normal intestinal motility (including phase III), and their loss interferes with electrical pacemaker activity, slow-wave propagation, and motor neurotransmission in the gut,[45–54] suggesting that altered ICC function may contribute to altered gut motility in IBS. It has yet to be conclusively demonstrated that changes in ICC are involved in IBS.

Postinfectious IBS

Over the last decade, it has been established that intestinal pathogens play a significant role in the development of IBS. Numerous studies have shown that IBS can be precipitated by an episode of acute gastroenteritis, and that up to 57% of subjects who otherwise had normal bowel function may continue to have altered bowel function for at least 6 years after recovering from the initial acute illness.[55] Based on 2 recent meta-analyses of this research, approximately 10% of subjects who have documented acute gastroenteritis develop IBS, with a summary odds ratio of 6 to 7 for PI-IBS.[16,17] As gastroenteritis is extremely common, so-called PI-IBS may in fact constitute a large proportion of IBS cases. Thus, reducing risk factors for IBS development after acute gastroenteritis may have an impact on the incidence of IBS.

Although the mechanisms of PI-IBS remain unclear, investigators have identified certain risk factors for the development of IBS after gastroenteritis. The 2 most significant of these are duration/severity of gastroenteritis and female sex.[56,57] Stress, manifest as recent traumatic life events, and a neurotic personality trait were also predictors of PI-IBS.[57] Evidence of low-grade inflammation is evident in PI-IBS patients. Rectal biopsies demonstrate mildly elevated intraepithelial lymphocytes and enteroendocrine cells that persisted 12 months after *Campylobacter jejuni* infection.[58] Increased rectal lymphocytes also occur in general IBS patients, but to a lesser degree.[59] Elevated expression of proinflammatory cytokine interleukin (IL)-1β was detected in *C jejuni* PI-IBS rectal biopsies[60] and in *Shigella* PI-IBS rectosigmoid and terminal ileum biopsies.[61] Thus, acute gastroenteritis may increase the risk of developing IBS in a susceptible individual through persistent low-grade activation of the gut immune system, or possibly through establishment of an intestinal dysbiosis, defined as an alteration of the composition of the gut flora. Animal infection models of PI-IBS will play a key role in characterizing the mechanistic pathways and underlying alterations in this process.

The discovery of PI-IBS has led to the development of several animal models. The most comprehensively studied model of PI-IBS developed by Canadian researchers uses *Trichinella spiralis*.[62] This model has now been well characterized.[32,63,64] As *T spiralis* is not a common pathogen in humans and is thus a rare cause of human IBS in the Western hemisphere, other models such as post–*C jejuni* are being developed. One rat model of *C jejuni* infection recapitulates many features of human

PI-IBS including altered stool form, bacterial overgrowth, and increased rectal lympho-cytes, observed 3 months after clearance of the initial acute infection.[65] In fact, some of the first descriptions of PI-IBS in humans stem from *C jejuni* gastroenteritis.

ROLE OF METHANOGENIC FLORA IN IBS

An important group of bacteria that colonize the gut are the methanogenic flora. This distinct group grows primarily under anaerobic conditions, and produces methane (CH_4) as a by-product of fermentation. Intestinal methane production has been linked to diseases such as C-IBS and diverticulosis.[66–69] The presence of significant methane production (seen even with fasting) is observed in 15% of normal controls, and is higher in subjects with conditions such as IBS.[34] Methanogenic archaebacteria are unique in that their metabolism increases in the presence of products from other bacteria,[70] and they use hydrogen and ammonia from other bacteria as a substrate for the production of methane.[71–73]

In studies of gut transit, methane has a physiologic effect. In IBS subjects, those with methane on breath test were noted to have constipation as a predominant symptom subtype (**Table 3**).[66,67] In addition, the amount of methane produced was related to the degree of constipation as measured by Bristol Stool Score and frequency of bowel movements.[67] This outcome is likely the direct effect of the methane gas,[74,75] as small intestinal methane infusion using an in vivo animal model leads to slowing of small intestinal transit by 69%.[76]

Antibiotic Treatment of IBS: Support for a Gut Flora Hypothesis

Although antibiotics will be discussed as a therapeutic approach to IBS in a later article, the role of antibiotics is important here because its benefit supports the concept of altered gut microflora. There are now 5 randomized controlled studies examining the effect of antibiotics in IBS, all of which have demonstrated significant improvement in primary outcome measures[34,40,41,77,78]; these are summarized in **Table 2**. The first of these studies used neomycin.[34] While neomycin demonstrated successful improvement in the primary outcome measure of the study, an important component of the result was that the antibiotic most improved the symptoms when subjects had normalization of their breath test findings. In fact, subjects with complete normalization of their breath test had a near 75% improvement in IBS. This finding is supported by another controlled study by Sharara and colleagues,[40] wherein subjects who were deemed responders to a course of the nonabsorbed antibiotic, rifaximin, had a greater reduction in breath hydrogen, indicating a reduction in intestinal flora. However, the most convincing of all these studies are the 2 latest phase 3 trials (TARGET 1 and TARGET 2).[40] In these studies, rifaximin was effective in improving IBS based on abdominal pain, stool consistency, bloating, and the primary outcome measure of global relief.

Although there is some remaining debate as to why antibiotics help improve IBS symptoms, these antibiotic approaches have provided support for the role of altered gut microflora in IBS.

Probiotics in IBS

If alterations in gut microbiota account for a large fraction of IBS, it seems reason-able that probiotics should restore a "healthy" gut microbiota and alleviate IBS symptoms. Unfortunately, the numerous controlled trials of probiotics in IBS have shown mixed results at best. These studies used a variety of probiotic species and strains, with heterogeneity of dosing regimens and clinical end points

Table 3
Support for the association between methanogens and constipation

Subjects	Total N	Methane N	Breath Test	Definition Positive Breath Test	Citation
32 IBS subjects	32	11	Not done	Breath methane concentration at least 1 ppm	Peled et al,[75] 1987
67 encopretic or constipated children, 40 healthy controls	107	35	Not done	Breath methane >3 ppm	Fiedorek et al,[74] 1990
120 C-IBS with positive lactulose breath test; 11 D-IBS with positive lactulose breath test	231	35	Lactulose	Breath methane >20 ppm within 90 min of lactulose	Pimentel et al,[34] 2003
12 C-IBS; 26 D-IBS; 12 IBS-like	50	12	Lactulose	Breath methane >20 ppm or any increase in concentration within 90 min of lactulose	Pimentel et al,[34] 2003
30 C-IBS; 149 D-IBS; 25 IBS-other	204	32	Glucose	Breath methane >20 ppm when baseline <10 ppm, or any increase of 12 ppm	Majewski et al,[100] 2007
224 IBS; 40 healthy controls	224	44	Lactulose	Breath methane $\geq$1 ppm at baseline or any time during test	Bratten et al,[101] 2008
31 C-IBS; 51 D-IBS; 48 IBS-mixed	130	35	Glucose	Methane excretion >10 ppm at baseline or after glucose	Parodi et al,[102] 2009
24 C-IBS; 23 D-IBS; 9 IBS-mixed/other	56	28	Lactulose	Any detection of methane >5 ppm	Hwang et al,[103] 2010
96 non-IBS chronic constipation; 106 controls	202	87	Glucose	Baseline methane $\geq$3 ppm	Attaluri et al,[104] 2010

(reviewed by Parkes and colleagues[79]). The data are strongest for *Bifidobacterium* and *Lactobacillus* strains. *Bifidobacterium infantis* 35624, *Lactobacillus salivarius* UCC4331, or placebo was given to 77 patients and after 8 weeks, the *B infantis* group had a significant reduction in composite IBS symptom scores and abdominal pain scores versus placebo ($P<.05$). In addition, a decrease in the ratio of IL-10/IL-12 cytokine expression in peripheral mononuclear cells suggested an additional anti-inflammatory effect that was not characterized further.[80] No significant benefit was noted with the *Lactobacillus* strain. A larger multicenter study of 362 women with IBS randomized them to receive *B infantis* (at a dose of 10^6, 10^8, or 10^{10} CFU daily) or placebo for 4 weeks followed by a 2-week washout. Only the middle dose led to statistically significant but modest improvements in abdominal pain, bloating/distention, and IBS composite scores at the end of treatment.[81] The unexpected dose response may have reflected poor capsule dissolution and subsequent lack of bioavailability of the higher-dose probiotic following ingestion. VSL#3 (a probiotic mixture of 8 species of *Bifidobacterium, Lactobacillus,* and *Streptococcus*) or placebo was given to 25 D-IBS patients for 8 weeks. No difference in the primary end point of global symptom relief or gastrointestinal transit was seen. However, the investigators observed a significant reduction in the secondary end point of abdominal bloating.[82] A larger follow-up study did not demonstrate a significant benefit for bloating, but noted a significant decrease in flatulence during the treatment period.[83]

More recently, 3 meta-analyses or systematic reviews identified a small overall beneficial effect of probiotics over placebo.[84–86] The investigators found the studies to be heterogeneous, and that funnel plot asymmetry suggested publication bias. However, several of the trials were of good quality, and these tended to show more modest treatment effects. The clinical trials, as well as animal and translational studies with probiotics, indicate that the myriad species and strains of probiotics are clearly unique, with different biochemical and physiologic effects and possibly highly specific interactions with the mucosal immune and neuroendocrine systems. Therefore, the benefits of one probiotic cannot be extrapolated to another strain without thorough studies. Fortunately, the safety profile and adverse event rate of probiotics has been good. Large, well-designed controlled trials are clearly needed to guide the future use of probiotics in treating IBS.

INFLAMMATION AND IBS

In the past 20 years there has been a growing appreciation of gut mucosal immunology and its role in IBS, particularly the role of lymphocytes, mast cells, and cytokines, which are now discussed.

Lymphocytic Infiltration

In a study of PI-IBS subjects, unprepped patients underwent sigmoidoscopy with rectal biopsy. The mucosal biopsies among these subjects demonstrated an increase in rectal lymphocytes as compared with healthy controls that persisted months after acute *Campylobacter* infection.[58] In the absence of understanding the mechanism of how gastroenteritis led to chronic altered patterns in bowel function, the persistence of low-level inflammation was provocative.

Another finding in examining subjects with IBS is the possibility of chronic inflammation of the enteric nervous system. In a seminal article, 10 D-IBS subjects with severe, refractory symptoms underwent a laparoscopic full-thickness biopsy of the small bowel. In this study, IBS subjects demonstrated evidence of excessive lymphocytes in the ganglia of the myenteric plexus.[87] This ambitious study suggested myenteritis to be present in selected IBS patients, which perhaps explains the visceral hypersensitivity that has been reported by several groups. However, this study is limited by its very small and highly selective study population.

Further evidence for T-cell activation and trafficking to the gut in IBS was demonstrated by Ohman and colleagues.[88] Peripheral blood lymphocyte expression of integrin beta-7 and endothelial cell expression of mucosal addressin cell adhesion molecule-1 (MAdCAM-1) was comparably elevated in patients with IBS and ulcerative colitis (UC) compared with asymptomatic controls, suggesting greater homing of lymphocytes to the gut mucosa.[88]

Mast Cells

Whether in the context of gut microflora or postulated food hypersensitivity, mast cells have been examined in IBS. The first description of altered mast cells in IBS by Weston and colleagues demonstrated elevation of mast cells in ileal biopsies. Since then, Barbara and colleagues[13] have conducted a series of studies examining the role of mast cells in IBS. In a major study, 44 IBS subjects were found to have elevated mucosal mast cells and tryptase in mucosal biopsies compared with controls. The extension of this study was that in deeper sections, there was a tendency for the mast cells to approximate enteric nerves (by <5 μm) in patients with greater abdominal pain. The elevation of small bowel mast cells was later confirmed by Guilarte and colleagues.[89] However, Barbara and colleagues[14] then used extracted material from IBS patients and applied this to a preparation of rat enteric nerves and increased afferent nerve activation. This more recent result has led these investigators to speculate that mast cells and their approximation to enteric nerves could serve to induce visceral hypersensitivity.

Innate Immunity

Another measure of inflammation and immune activation is the balance between proinflammatory and anti-inflammatory cytokines. Although the data on cytokines have been limited to date, a provocative finding in the examination of cytokines in IBS was made during the study of the probiotic B infantis.[80] Specifically, this group found a low IL-10:IL-12 ratio at baseline in IBS. This ratio was normalized with the administration of the B infantis. The difficulty with this study is that the investigators do not state all the cytokines measured. Furthermore, the ratio of these 2 cytokines as a measure of the "inflammatory state" is unconventional. Finally, this same group has since not found this profile in their more comprehensive cytokine studies. Specifically, a recently published study by Scully and colleagues[90] demonstrated in a large group of IBS subjects that IL-6 and IL-8 were elevated in IBS patients without comorbidities, but not IL-10 or IL-12. Furthermore, IBS with coexisting fibromyalgia, chronic fatigue syndrome, or premenstrual dystrophic disorder were associated with the same profile. However, tumor necrosis factor-α (TNF-α) and IL-1β were also noted to be elevated. Similarly, Liebregts and colleagues[91] demonstrated increased IL-6, IL-1β, and TNF-α levels in D-IBS patients compared with healthy controls, patients with mixed IBS, and C-IBS patients. Rectosigmoid and terminal ileal mucosal tissue from PI-IBS patients have also demonstrated elevated levels of proinflammatory cytokine IL-1β mRNA in 2 studies.

Gut Microbiota and Inflammation

Alterations in the gut microflora are associated with IBS, and studies outlined in this review point to the altered flora as a key determinant in pathogenesis. The near consistent finding of low-grade inflammation and intestinal immune activation in IBS, and PI-IBS in particular, may be driven by the gut flora, just as inflammatory bowel disease (IBD) mucosal inflammation is thought to be the result of microbial stimulation of a dysregulated immune system in a genetically susceptible host. This proposed mechanism for IBD is supported by the absence of intestinal inflammation in various germ-free animal models.[92] In that case, might IBS simply reside within a spectrum of intestinal inflammation, bound by IBD at one end and normal mucosa at the other?[93] Genetic susceptibility to IBS may manifest in exaggerated or prolonged low-grade inflammatory responses, psychological vulnerabilities, and/or neurochemical alterations. While most of this discussion of IBS pathogenesis is still rather speculative, the evidence for an activated immune system in IBS is ever increasing. However, the level of lymphocyte elevation seen by Spiller and colleagues[57] of little over 1 additional lymphocyte per 100 epithelial cells, although statistically significant compared with controls, had questionable impact in a subject with already concurrent diarrhea. Was the diarrhea causing the subtle inflammation or is this part of the mechanism of PI-IBS? Further work remains to be done to determine the relevance of this finding.

Of interest, the gut appears to demonstrate a response to gut flora through another pathway. Defensins are innate proteins thought to control intestinal flora through antimicrobial properties. Langhorst and colleagues[94] used enzyme-linked immunosorbent assay to measure fecal levels of this antimicrobial peptide; levels in the colon were detected by immunohistochemistry. Surprisingly, D-IBS and UC patients had elevated fecal β-defensin–2, 72.9 ng/g and 104.9 ng/g, respectively, compared with healthy controls (31.0 ng/g) ($P<.005$). This result may provide further indirect support for a microbial immune interaction.

Anti-Inflammatory Therapy

Despite the evidence for chronic low-grade mucosal inflammation in IBS and PI-IBS, anti-inflammatory therapies have been disappointing in treating symptoms and providing compelling support for the significance of this inflammation in IBS. A placebo-controlled, double-blind, randomized 3-week trial using prednisolone to treat PI-IBS did not improve symptom severity even though a drop in rectal T cells was noted in this underpowered study.[95] Data on the anti-inflammatory drug mesalazine appear promising, but only one study has appeared as a full peer-reviewed article; treated patients in this blinded, randomized controlled trial (RCT) had improved symptoms and decreased mast cells compared with placebo-treated participants.[96] Finally, the use of the mast cell stabilizer ketotifen was associated with improved IBS symptoms and reduced visceral hypersensitivity in a blinded RCT,[97] but larger studies are needed to confirm the effect of an anti-inflammatory approach as regards IBS.

SUMMARY

In the last decade, there has been a significant acceleration in our understanding of gut flora as it pertains to IBS. The preceding sections of this review point to qualitative and quantitative alterations in the gut microflora to be strongly associated with IBS. While specific alterations of stool flora have been demonstrated, these results are difficult to interpret because of a lack of diet control in this research.

Evidence is also accumulating, using direct and indirect testing, that a proportion of IBS subjects may have small intestinal bacterial overgrowth. The evidence for altered gut microflora is supported by an ever increasing list of large randomized controlled studies demonstrating the efficacy of antibiotics in IBS.

Two interesting areas in the study of gut microbes and IBS are the association between methanogenic organisms and constipation in IBS (see **Table 3**), and the role of acute gastroenteritis in the precipitation of IBS. In the case of methane and methanogenic microbes, it appears that methane gas produced by these organisms contributes to a slowing of intestinal transit, which may be responsible for the constipation. In the case of PI-IBS, there is a clear cause-and-effect relationship between acute infection in the gastrointestinal tract and the development of IBS. This breakthrough has led to the development of several animal models in an attempt to characterize the mechanisms of this process.

While there is a growing body of literature examining gut inflammation in IBS, such literature is in its early stages. Mast cells may have an important role in IBS but that role remains to be determined, as studies on cellular infiltrates and cytokines are at this time inconsistent and need validation. Given the complex disease heterogeneity and pathophysiology that is IBS, it is likely unrealistic that any one therapeutic approach, whether antibiotic, probiotic, or anti-inflammatory, will achieve broad efficacy unless patients are first carefully selected and stratified for their underlying pathophysiologic mechanism of IBS.

REFERENCES

1. Drossman DA, Sandler RS, McKee DC, et al. Bowel patterns among subjects not seeking health care. Use of a questionnaire to identify a population with bowel dysfunction. Gastroenterology 1982;83(3):529–34.
2. Thompson WG, Heaton KW. Functional bowel disorders in apparently healthy people. Gastroenterology 1980;79(2):283–8.
3. The burden of gastrointestinal diseases. Bethesda (MD): American Gastroenterological Association; 2001.
4. Lackner JM, Gudleski GD, Zack MM, et al. Measuring health-related quality of life in patients with irritable bowel syndrome: can less be more? Psychosom Med 2006;68(2):312–20.
5. Whitehead WE, Crowell MD, Robinson JC, et al. Effects of stressful life events on bowel symptoms: subjects with irritable bowel syndrome compared with subjects without bowel dysfunction. Gut 1992;33(6):825–30.
6. Silverman DH, Munakata JA, Ennes H, et al. Regional cerebral activity in normal and pathological perception of visceral pain. Gastroenterology 1997;112(1): 64–72.
7. Whitehead WE, Holtkotter B, Enck P, et al. Tolerance for rectosigmoid distention in irritable bowel syndrome. Gastroenterology 1990;98(5 Pt 1):1187–92.
8. Mayer EA, Raybould HE. Role of visceral afferent mechanisms in functional bowel disorders. Gastroenterology 1990;99(6):1688–704.
9. Drossman DA, Li Z, Andruzzi E, et al. U.S. householder survey of functional gastrointestinal disorders. Prevalence, sociodemography, and health impact. Dig Dis Sci 1993;38(9):1569–80.
10. Bond JH Jr, Engel RR, Levitt MD. Factors influencing pulmonary methane excretion in man. An indirect method of studying the in situ metabolism of the methane-producing colonic bacteria. J Exp Med 1971;133(3):572–88.
11. Savage DC. Microbial ecology of the gastrointestinal tract. Annu Rev Microbiol 1977;31:107–33.
12. Simon GL, Gorbach SL. Intestinal flora in health and disease. Gastroenterology 1984;86(1):174–93.
13. Barbara G, De Giorgio R, Stanghellini V, et al. New pathophysiological mechanisms in irritable bowel syndrome. Aliment Pharmacol Ther 2004;20(Suppl 2):1–9.
14. Barbara G, Wang B, Stanghellini V, et al. Mast cell-dependent excitation of visceral-nociceptive sensory neurons in irritable bowel syndrome. Gastroenterology 2007;132(1):26–37.

15. Floch MH. Bile salts, intestinal microflora and enterohepatic circulation. Dig Liver Dis 2002;34(Suppl 2):S54–7.

16. Halvorson HA, Schlett CD, Riddle MS. Postinfectious irritable bowel syndrome—a meta-analysis. Am J Gastroenterol 2006;101(8):1894–9 [quiz: 1942].

17. Thabane M, Kottachchi DT, Marshall JK. Systematic review and meta-analysis: the incidence and prognosis of post-infectious irritable bowel syndrome. Aliment Pharmacol Ther 2007;26(4):535–44.

18. Abrams GD, Bishop JE. Effect of the normal microbial flora on gastrointestinal motility. Proc Soc Exp Biol Med 1967;126(1):301–4.

19. Iwai H, Ishihara Y, Yamanaka J, et al. Effects of bacterial flora on cecal size and transit rate of intestinal contents in mice. Jpn J Exp Med 1973;43(4):297–305.

20. Caenepeel P, Janssens J, Vantrappen G, et al. Interdigestive myoelectric complex in germ-free rats. Dig Dis Sci 1989;34(8):1180–4.

21. Husebye E, Hellstrom PM, Midtvedt T. Intestinal microflora stimulates myoelectric activity of rat small intestine by promoting cyclic initiation and aboral propagation of migrating myoelectric complex. Dig Dis Sci 1994;39(5):946–56.

22. Husebye E, Hellstrom PM, Sundler F, et al. Influence of microbial species on small intestinal myoelectric activity and transit in germ-free rats. Am J Physiol Gastrointest Liver Physiol 2001;280(3):G368–80.

23. Hooper LV, Gordon JI. Commensal host-bacterial relationships in the gut. Science 2001;292(5519):1115–8.

24. Malinen E, Rinttila R, Kajander K, et al. Analysis of the fecal microbiota of irritable bowel syndrome patients and healthy controls with real-time PCR. Am J Gastroenterol 2005;100(2):373–82.

25. Si JM, Yu YC, Fan YJ, et al. Intestinal microecology and quality of life in irritable bowel syndrome patients. World J Gastroenterol 2004;10(12):1802–5.

26. Kerckhoffs AP, Samsom M, van der Res ME, et al. Lower Bifidobacteria counts in both duodenal mucosa-associated and fecal microbiota in irritable bowel syndrome patients. World J Gastroenterol 2009;15(23):2887–92.

27. Tana C, Umesaki Y, Imaoka A, et al. Altered profiles of intestinal microbiota and organic acids may be the origin of symptoms in irritable bowel syndrome. Neurogastroenterol Motil 2009;22(5):512–9, e114–5.

28. Rousseaux C, Thuru X, Gelot A, et al. *Lactobacillus acidophilus* modulates intestinal pain and induces opioid and cannabinoid receptors. Nat Med 2007;13(1):35–7.

29. Gudmand-Hoyer E, Riis P, Wulff HR. The significance of lactose malabsorption in the irritable colon syndrome. Scand J Gastroenterol 1973;8(3):273–8.

30. Vernia P, Marinaro V, Argnani F, et al. Self-reported milk intolerance in irritable bowel syndrome: what should we believe? Clin Nutr 2004;23(5):996–1000.

31. Kassinen A, Krogius-Kurikka L, Makivuokko H, et al. The fecal microbiota of irritable bowel syndrome patients differs significantly from that of healthy subjects. Gastroenterology 2007;133(1):24–33.

32. Bercík P, Wang L, Verdu EF, et al. Visceral hyperalgesia and intestinal dysmotility in a mouse model of postinfective gut dysfunction. Gastroenterology 2004;127(1):179–87.

33. Pimentel M, Chow EJ, Lin HC. Eradication of small intestinal bacterial overgrowth reduces symptoms of irritable bowel syndrome. Am J Gastroenterol 2000;95(12):3503–6.

34. Pimentel M, Chow EJ, Lin HC. Normalization of lactulose breath testing correlates with symptom improvement in irritable bowel syndrome. A double-blind, randomized, placebo-controlled study. Am J Gastroenterol 2003;98(2):412–9.

35. Ford AC, Spiegel BM, Talley NJ, et al. Small intestinal bacterial overgrowth in irritable bowel syndrome: systematic review and meta-analysis. Clin Gastroenterol Hepatol 2009;7(12):1279–86.
36. Shah ED, Basseri RJ, Chong K, et al. Abnormal breath testing in IBS: a meta-analysis. Dig Dis Sci 2010;55(9):2441–9.
37. Posserud I, Stotzer PO, Bjornsson ES, et al. Small intestinal bacterial overgrowth in patients with irritable bowel syndrome. Gut 2007;56(6):802–8.
38. Pimentel M, Park S, Mirocha J, et al. The effect of a nonabsorbed oral antibiotic (rifaximin) on the symptoms of the irritable bowel syndrome: a randomized trial. Ann Intern Med 2006;145(8):557–63.
39. Lembo A. Rifaximin for the treatment of diarrhea-associated irritable bowel syndrome: short term treatment leading to long term sustained response, efficacy of co-primary endpoints: adequate relief/control of global IBS symptoms and IBS-associated bloating. San Diego (CA): Digestive Disease Week; 2008.
40. Pimentel M, Lembo A, Chey WD, et al. Rifaximin therapy for patients with irritable bowel syndrome without constipation. N Engl J Med 2011;364:22–32.
41. Sharara AI, Aoun E, Abdul-Baki H, et al. A randomized double-blind placebo-controlled trial of rifaximin in patients with abdominal bloating and flatulence. Am J Gastroenterol 2006;101(2):326–33.
42. Szurszewski JH. A migrating electric complex of canine small intestine. Am J Physiol 1969;217(6):1757–63.
43. Vantrappen G, Janssens J, Hellemans J, et al. The interdigestive motor complex of normal subjects and patients with bacterial overgrowth of the small intestine. J Clin Invest 1977;59(6):1158–66.
44. Nieuwenhuijs VB, Verheem A, van Dujvenbode-Beumer H, et al. The role of interdigestive small bowel motility in the regulation of gut microflora, bacterial overgrowth, and bacterial translocation in rats. Ann Surg 1998;228(2):188–93.
45. Sarna SK. Are interstitial cells of Cajal plurifunction cells in the gut? Am J Physiol Gastrointest Liver Physiol 2008;294(2):G372–90.
46. Der-Silaphet T, Malysz J, Hagel S, et al. Interstitial cells of Cajal direct normal propulsive contractile activity in the mouse small intestine. Gastroenterology 1998;114(4):724–36.
47. Malysz J, Thuneberg L, Mikkelsen HB, et al. Action potential generation in the small intestine of W mutant mice that lack interstitial cells of Cajal. Am J Physiol 1996;271(3 Pt 1):G387–99.
48. Langton P, Ward SM, Carl A, et al. Spontaneous electrical activity of interstitial cells of Cajal isolated from canine proximal colon. Proc Natl Acad Sci U S A 1989;86(18):7280–4.
49. Ordog T, Ward SM, Sanders KM. Interstitial cells of Cajal generate electrical slow waves in the murine stomach. J Physiol 1999;518(Pt 1):257–69.
50. Streutker CJ, Huizinga JD, Campbell F, et al. Loss of CD117 (c-kit)- and CD34-positive ICC and associated CD34-positive fibroblasts defines a subpopulation of chronic intestinal pseudo-obstruction. Am J Surg Pathol 2003;27(2):228–35.
51. Vanderwinden JM, Liu H, De Laet MH, et al. Study of the interstitial cells of Cajal in infantile hypertrophic pyloric stenosis. Gastroenterology 1996;111(2):279–88.
52. Ordog T, Takayama I, Cheung WK, et al. Remodeling of networks of interstitial cells of Cajal in a murine model of diabetic gastroparesis. Diabetes 2000;49(10):1731–9.
53. Bassotti G, Villanacci V, Maurer CA, et al. The role of glial cells and apoptosis of enteric neurones in the neuropathology of intractable slow transit constipation. Gut 2006;55(1):41–6.

54. Torihashi S, Ward SM, Nishikawa M, et al. c-kit-dependent development of inter-stitial cells and electrical activity in the murine gastrointestinal tract. Cell Tissue Res 1995;280(1):97–111.
55. Neal KR, Barker L, Spiller RC. Prognosis in post-infective irritable bowel syndrome: a six year follow up study. Gut 2002;51(3):410–3.
56. Neal KR, Hebden J, Spiller R. Prevalence of gastrointestinal symptoms six months after bacterial gastroenteritis and risk factors for development of the irritable bowel syndrome: postal survey of patients. BMJ 1997;314(7083):779–82.
57. Gwee KA, Leong YL, Graham C, et al. The role of psychological and biological factors in postinfective gut dysfunction. Gut 1999;44(3):400–6.
58. Spiller RC, Jenkins D, Thornley JP, et al. Increased rectal mucosal enteroendo-crine cells, T lymphocytes, and increased gut permeability following acute Campylobacter enteritis and in post-dysenteric irritable bowel syndrome. Gut 2000;47(6):804–11.
59. Dunlop SP, Jenkins D, Spiller RC. Distinctive clinical, psychological, and histo-logical features of postinfective irritable bowel syndrome. Am J Gastroenterol 2003;98(7):1578–83.
60. Gwee KA, Collins SM, Read NW, et al. Increased rectal mucosal expression of interleukin 1beta in recently acquired post-infectious irritable bowel syndrome. Gut 2003;52(4):523–6.
61. Wang LH, Fang XC, Pan GZ. Bacillary dysentery as a causative factor of irritable bowel syndrome and its pathogenesis. Gut 2004;53(8):1096–101.
62. Adam B, Liebregts T, Gschossmann JM, et al. Severity of mucosal inflammation as a predictor for alterations of visceral sensory function in a rat model. Pain 2006;123(1/2):179–86.
63. Bradesi S, Kokkotou E, Simeonidis S, et al. The role of neurokinin 1 receptors in the maintenance of visceral hyperalgesia induced by repeated stress in rats. Gastroenterology 2006;130(6):1729–42.
64. Barbara G, Vallance BA, Collins SM. Persistent intestinal neuromuscular dysfunction after acute nematode infection in mice. Gastroenterology 1997; 113(4):1224–32.
65. Pimentel M, Chatterjee S, Chang C, et al. A new rat model links two contempo-rary theories in irritable bowel syndrome. Dig Dis Sci 2008;53(4):982–9.
66. Pimentel M, Mayer AG, Park S, et al. Methane production during lactulose breath test is associated with gastrointestinal disease presentation. Dig Dis Sci 2003;48(1):86–92.
67. Chatterjee S, Park S, Low K, et al. The degree of breath methane production in IBS correlates with the severity of constipation. Am J Gastroenterol 2007;102(4): 837–41.
68. Weaver GA, Krause JS, Miller TL, et al. Incidence of methanogenic bacteria in a sigmoidoscopy population: an association of methanogenic bacteria and diverticulosis. Gut 1986;27(6):698–704.
69. Haines A, Metz G, Dilawari J, et al. Breath-methane in patients with cancer of the large bowel. Lancet 1977;2(8036):481–3.
70. Jones WJ, Nagle DP Jr, Whitman WB. Methanogens and the diversity of archae-bacteria. Microbiol Rev 1987;51(1):135–77.
71. McKay LF, Holbrook WP, Eastwood MA. Methane and hydrogen production by human intestinal anaerobic bacteria. Acta Pathol Microbiol Immunol Scand B 1982;90(3):257–60.
72. Blaut M. Metabolism of methanogens. Antonie Van Leeuwenhoek 1994;66(1–3): 187–208.

73. Gibson GR, Cummings JH, Macfarlane GT, et al. Alternative pathways for hydrogen disposal during fermentation in the human colon. Gut 1990;31(6): 679–83.
74. Fiedorek SC, Pumphrey CL, Casteel HB. Breath methane production in children with constipation and encopresis. J Pediatr Gastroenterol Nutr 1990;10(4): 473–7.
75. Peled Y, Weinberg D, Hallak A, et al. Factors affecting methane production in humans. Gastrointestinal diseases and alterations of colonic flora. Dig Dis Sci 1987;32(3):267–71.
76. Pimentel M, Lin HC, Enayati P, et al. Methane, a gas produced by enteric bacteria, slows intestinal transit and augments small intestinal contractile activity. Am J Physiol Gastrointest Liver Physiol 2006;290(6):G1089–95.
77. Pimentel M, Park S, Kane SV, et al. Rifaximin, a non-absorbable antibiotic improves the symptoms of irritable bowel syndrome: a randomized, double-blind, placebo-controlled study. Ann Intern Med 2006;145:557–63.
78. Lembo A, Zakko SF, Ferreira NL, et al. T1390 Rifaximin for the treatment of diarrhea-associated irritable bowel syndrome: short term treatment leading to long term sustained response. Gastroenterology 2008;134(4 Suppl 1):A-545.
79. Parkes GC, Sanderson JD, Whelan K. Treating irritable bowel syndrome with probiotics: the evidence. Proc Nutr Soc 2010;69(2):187–94.
80. O'Mahony L, McCarthy J, Kelly P, et al. Lactobacillus and bifidobacterium in irritable bowel syndrome: symptom responses and relationship to cytokine profiles. Gastroenterology 2005;128(3):541–51.
81. Whorwell PJ, Altringer L, Morel J, et al. Efficacy of an encapsulated probiotic *Bifidobacterium infantis* 35624 in women with irritable bowel syndrome. Am J Gastroenterol 2006;101(7):1581–90.
82. Kim HJ, Camilleri M, McKinzie S, et al. A randomized controlled trial of a probiotic, VSL#3, on gut transit and symptoms in diarrhoea-predominant irritable bowel syndrome. Aliment Pharmacol Ther 2003;17(7):895–904.
83. Kim HJ, Vasquez Roque MI, Camilleri M, et al. A randomized controlled trial of a probiotic combination VSL# 3 and placebo in irritable bowel syndrome with bloating. Neurogastroenterol Motil 2005;17(5):687–96.
84. McFarland LV, Dublin S. Meta-analysis of probiotics for the treatment of irritable bowel syndrome. World J Gastroenterol 2008;14(17):2650–61.
85. Moayyedi P, Ford AC, Talley NJ, et al. The efficacy of probiotics in the treatment of irritable bowel syndrome: a systematic review. Gut 2010;59(3):325–32.
86. Brenner DM, Moeller MJ, Chey WD, et al. The utility of probiotics in the treatment of irritable bowel syndrome: a systematic review. Am J Gastroenterol 2009; 104(4):1033–49 [quiz: 1050].
87. Tornblom H, Lindberg G, Nyberg B, et al. Full-thickness biopsy of the jejunum reveals inflammation and enteric neuropathy in irritable bowel syndrome. Gastroenterology 2002;123(6):1972–9.
88. Ohman L, Isaksson S, Lungren A, et al. A controlled study of colonic immune activity and beta7+ blood T lymphocytes in patients with irritable bowel syndrome. Clin Gastroenterol Hepatol 2005;3(10):980–6.
89. Guilarte M, Santos J, deTorres I, et al. Diarrhoea-predominant IBS patients show mast cell activation and hyperplasia in the jejunum. Gut 2007;56(2):203–9.
90. Scully P, McKernan DP, Keohane J, et al. Plasma cytokine profiles in females with irritable bowel syndrome and extra-intestinal co-morbidity. Am J Gastroenterol 2010;105(10):2235–43.

91. Liebregts T, Adam B, Bredack C, et al. Immune activation in patients with irritable bowel syndrome. Gastroenterology 2007;132(3):913–20.
92. Sartor RB. Microbial influences in inflammatory bowel diseases. Gastroenterology 2008;134(2):577–94.
93. Parkes GC, Brostoff J, Whelen K, et al. Gastrointestinal microbiota in irritable bowel syndrome: their role in its pathogenesis and treatment. Am J Gastroenterol 2008;103(6):1557–67.
94. Langhorst J, Junge A, Rueffer A, et al. Elevated human beta-defensin-2 levels indicate an activation of the innate Immune system in patients with irritable bowel syndrome. Am J Gastroenterol 2009;104(2):404–10.
95. Dunlop SP, Jenkins D, Neal KR, et al. Randomized, double-blind, placebo-controlled trial of prednisolone in post-infectious irritable bowel syndrome. Aliment Pharmacol Ther 2003;18(1):77–84.
96. Corinaldesi R, Stanghellini V, Cremon C, et al. Effect of mesalazine on mucosal immune biomarkers in irritable bowel syndrome: a randomized controlled proof-of-concept study. Aliment Pharmacol Ther 2009;30(3):245–52.
97. Klooker TK, Braak B, Koopman KE, et al. The mast cell stabiliser ketotifen decreases visceral hypersensitivity and improves intestinal symptoms in patients with irritable bowel syndrome. Gut 2010;59(9):1213–21.
98. Matto J, Manuksela L, Kajander K, et al. Composition and temporal stability of gastrointestinal microbiota in irritable bowel syndrome—a longitudinal study in IBS and control subjects. FEMS Immunol Med Microbiol 2005;43(2):213–22.
99. Maukonen J, Matto J, Satokari R, et al. PCR DGGE and RT-PCR DGGE show diversity and short-term temporal stability in the *Clostridium coccoides-Eubacterium* rectale group in the human intestinal microbiota. FEMS Microbiol Ecol 2006;58(3):517–28.
100. Majewski M, McCallum RW. Results of small intestinal bacterial overgrowth testing in irritable bowel syndrome patients: clinical profiles and effects of antibiotic trial. Adv Med Sci 2007;52:139–42.
101. Bratten JR, Spanier J, Jones MP. Lactulose breath testing does not discriminate patients with irritable bowel syndrome from healthy controls. Am J Gastroenterol 2008;103(4):958–63.
102. Parodi A, Dulbecco P, Savarino E, et al. Positive glucose breath testing is more prevalent in patients with IBS-like symptoms compared with controls of similar age and gender distribution. J Clin Gastroenterol 2009;43(10):962–6.
103. Hwang L, Low K, Khoshini R, et al. Evaluating breath methane as a diagnostic test for constipation-predominant IBS. Dig Dis Sci 2010;55(2):398–403.
104. Attaluri A, Jackson M, Valestin J, et al. Methanogenic flora is associated with altered colonic transit but not stool characteristics in constipation without IBS. Am J Gastroenterol 2010;105(6):1407–11.

Symptom-Based Diagnostic Criteria for Irritable Bowel Syndrome: the More Things Change, the More They Stay the Same

Paul Moayyedi, MB ChB, PhD, MPH, FRCP, FRCPC, AGAF[a],*,
Alexander C. Ford, MD, MRCP[b]

KEYWORDS

• IBS • Diagnostic accuracy • Rome criteria • Manning criteria

Medical students are taught that 90% of all diagnoses are made through the careful assessment of the patients' symptoms. This methodology was probably true in the past, but clinicians now rely heavily on techniques such as endoscopy or radiology before making a definitive diagnosis of organic disease. Indeed, most gastroenterologists would require endoscopic confirmation before labeling a patient as having peptic ulcer disease and would make a diagnosis of Crohn disease based on small bowel radiology or colonoscopy. However, the most common causes of symptoms of the gastrointestinal (GI) tract are functional, and most GI investigations are normal. It is therefore important that clinicians obtain a thorough history so that the disorder of the patient can be accurately defined. Gastroenterologists seem to be aware of this method, because office visits are longer than that for primary care providers, particularly for those patients diagnosed with irritable bowel syndrome (IBS).[1] However, community gastroenterologists and primary care providers still think that IBS is a diagnosis of exclusion, whereas IBS experts are more likely to make a positive diagnosis.[2] This scenario suggests that experts are more confident on the accuracy of symptoms in diagnosing IBS.

[a] Division of Gastroenterology, Farncombe Family Digestive Health Research Institute, Department of Medicine, McMaster University Medical Centre, 1200 Main Street West, HSC Room 4W8E, Hamilton, ON, L8N 3Z5 Canada
[b] University of Leeds, Leeds Gastroenterology Institute, Room 230, D Floor, Clarendon Wing, Leeds General Infirmary, Great George Street, Leeds, LS1 3EX, UK
* Corresponding author.
E-mail address: moayyep@mcmaster.ca

Gastroenterol Clin N Am 40 (2011) 87–103
doi:10.1016/j.gtc.2010.12.007
0889-8553/11/$ – see front matter © 2011 Elsevier Inc. All rights reserved.

gastro.theclinics.com

The rigorous evaluation of symptoms that identify patients with IBS started with the criteria identified by Manning and colleagues.[3] Researchers then developed more complex models that relied on symptoms and simple investigations to diagnose IBS.[4] From an academic perspective, the field was still in disarray, with researchers recruiting subjects using a variety of definitions of IBS. This scenario made it difficult to compare studies because it was unclear as to what type of patient was being evaluated. Progress came with the Rome Foundation, which brought together a group of experts to reach a consensus on the appropriate definition of IBS. There have been 3 iterations[5–7] of Rome Foundation's symptom-based definitions of IBS and these have been predominantly used in research studies evaluating functional GI disorders; they have also been used to help manage IBS in clinical practice.[8–10] Although the Rome criteria have undoubtedly brought order to functional GI research, the question remains as to their accuracy in diagnosis[11] and whether they are any better than the previous symptom-based criteria.

ACCURACY OF SYMPTOM-BASED CRITERIA FOR IBS

The authors have updated their previous systematic review[12] addressing this issue searching MEDLINE (1950–October 2010) and EMBASE (1908–October 2010) using a predefined search strategy.[12] No new studies were eligible for the review, but a further systematic review[13] that also evaluated the accuracy of symptom-based criteria in IBS has been published subsequently. This review identified 15 more studies than that of the authors', so it is important to establish the differences between the 2 systematic reviews. It has been shown that there can be errors in systematic reviews of IBS that can change the interpretation of the data.[14] It is therefore important that the researchers account for any discrepancy between these 2 systematic reviews. The systematic review of the authors[12] required imaging of the colon with colonoscopy, barium enema, or computed tomographic colography to exclude organic disease. One article[15] included in the systematic review by Jellema and colleagues[13] investigated patients with flexible sigmoidoscopy only and was therefore excluded from the review. A study[16] was excluded that just compared Rome I with Rome II criteria without a gold standard for diagnosing IBS that was included by Jellema and colleagues. One study[17] included by Jemella and colleagues was excluded by the authors' review because data to provide sensitivity and specificity could not be extracted. The authors excluded 3 papers[18–20] that evaluated scoring models that separated organic from any functional GI disease but were not specifically designed to identify patients with IBS. Also, the review excluded 9 studies[21–29] that enrolled patients with both upper and lower GI symptoms (the 2 types of symptoms could not be separated in the review). This exclusion is because the main question is whether symptom-based criteria can identify patients with IBS in subjects with lower GI symptoms, not any GI symptom (eg, it was anticipated that the criteria could easily distinguish a patient with gastroesophageal reflux disease from a patient with IBS).

The 10 studies assessing 2355 patients with lower GI symptoms[3,4,30–37] included in the original review were reanalyzed to evaluate the diagnostic utility of symptom-based criteria in identifying patients with IBS. The study characteristics are described in **Table 1**. Individual symptoms perform poorly in identifying patients with IBS (**Table 2**),[12] so it is important to consider symptom complexes when making the diagnosis. Studies investigated the accuracy of Manning criteria (**Box 1**), Rome I criteria (see **Box 1**), and statistical models (**Box 2**). There were 4 studies[3,30–32] that evaluated 574 patients reporting on the accuracy of Manning criteria. Sensitivity varied between 66% and 90%, with specificity between 56% and 87% (**Fig. 1**). One study[37] involving

602 participants evaluated the Rome I criteria and reported a sensitivity of 71% and specificity of 85%. The Kruis model was evaluated in 4 studies[4,32–34] in 1171 patients, and sensitivities ranged between 56% and 83%, with specificities between 65% and 97% (see **Fig. 1**). The accuracy of other statistical models was investigated by 4 studies[33–36] (1 study[33] evaluated a different scoring system of the Kruis model) in 863 patients. Sensitivity varied between 76% and 91%, with specificity between 53% and 100% (see **Fig. 1**).

Overall, when summary receiver operator curves (SROCs) were created, statistical models were more accurate than symptom-based criteria in diagnosing IBS (**Fig. 2**). There were no major differences between Kruis criteria or the other type of models, and there was also no difference between Rome I and Manning criteria (**Fig. 3**). These results need to be treated with caution because there are too few studies to accurately construct SROCs.[38] Furthermore, there is the issue of an absence of a gold standard to diagnose IBS. The studies in this review used the normal result of lower bowel investigations and clinical opinion to diagnose IBS. However, clinicians may not be able to distinguish between different functional bowel diseases, and there was also variation in what diseases were considered "organic," with some studies defining diverticular disease, for example, as an organic disorder.[12] This imprecise reference standard may mean that the accuracy of methods of diagnosing IBS is underestimated. Furthermore, models that were generated from complex statistical analysis of datasets may overestimate accuracy because the models were constructed to best fit the data retrospectively, and when tested prospectively, their accuracy may be reduced. This finding was observed when the Kruis model[4] was tested prospectively.[33,34]

The overall accuracy of symptom-based criteria in diagnosing IBS is therefore unclear, although there seems to be room for improvement, with only modest sensitivity and specificity compared with clinical opinion after lower GI tract investigation. Despite this limitation, symptom-based diagnostic criteria have become the gold standard method for making a positive diagnosis of IBS in both primary and secondary care,[39–41] rather than exhaustive investigation to exclude an underlying organic cause. This approach is endorsed by the recently updated management guidelines from both the American College of Gastroenterology and the British Society of Gastroenterology. However, the use of such diagnostic criteria to reach a diagnosis of IBS has advantages and disadvantages for both patients and clinicians.

Pros and Cons of Symptom-based Diagnostic Criteria

As previously mentioned, the presence of individual symptoms, such as lower abdominal pain, mucus per rectum, tenesmus, change in stool pattern, and bloating, alone are insufficiently accurate to diagnose IBS (see **Table 2**).[12] In reality, physicians rarely use a single item from the clinical history to formulate a diagnosis and are more likely to combine various items together. In addition, at the time of writing, there is no accurate biomarker for IBS.[42] Using a symptom-based approach to define its presence is therefore a useful strategy for doctors consulting with a patient with symptoms suggestive of IBS, to maximize the likelihood of reaching the correct diagnosis, and minimize uncertainty. The groups of symptoms that together make up these diagnostic criteria cluster together and demonstrate statistically significant associations with each other in community-based factor analysis studies.[10,43–45] These observations lend weight to the biologic plausibility of IBS as a distinct clinical entity and this, together with their use to help make a positive diagnosis of the condition, may provide reassurance to the patient, and reduce the feeling that they are being told

Table 1
Characteristics of included studies in the systematic review of diagnostic accuracy of symptoms in IBS

Refs.	Country	Total Number	Proportion IBS (%)	Method of Assessment	Type of Patient	Setting	Assessors Blinded?
3	England	65	49	Symptom-based criteria	Referred to outpatient clinic with lower GI symptoms; unclear who referred	Gastroenterology and surgical clinic in a single hospital	Yes
4	Germany	317	34	Statistical model	Referred to outpatient clinic with lower GI symptoms by external physician	Internal medicine clinic in a single hospital	Yes
30	Korea	74	78	Symptom-based criteria	Referred to outpatient clinic with lower GI symptoms; unclear who referred	Internal medicine clinic in a single hospital	Yes
31	India	88	74	Symptom-based criteria	Referred to outpatient clinic with lower GI symptoms; unclear who referred	Gastroenterology clinic in a single hospital	Unclear
32	Turkey	347	48	Symptom-based criteria and statistical model	Referred to outpatient clinic with lower GI symptoms; unclear who referred	Gastroenterology clinic and internal medicine clinic in 2 hospitals	Yes
33	Italy	253	21	Statistical model	Referred to outpatient clinic with lower GI symptoms by PCP	Gastroenterology clinic in a single hospital	Yes

34	Italy	254	60	Statistical model	Consulted PCP or referred to outpatient clinic with lower GI symptoms	14 PCPs and a gastroenterology clinic in a single hospital	Yes
35	India	75	73	Statistical model	Referred to outpatient clinic with lower GI symptoms, unclear who referred	Gastroenterology clinic in a single hospital	Yes
36	Australia	280	76	Statistical model	Referred to outpatient clinic with lower GI symptoms by PCP primarily and also by surgeons and internists	Gastroenterology clinic in a single hospital	Yes
37	England	602	56	Symptom-based criteria	Referred to outpatient clinic with lower GI symptoms by PCP	Gastroenterology clinic in a single hospital	Yes

Abbreviations: GI, gastrointestinal; PCP, primary care provider.

Data from Ford AC, Talley NJ, Veldhuyzen van Zanten SJ, et al. Will the history and physical examination help establish that irritable bowel syndrome is causing this patient's lower gastrointestinal tract symptoms? JAMA 2008;300:1793–805.

Table 2
Accuracy of individual symptoms for the diagnosis of IBS

Symptom Item	Refs.	Sensitivity (95% CI)	Specificity (95% CI)	Positive Likelihood Ratio (95% CI)	Negative Likelihood Ratio (95% CI)
Lower abdominal pain	3	0.97 (0.84–1.0)	0.09 (0.02–0.24)	1.1 (0.92–1.3)	0.34 (0.05–2.3)
	4	0.96 (0.91–0.99)	0.45 (0.39–0.52)	1.8 (1.6–2.0)	0.08 (0.03–0.20)
	33	0.87 (0.74–0.94)	0.36 (0.29–0.43)	1.4 (1.1–1.6)	0.38 (0.18–0.73)
	36	0.80 (0.74–0.85)	0.33 (0.22–0.46)	1.2 (1.0–1.5)	0.60 (0.40–0.94)
Mucus per rectum	3	0.47 (0.29–0.65)	0.79 (0.61–0.91)	2.2 (1.1–4.7)	0.67 (0.45–0.96)
	30	0.19 (0.10–0.31)	0.81 (0.54–0.96)	1.0 (0.36–3.2)	1.0 (0.80–1.4)
	31	0.78 (0.67–0.88)	0.35 (0.1–0.57)	1.2 (0.92–1.8)	0.62 (0.31–1.3)
	36	0.36 (0.29–0.42)	0.65 (0.52–0.76)	1.0 (0.71–1.5)	0.99 (0.82–1.2)
Incomplete evacuation	3	0.59 (0.41–0.76)	0.67 (0.48–0.82)	1.8 (1.0–3.2)	0.61 (0.37–0.97)
	30	0.78 (0.65–0.87)	0.31 (0.11–0.59)	1.1 (0.85–1.8)	0.72 (0.33–1.8)
	31	0.85 (0.74–0.92)	0.35 (0.16–0.57)	1.3 (1.0–1.9)	0.44 (0.21–0.99)
	36	0.72 (0.66–0.78)	0.42 (0.30–0.55)	1.3 (1.0–1.6)	0.65 (0.46–0.94)
Looser stools at onset of pain	3	0.81 (0.63–0.93)	0.73 (0.54–0.88)	3.0 (1.7–5.8)	0.26 (0.12–0.52)
	30	0.59 (0.45–0.71)	0.63 (0.35–0.85)	1.6 (0.89–3.3)	0.66 (0.42–1.2)
	31	0.48 (0.35–0.60)	0.87 (0.66–0.97)	3.7 (1.4–11)	0.60 (0.45–0.82)
	36	0.50 (0.43–0.57)	0.70 (0.57–0.80)	1.7 (1.2–2.5)	0.72 (0.59–0.90)
More frequent stools at onset of pain	3	0.74 (0.55–0.88)	0.70 (0.51–0.85)	2.5 (1.5–4.6)	0.37 (0.19–0.67)
	30	0.57 (0.43–0.70)	0.69 (0.41–0.89)	1.8 (0.96–4.1)	0.63 (0.41–1.0)
	31	0.35 (0.24–0.48)	0.91 (0.72–0.99)	4.1 (1.3–15)	0.71 (0.56–0.92)
	36	0.51 (0.44–0.58)	0.62 (0.49–0.74)	1.3 (0.98–1.9)	0.79 (0.63–1.0)
Pain relieved by defecation	3	0.71 (0.52–0.86)	0.70 (0.51–0.85)	2.4 (1.4–4.4)	0.41 (0.22–0.72)
	30	0.59 (0.45–0.71)	0.69 (0.41–0.89)	1.9 (1.0–4.2)	0.60 (0.39–1.0)
	31	0.66 (0.53–0.77)	0.57 (0.34–0.77)	1.5 (0.99–2.6)	0.60 (0.37–1.0)
	36	0.55 (0.48–0.62)	0.67 (0.54–0.78)	1.7 (1.2–2.4)	0.67 (0.54–0.86)
Patient reported visible abdominal distension	3	0.59 (0.41–0.76)	0.79 (0.61–0.91)	2.8 (1.4–5.8)	0.52 (0.32–0.78)
	30	0.40 (0.27–0.53)	0.63 (0.35–0.85)	1.1 (0.57–2.3)	0.97 (0.67–1.6)
	31	0.22 (0.12–0.33)	0.87 (0.66–0.97)	1.7 (0.59–5.1)	0.90 (0.75–1.2)

Abbreviation: CI, confidence interval.
Data from Ford AC, Talley NJ, Veldhuyzen van Zanten SJ, et al. Will the history and physical examination help establish that irritable bowel syndrome is causing this patient's lower gastrointestinal tract symptoms? JAMA 2008;300:1793–805.

Box 1
Summary of symptom-based criteria for diagnosing IBS

Manning criteria[3]

Symptom duration not defined

Number of symptoms required for diagnosis also not defined but more than 3 generally used

- Abdominal pain relieved by defecation
- More frequent stools with the onset of abdominal pain
- Looser stools with the onset of abdominal pain
- Visible abdominal distension reported by patient
- Incomplete evacuation
- Passage of mucus per rectum

Rome I criteria[5]

Symptoms present for at least 3 months. Patient must experience abdominal pain or discomfort relieved with defecation or associated with a change in stool frequency or consistency. In addition, there should be at least 2 of the following features for 25% of days or more:

- Altered stool frequency
- Altered stool form
- Altered stool passage
- Bloating or distension
- Passage of mucus per rectum

Rome II criteria[6]

Symptoms present for at least 12 weeks in 1 year (need not be consecutive). Patient must experience abdominal pain with at least 2 of the following features:

- Relieved by defecation
- Onset of pain associated with change in stool frequency
- Onset of pain associated with change in stool form

Rome III criteria[7]

Symptoms present for at least 3 days per month in the last 3 months (with symptom onset at least 6 months previously) with at least 2 of the following features:

- Pain improved with defecation
- Onset of pain associated with change in stool frequency
- Onset of pain associated with change in stool form

---

that either there is nothing wrong with them or there is no detectable explanation for their symptoms.

The use of symptom-based diagnostic criteria to make the diagnosis of IBS, without the need for recourse to numerous invasive investigations, is also of benefit to the health service. There is no conclusive evidence that this approach is cost-effective,[46] but it should discourage physicians from overinvestigating young patients who are otherwise well and clearly meet these criteria and in whom the diagnostic yield of

Box 2
Summary of statistical models for diagnosing IBS

Kruis and colleagues[4]

Score greater than 44 defined as IBS

Item		Score
1	At least 1 of the following: abdominal pain, flatulence, change in bowel habit	+34
2	Symptoms for more than 2 years	+16
3	Abdominal pain described as burning, cutting, very strong, terrible, feeling of pressure, dull, boring, or not so bad[a]	+23
4	Alternating constipation and diarrhea	+14
5	History or physical pathognomonic for any diagnosis other than IBS	−47
6	ESR>20 mm/2 h	−13
7	Leucocytosis>10,000/cm^3	−50
8	Hemoglobin low (<12 g% female, <14 g% male)	−98
9	History of blood in stool	−98

[a] Scored only if 1 statement in the first line or more than 2 statements in total endorsed.

Bellentani and colleagues[34]

Score less than 0 defined as IBS

Item		Score
1	Visible distension of the abdomen	−39
2	First-degree relatives have colitis	−35
3	Have a feeling of distension	−34
4	Suffer from flatulence	−33
5	Suffer from irregularities of bowel movements	−26
6	ESR>17 mm/h	+134
7	History of blood in the stool	+112
8	Age>45 years	+95
9	Leucocytosis>10,000/cm^3	+85
10	Fever between 37°C and 38°C	+74
11	History of cancer in first-degree relatives	+33

Mazumdar and colleagues[35]

Score less than 0 defined as IBS

Item		Score Present	Absent
1	Abdominal pain	+3	−9
2	Early morning abdominal pain	+15	−2
3	Postprandial abdominal pain	−5	+3
4	Poorly localized pain	+14	−30
5	Food aggravating pain	+17	−11

6	Pain relieved after flatus or defecation	+2	−10
7	Nocturnal diarrhea	−24	+4
8	Alternating constipation/diarrhea	+16	−5
9	Repeated attempts to pass stool	+14	−9
10	Straining at defecation	+11	−5
11	Feeling of incomplete evacuation	+11	−9
12	Food precipitating bowel movement	+12	−10
13	Stress factor	+12	−5
14	Excess mucus in stool	+10	−30
15	Blood in stool	−4	+6
16	Blood uniformly mixed with stool	−37	+21
17	Blood after stool	+30	−18
18	Gas bloat/belching	+25	−4
19	Borborygmi	+8	−4

Hammer and colleagues[36]

Model not defined. Only odds ratios given. Odds ratio less than 1 is more indicative of IBS.

Item		Odds Ratio (95% CI)
1	Age>50 years	2.96 (1.47–5.94)
2	Female sex	0.43 (0.22–0.86)
3	Blood on toilet paper	2.19 (1.06–4.52)
4	Severe pain	0.85 (0.42–1.74)
5	Pain>6 times in past year	0.21 (0.08–0.52)
6	Radiating pain	0.38 (0.16–0.88)
7	Pain/looser bowel movements	0.47 (0.23–0.96)
8	Diarrhea	2.69 (1.03–7.02)
9	Acid reflux	0.36 (0.13–0.98)

such investigations are likely to be low. Theoretically, this approach would save the US health service US $364 per patient with IBS.[2] There is some evidence from longitudinal studies that once a diagnosis of IBS is reached it is unlikely to be revised after further investigations of the GI tract for the same symptoms in the future,[47] and that the subsequent detection of a missed diagnosis of organic disease, which may have been the underlying explanation for the patient's original presentation with symptoms, is unlikely.[48]

The standardization of the criteria used to define IBS, and the creation of distinct subgroups according to the predominant symptom reported by the individual, is also helpful. Firstly, this standardization allows the recruitment of homogeneous groups of participants into clinical trials of therapies for the disorder, thus allowing the results to be applied to similar patients encountered in normal clinical practice. Secondly, it means that therapy can be tailored according to the predominant symptom reported by the patient, as has been the case in recent years with the development and testing of drugs such as alosetron, tegaserod, lubiprostone, and linaclotide.[49–52] Thirdly, it allows the investigation of subgroups of patients according to predominant symptom to better understand the pathophysiologies and causative

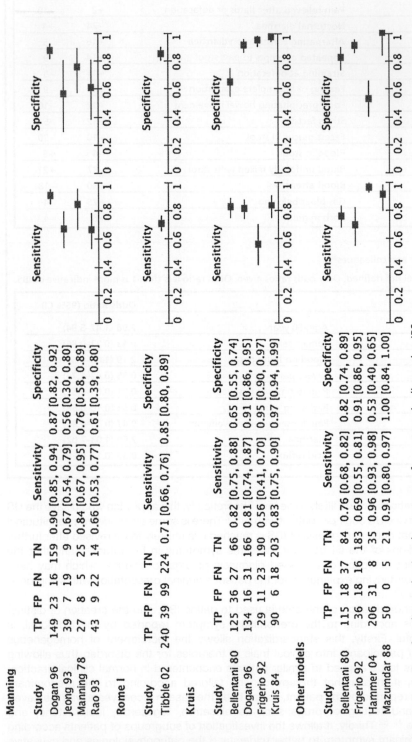

Manning

Study	TP	FP	FN	TN	Sensitivity	Specificity
Dogan 96	149	23	16	159	0.90 [0.85, 0.94]	0.87 [0.82, 0.92]
Jeong 93	39	7	19	9	0.67 [0.54, 0.79]	0.56 [0.30, 0.80]
Manning 78	27	8	5	25	0.84 [0.67, 0.95]	0.76 [0.58, 0.89]
Rao 93	43	9	22	14	0.66 [0.53, 0.77]	0.61 [0.39, 0.80]

Rome I

Study	TP	FP	FN	TN	Sensitivity	Specificity
Tibble 02	240	39	99	224	0.71 [0.66, 0.76]	0.85 [0.80, 0.89]

Kruis

Study	TP	FP	FN	TN	Sensitivity	Specificity
Bellentani 80	125	36	27	66	0.82 [0.75, 0.88]	0.65 [0.55, 0.74]
Dogan 96	134	16	31	166	0.81 [0.74, 0.87]	0.91 [0.86, 0.95]
Frigerio 92	29	11	23	190	0.56 [0.41, 0.70]	0.95 [0.90, 0.97]
Kruis 84	90	6	18	203	0.83 [0.75, 0.90]	0.97 [0.94, 0.99]

Other models

Study	TP	FP	FN	TN	Sensitivity	Specificity
Bellentani 80	115	18	37	84	0.76 [0.68, 0.82]	0.82 [0.74, 0.89]
Frigerio 92	36	18	16	183	0.69 [0.55, 0.81]	0.91 [0.86, 0.95]
Hammer 04	206	31	8	35	0.96 [0.93, 0.98]	0.53 [0.40, 0.65]
Mazumdar 88	50	0	5	21	0.91 [0.80, 0.97]	1.00 [0.84, 1.00]

Fig. 1. Forest plot of studies evaluating the accuracy of symptoms in diagnosing IBS.

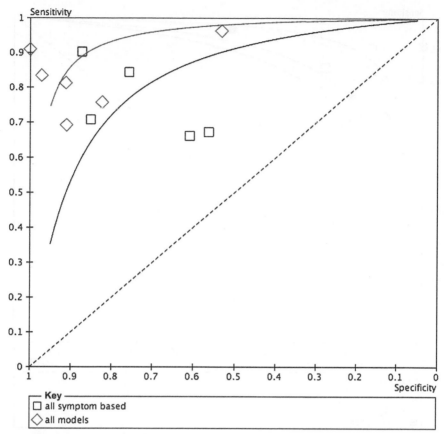

Fig. 2. SROC of diagnostic accuracy of statistical models versus symptom-based criteria for diagnosing IBS.

mechanisms that may cause IBS,[53–55] enabling the development of new therapies targeting these abnormalities, rather than treating the condition as one amorphous disorder.

Despite these advantages, the use of symptom-based diagnostic criteria in making a diagnosis of IBS also has limitations. As has been shown, the utility of such criteria in clinical practice is limited. In addition, in the absence of a true reference standard with which to compare the criteria, other than negative lower GI investigations, their accuracy remains speculative. In some patients presenting with symptoms that meet these criteria, an organic diagnosis is therefore missed, which may prompt the physician and patient to ignore recommendations for a positive diagnosis to be made to minimize the risk of this oversight occurring. Indeed, there are several recent studies that suggest that organic conditions, such as celiac disease,[56] small intestinal bacterial overgrowth,[57] bile acid malabsorption,[58] and exocrine pancreatic insufficiency,[59] are more common in individuals meeting diagnostic criteria for IBS than in asymptomatic individuals. However, it may seem that organic findings in lower GI endoscopy are no more common in patients with IBS than in controls without IBS.[60]

The Rome criteria[6] have become increasingly important over the last 10 years, particularly from a research perspective. However, a further limitation of such

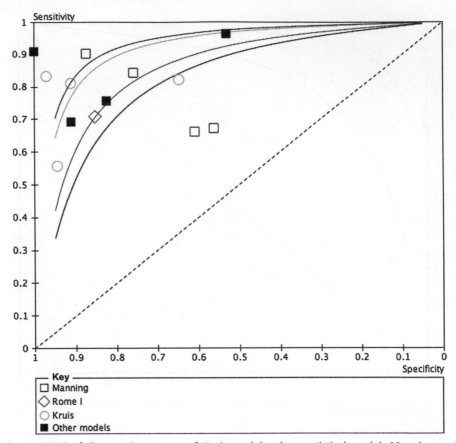

Fig. 3. SROC of diagnostic accuracy of Kruis model, other statistical models Manning and Rome I criteria for diagnosing IBS.

diagnostic criteria is that studies validating any of the iterations of the Rome criteria are scarce.[61] The authors have shown that there is only 1 study that has rigorously validated Rome I criteria[37] and data to support the accuracy of Rome II and Rome II are sparse.[10,12] Despite lack of sufficient data, investigators conducting research in any aspect of IBS are expected to use these criteria or risk criticism of their study design and methodology. Unquestioning acceptance of this situation runs the risk of stifling useful research in IBS diagnostics in the future.

In addition, it is argued that although the Rome criteria are useful to select patients for clinical trials, they are less relevant to physicians in primary care because the criteria have been developed primarily by gastroenterologists in secondary or tertiary care. A consensus panel suggested that existing diagnostic criteria were not sufficiently broad for use in primary care,[62] and surveys demonstrate that few primary care physicians are aware of, or use, any of the existing diagnostic criteria to diagnose IBS.[63] As this is the setting where most patients present, are diagnosed, and are treated, the ethos behind the use of such criteria to make the diagnosis of IBS is called into question.

One final issue that limits the usefulness of these criteria is the degree of overlap with other functional GI disorders and their lack of stability over time. The prevalence of IBS is higher in individuals with symptoms suggestive of dyspepsia or gastroesophageal reflux disease than in individuals without these symptoms. In a recent meta-analysis the prevalence of IBS was 8-fold higher in individuals with dyspepsia, and there was considerable overlap between the 2 conditions,[64] no matter which of the various available symptom-based diagnostic criteria for each were used to define their presence. During follow-up, individuals with IBS often experience a flux in their symptoms. Predominant stool pattern reported by the patient may change,[65] or the symptoms alter to such an extent that the individual no longer meets diagnostic criteria for IBS but does meet criteria for one of the other functional GI disorders, such as dyspepsia, gastroesophageal reflux disease, or chronic idiopathic constipation.[66–69] This finding calls into question potentially artificial divisions between these conditions, and the fact that some therapies, such as antidepressants,[70] agents acting on the 5-hydroxytryptamine receptor,[71,72] or the guanylate cyclase receptor[73] seem to be of benefit in more than 1 of the functional GI disorders reinforces the potential for common mechanisms in their pathophysiology.

SUMMARY

There have been several changes to symptom-based criteria defining IBS over the past 20 years through the efforts of the Rome Foundation, which has brought more consistency to the type of patients who participate in IBS research studies. However, to paraphrase the French proverb *plus ça change, plus c'est la même chose*, although much has changed, much has stayed the same. There has been little research into the diagnostic accuracy of Rome II and Rome III criteria and it is not clear whether they are any more accurate than more traditional symptom-based criteria such as that described by Manning and colleagues[3] more than 30 years ago. Community gastroenterologists can therefore be forgiven for still treating IBS as a diagnosis of exclusion. Perhaps the Rome criteria are trying to achieve too much. These definitions may be useful for including patients in research studies but may not be rigorous enough to exclude organic disease. This drawback may not matter in the context of a research trial because patients often have to have exhaustive investigations. In clinical practice however, there may need to be a more exhaustive set of questions completed before the physician can make a positive diagnosis of IBS. The answer could lie with studies that have evaluated statistical models to diagnose IBS. There have been several different questionnaires proposed (see **Box 2**) but some common themes seem to emerge from them. Rather than just focusing on IBS symptoms, they also look at demographic factors such as age and gender. They also look at selected alarm features,[74] such as blood mixed with the stool. Also, they evaluate other disorders, such as acid reflux,[36] that may be associated with IBS and may support the diagnosis, if present. Further work in this area is needed if we are to gain insights that will truly help clinicians to confidently diagnose IBS.

REFERENCES

1. Ananthakrishnan AN, McGinley EL, Saeian K. Length of office visits for gastrointestinal disease: impact of physician specialty. Am J Gastroenterol 2010;105:1719–25.
2. Spiegel BM, Farid M, Esrailian E, et al. Is irritable bowel syndrome a diagnosis of exclusion? a survey of primary care providers, gastroenterologists, and IBS experts. Am J Gastroenterol 2010;105:848–58.
3. Manning AP, Thompson WG, Heaton KW, et al. Towards a positive diagnosis of the irritable bowel. BMJ 1978;2(6138):653–4.

4. Kruis W, Thieme C, Weinzierl M, et al. A diagnostic score for the irritable bowel syndrome. Its value in the exclusion of organic disease. Gastroenterology 1984;87:1–7.
5. Drossman DA, Thompson WG, Talley NJ. Identification of sub-groups of functional gastrointestinal disorders. Gastroenterol Int 1990;3:159–72.
6. Thompson WG, Longstreth GF, Drossman DA, et al. Functional bowel disorders and functional abdominal pain. Gut 1999;45(Suppl II):II43–7.
7. Longstreth GF, Thompson WG, Chey WD, et al. Functional bowel disorders. Gastroenterology 2006;130:1480–91.
8. Drossman DA. Rome foundation diagnostic algorithms. Preface. Am J Gastroenterol 2010;105:741–2.
9. Kellow JE. Introduction: a practical evidence-based approach to the diagnosis of the functional gastrointestinal disorders. Am J Gastroenterol 2010;105:743–6.
10. Spiller RC. Bowel disorders. Am J Gastroenterol 2010;105:775–85.
11. Whitehead WE, Drossman DA. Validation of symptom-based diagnostic criteria for irritable bowel syndrome: a critical review. Am J Gastroenterol 2010;105:814–20.
12. Ford AC, Talley NJ, Veldhuyzen van Zanten SJ, et al. Will the history and physical examination help establish that irritable bowel syndrome is causing this patient's lower gastrointestinal tract symptoms? JAMA 2008;300:1793–805.
13. Jellema P, van der Windt DA, Chellevis FG, et al. Systematic review: accuracy of symptom-based criteria for diagnosis of irritable bowel syndrome in primary care. Aliment Pharmacol Ther 2009;30:695–706.
14. Ford AC, Guyatt GH, Talley NJ, et al. Errors in the conduct of systematic reviews of pharmacological interventions for irritable bowel syndrome. Am J Gastroenterol 2010;105:280–8.
15. Vanner SJ, Depew WT, Paterson WG, et al. Predictive value of the Rome criteria for diagnosing the irritable bowel syndrome. Am J Gastroenterol 1999;94:2912–7.
16. Banerjee R, Choung OW, Gupta R, et al. Rome I criteria are more sensitive than Rome II for diagnosis of irritable bowel syndrome in Indian patients. Indian J Gastroenterol 2005;24:164–6.
17. Kapoor KK, Nigam P, Rastogi CK, et al. Clinical profile of irritable bowel syndrome. Indian J Gastroenterol 1985;4:15–6.
18. Orient JO, Kettel LJ, Lim J. A test of a linear discriminant for identifying low-risk abdominal pain. Med Decis Making 1985;5:77–87.
19. Orient JO. Evaluation of abdominal pain: clinicians' performance compared with three protocols. South Med J 1986;79:793–9.
20. Wasson JH, Sox HC Jr, Sox CH. The diagnosis of abdominal pain in ambulatory male patients. Med Decis Making 1981;1:215–24.
21. Hammer J, Talley NJ. Value of different diagnostic criteria for the irritable bowel syndrome among men and women. J Clin Gastroenterol 2008;42:160–6.
22. Poynard T, Couturier D, Frexinos J, et al. French experience of Manning's criteria in the irritable bowel syndrome. Eur J Gastroenterol Hepatol 1992;4:747–52.
23. Chalubinski K, Brunner H. [Positive diagnosis of irritable colon: a scored chart or standardized anamnesis?] Wien Klin Wochenschr 1987;99:819–24 [in German].
24. Mohamed AS, Khan BA. A more positive diagnosis of irritable bowel syndrome in Saudi patients. Ann Saudi Med 1999;19:459–61.
25. Mouzas IA, Fragkiadakis N, Moschandreas J, et al. Validation and results of a questionnaire for functional bowel disease in out-patients. BMC Public Health 2002;2:8.
26. Talley NJ, Phillips SF, Melton J III, et al. A patient questionnaire to identify bowel disease. Ann Intern Med 1989;111:671–4.

27. Enck P, Whitehead WE, Schuster MM, et al. Psychosomatic aspects of irritable bowel syndrome. Specificity of clinical symptoms, psychopathological features and motor activity of the rectosigmoid. Dtsch Med Wochenschr 1988;113: 459–62.
28. Starmans R, Muris JW, Fijten GH, et al. The diagnostic value of scoring models for organic and non-organic gastrointestinal disease, including the irritable-bowel syndrome. Med Decis Making 1994;14:208–16.
29. Talley NJ, Phillips SF, Melton LJ, et al. Diagnostic value of the Manning criteria in irritable bowel syndrome. Gut 1990;31:77–81.
30. Jeong H, Lee HR, Yoo BC, et al. Manning criteria in irritable bowel syndrome: its diagnostic significance. Korean J Intern Med 1993;8:34–9.
31. Rao KP, Gupta S, Jain AK, et al. Evaluation of Manning's criteria in the diagnosis of irritable bowel syndrome. J Assoc Physicians India 1993;41:357–63.
32. Dogan UB, Unal S. Kruis scoring system and Manning's criteria in diagnosis of irritable bowel syndrome: is it better to use combined? Acta Gastroenterol Belg 1996;59:225–8.
33. Frigerio G, Beretta A, Orsenigo G, et al. Irritable bowel syndrome. Still far from a positive diagnosis. Dig Dis Sci 1992;37:164–7.
34. Bellentani S, Baldoni P, Petrella S, et al. A simple score for the identification of patients at high risk of organic diseases of the colon in the family doctor consulting room. The Local IBS Study Group. Fam Pract 1990;7:307–12.
35. Mazumdar TN, Prasad KV, Bhat PV. Formulation of a scoring chart for irritable bowel syndrome (IBS): a prospective study. Indian J Gastroenterol 1988;7.101–2.
36. Hammer J, Eslick GD, Howell SC, et al. Diagnostic yield of alarm features in irritable bowel syndrome and functional dyspepsia. Gut 2004;53:666–72.
37. Tibble JA, Sigthorsson G, Foster R, et al. Use of surrogate markers of inflammation and Rome criteria to distinguish organic from nonorganic intestinal disease. Gastroenterology 2002;123:450–60.
38. Jones CM, Athanasiou T. Summary receiver operating characteristic curve analysis techniques in the evaluation of diagnostic tests. Ann Thorac Surg 2005;79: 16–20.
39. Brandt LJ, Chey WD, Foxx-Orenstein AE, et al. An evidence-based systematic review on the management of irritable bowel syndrome. Am J Gastroenterol 2009;104(Suppl I):S8–35.
40. National Institute for Health and Clinical Excellence. Irritable bowel syndrome in adults: diagnosis and management of irritable bowel syndrome in primary care. Availale at: http://guidance.nice.org.uk/CG61/NICEGuidance/pdf/English. Accessed January 21, 2011.
41. Spiller R, Aziz Q, Creed F, et al. Guidelines on the irritable bowel syndrome: mechanisms and practical management. Gut 2007;56:1770–98.
42. Lembo AJ, Neri B, Tolley J, et al. Use of serum biomarkers in a diagnostic test for irritable bowel syndrome. Aliment Pharmacol Ther 2009;29:834–42.
43. Whitehead WE, Crowell MD, Bosmajian L, et al. Existence of irritable bowel syndrome supported by factor analysis of symptoms in two community samples. Gastroenterology 1990;98:336–40.
44. Taub E, Cuevas JL, Cook EW, et al. Irritable bowel syndrome defined by factor analysis. Gender and race comparisons. Dig Dis Sci 1995;40:2647–55.
45. Talley NJ, Boyce P, Jones M. Identification of distinct upper and lower gastrointestinal symptom groupings in an urban population. Gut 1998;42:690–5.
46. Martin R, Barron JJ, Zacker C. Irritable bowel syndrome: toward a cost-effective management approach. Am J Manag Care 2001;7:S268–75.

47. Adeniji OA, Barnett CB, Di Palma JA. Durability of the diagnosis of irritable bowel syndrome based on clinical criteria. Dig Dis Sci 2004;49:572–4.

48. Owens DM, Nelson DK, Talley NJ. The irritable bowel syndrome: long-term prognosis and the physician-patient interaction. Ann Intern Med 1995;122: 107–12.

49. Camilleri M, Northcutt AR, Kong S, et al. Efficacy and safety of alosetron in women with irritable bowel syndrome: a randomised, placebo-controlled trial. Lancet 2000;355:1035–40.

50. Chey WD, Pare P, Viegas A, et al. Tegaserod for female patients suffering from IBS with mixed bowel habits or constipation: a randomized controlled trial. Am J Gastroenterol 2008;103:1217–25.

51. Johanson JF, Drossman DA, Panas R, et al. Clinical trial: phase 2 study of lubiprostone for irritable bowel syndrome with constipation. Aliment Pharmacol Ther 2008;27:685–96.

52. Johnston JM, Kurtz CB, MacDougall JE, et al. Linaclotide improves abdominal pain and bowel habits in a phase IIb study of patients with irritable bowel syndrome with constipation. Gastroenterology 2010;139(6):1877–86, e2.

53. Zhou Q, Souba WW, Croce CM, et al. MicroRNA-29a regulates intestinal membrane permeability in patients with irritable bowel syndrome. Gut 2010;59: 775–84.

54. Marciani L, Cox EF, Hoad CL, et al. Postprandial changes in small bowel water content in healthy subjects and patients with irritable bowel syndrome. Gastroenterology 2010;138:469–77.

55. Abrahamsson H, Ostlund-Lindqvist AM, Nilsson R, et al. Altered bile acid metabolism in patients with constipation-predominant irritable bowel syndrome and functional constipation. Scand J Gastroenterol 2008;43:1483–8.

56. Ford AC, Chey WD, Talley NJ, et al. Yield of diagnostic tests for celiac disease in subjects with symptoms suggestive of irritable bowel syndrome: systematic review and meta-analysis. Arch Intern Med 2009;169:651–8.

57. Ford AC, Spiegel BM, Talley NJ, et al. Small intestinal bacterial overgrowth in irritable bowel syndrome: systematic review and meta-analysis. Clin Gastroenterol Hepatol 2009;7:1279–86.

58. Wedlake L, A'Hern R, Russell D, et al. Systematic review: the prevalence of idiopathic bile acid malabsorption as diagnosed by SeHCAT scanning in patients with diarrhoea-predominant irritable bowel syndrome. Aliment Pharmacol Ther 2009;30:707–17.

59. Leeds JS, Hopper AD, Sidhu R, et al. Some patients with irritable bowel syndrome may have exocrine pancreatic insufficiency. Clin Gastroenterol Hepatol 2010;8:433–8.

60. Chey WD, Nojkov B, Rubenstein JH, et al. The yield of colonoscopy in patients with non-constipated irritable bowel syndrome: results from a prospective, controlled US trial. Am J Gastroenterol 2010;105:859–65.

61. Molinder HK, Kjellstrom L, Nylin HB, et al. Doubtful outcome of the validation of the Rome II questionnaire: validation of a symptom based diagnostic tool. Health Qual Life Outcomes 2009;7:106.

62. Rubin G, de Wit N, Meineche-Schmidt V, et al. The diagnosis of IBS in primary care: consensus development using nominal group technique. Fam Pract 2006;23:687–92.

63. Thompson WG, Heaton KW, Smyth GT, et al. Irritable bowel syndrome: the view from general practice. Eur J Gastroenterol Hepatol 1997;9:689–92.

64. Ford AC, Marwaha A, Lim A, et al. Systematic review and meta-analysis of the prevalence of irritable bowel syndrome in individuals with dyspepsia. Clin Gastroenterol Hepatol 2010;8:401–9.

65. Drossman DA, Morris CB, Hu Y, et al. A prospective assessment of bowel habit in irritable bowel syndrome in women: defining an alternator. Gastroenterology 2005;128:580–9.

66. Agreus L, Svardsudd K, Talley NJ, et al. Natural history of gastroesophageal reflux disease and functional abdominal disorders. Am J Gastroenterol 2001;96: 2905–14.

67. Ford AC, Forman D, Bailey AG, et al. Fluctuation of gastrointestinal symptoms in the community: a 10-year longitudinal follow-up study. Aliment Pharmacol Ther 2008;28:1013–20.

68. Halder SLS, Locke GR III, Schleck CD, et al. Natural history of functional gastrointestinal disorders: a 12-year longitudinal population-based study. Gastroenterology 2007;133:799–807.

69. Wong RK, Palsson O, Turner MJ, et al. Inability of the Rome III criteria to distinguish functional constipation from constipation-subtype irritable bowel syndrome. Am J Gastroenterol 2010;105:2228–34.

70. Ford AC, Talley NJ, Schoenfeld PS, et al. Efficacy of antidepressants and psychological therapies in irritable bowel syndrome: systematic review and meta-analysis. Gut 2009;58:367–78.

71. Ford AC, Brandt LJ, Young C, et al. Efficacy of 5-HT$_3$ antagonists and 5-HT$_4$ agonists in irritable bowel syndrome: systematic review and meta-analysis. Am J Gastroenterol 2009;104:1831–43.

72. Vakil N, Laine L, Talley NJ, et al. Tegaserod treatment for dysmotility-like functional dyspepsia: results of two randomized, controlled trials. Am J Gastroenterol 2008;103:1906–19.

73. Lembo AJ, Kurtz CB, MacDougall JE, et al. Efficacy of linaclotide for patients with chronic constipation. Gastroenterology 2010;138:886–95.

74. Whitehead WE, Palsson OS, Feld AD, et al. Utility of red flag symptom exclusions in the diagnosis of irritable bowel syndrome. Aliment Pharmacol Ther 2006;24: 137–46.

The Role of Diagnostic Testing in Irritable Bowel Syndrome

David L. Furman, MD[a], Brooks D. Cash, MD[a,b,c],*

KEYWORDS

- Irritable bowel syndrome • Rome criteria
- Celiac disease • Colonoscopy • Diagnosis

The irritable bowel syndrome (IBS) is one of the most common conditions encountered in general medical practices.[1,2] It has been estimated that IBS is responsible for 2.4 million to 3.5 million physician visits per year and represents 12% of primary care and 28% of gastroenterological referrals.[3] Although IBS has a variety of presentations and symptoms that can differ among patients with the condition, this condition can be broadly characterized as the presence of abdominal pain or discomfort associated with altered bowel movement form and/or bowel movement frequency.

For a variety of reasons, clinicians often struggle to arrive at a confident diagnosis of IBS. The differential diagnosis in patients with symptoms suggestive of IBS is broad (**Box 1**), and there is no reliable biologic marker for this condition. Because it is so common, the classic clinical symptoms of abdominal pain or discomfort associated with alterations in bowel function are readily recognizable to most physicians. In a 2006 survey, 53% of family practitioners, 63% of general internists, and 24% of gastroenterologists reported feeling "very comfortable" at making the diagnosis of IBS at the first visit.[4] However, in another survey, 75% of clinicians indicated that they believed the diagnosis of IBS was one that could be made only after exclusion of organic disease.[5]

Over the past 30 years, several groups have attempted to develop symptom-based criteria to guide researchers and clinicians in identifying patients with IBS. Multiple

The opinions and assertions contained herein are the sole views of the authors and should not be construed as official or as representing the views of the US Navy, Department of Defense, or Department of Veteran Affairs.

Disclosure: Dr Cash has served as a consultant to Prometheus Laboratories.

[a] Gastroenterology Service, National Naval Medical Center, 8901 Wisconsin Avenue, Bethesda, MD 20889-5000, USA

[b] Uniformed Services University of the Health Sciences, 4301 Jones Bridge Road, Bethesda, MD 20814, USA

[c] National Naval Medical Center, 8901 Wisconsin Avenue, Bethesda, MD 20889-5000, USA

* Corresponding author. National Naval Medical Center, 8901 Wisconsin Avenue, Bethesda, MD 20889-5000.

E-mail address: brooks.cash@med.navy.mil

Gastroenterol Clin N Am 40 (2011) 105–119
doi:10.1016/j.gtc.2010.12.001
0889-8553/11/$ – see front matter. Published by Elsevier Inc.

Box 1
Differential diagnosis of suspected IBS

IBS

Celiac disease

Disaccharide maldigestion

Food intolerance

Small intestine bacterial overgrowth

Bile acid malabsorption

Chronic pancreatitis

Enteric neuropathy or myopathy

Gastrointestinal infection

Inflammatory bowel disease (IBD)

Thyroid dysfunction (hyper or hypo)

Malignancy

Metabolic disease

Medication side effects

Other functional gastrointestinal disorders

symptom-based criteria (**Table 1**) have been developed, including the Manning, Rome I, Rome II, and Rome III criteria.[6–9] In particular, the Rome criteria, developed by multinational working groups, provide a uniform framework for the selection of patients in diagnostic and therapeutic trials of IBS. However, in recent years, the application of these criteria to patients in clinical practice has been encouraged.[10,11] The Rome III criteria for IBS include at least 12 weeks (which need not be consecutive), in the preceding 12 months, of abdominal discomfort or pain that is accompanied by at least 2 of the following 3 symptoms: the abdominal discomfort or pain is (1) relieved with defecation, (2) associated with a change in the frequency of defecation, and/or (3) associated with a change in the form or appearance of the stool.[9] Several studies have found the Rome criteria to be quite specific for IBS.[12] The Rome III criteria have the advantage of being easier to recall and use than the older versions of the Rome criteria. However, recent studies suggest that there are differences in sensitivity and specificity among the various vintages of the Rome criteria, likely because of the more restrictive temporal pain requirements with Rome II and III.[13,14] Generally speaking, most patients who fulfill IBS criteria actually do suffer with IBS, but because the condition is so common and so protean, there are likely many patients who do not strictly fulfill symptom-based criteria but ultimately end up with a diagnosis of IBS.

DIAGNOSIS OF IBS

The Rome Committee on Functional Gastrointestinal Disorders and other IBS authorities recommend that selected diagnostic tests be performed as part of the routine evaluation of patients with suspected IBS.[15,16] These tests include serum and stool studies, as well as colonic visualization, to exclude important organic gastrointestinal diseases.[17] Others propose a limited screen for disorders that may masquerade as IBS, such as celiac disease.[18] Recently the necessity of these evaluations has been

Table 1
Symptom-based criteria for the diagnosis of IBS

Manning	Rome I	Rome II	Rome III
Abdominal pain relieved by defecation	>12 wk of continuous or recurrent symptoms of abdominal pain or discomfort:	>12 wk, which need not be consecutive, in the preceding 12 mo, of abdominal discomfort or pain that has 2 or more of 3 features:	Recurrent abdominal pain or discomfort at least 3 d/mo for past 3 mo, with symptom onset >6 mo before diagnosis, associated with 2 or more of the following:
Looser stools with the onset of pain	1. Relieved with defecation or	Relieved with defecation	Improvement with defecation
More frequent stools with the onset of pain	2. Associated with change in frequency of stool or	Onset associated with change in stool frequency	Onset associated with a change in frequency of stool
Abdominal distention	3. Associated with a change in consistency of stool	Onset associated with a change in form (appearance) of stool	Onset associated with a change in stool form (appearance)
Passage of mucus in stools	Two or more of the following, at least on one-fourth of occasions or days:		
Sensation of incomplete evacuation	1. Altered stool frequency		
	2. Altered stool form		
	3. Passage of mucus		
	4. Bloating or feeling of abdominal distention		

questioned.[19] The most recent guidelines on the evaluation of IBS, published by the American College of Gastroenterology (ACG) IBS Task Force, encourage clinicians to make a positive diagnosis of IBS based on a thorough history, using symptom-based criteria and considering the presence or absence of specific alarm features such as rectal bleeding or unintended weight loss.[20] In the absence of alarm features, the Task Force does not recommend the routine use of diagnostic imaging studies, blood tests, or stool studies to exclude less-common organic diseases in the evaluation of a patient with typical IBS symptoms.[20]

Ostensibly, the performance of a diagnostic test should alter clinicians' estimate of the pretest probability of a disease so that they may be reasonably assured that the disease being considered is either present or absent based on the results of the diagnostic test. In the case of IBS, diagnostic tests are performed to exclude organic diseases that may have similar presenting symptoms and in doing so serve to reassure the clinician and patient that the diagnosis of IBS is correct. IBD, colorectal cancer (CRC), systemic hormonal disturbances, enteric infections, and malabsorptive diseases such as celiac disease are of greatest concern to the clinician faced with a patient with symptoms suggestive of IBS. Prevalence rates (pretest probability) for many of these conditions in patients with suspected IBS and non-IBS controls/population norms are presented in **Table 2**. These values are subject to regional and demographic variations that, when individualized, could affect the decision to pursue diagnostic tests to exclude certain conditions.

Screening patients first for alarming clinical or historical features such as unintended weight loss of more than 4.5 kg (10 lb), fevers or chills, high-volume ($\geq$300 mL/d) diarrhea, nocturnal diarrhea, family history of gastrointestinal malignancy, IBD, celiac disease, or older age ($\geq$50 years) at onset of IBS symptoms is thought to identify those patients at a greater risk of harboring an occult disease, rather than IBS alone, as a basis for their gastrointestinal symptoms, thereby justifying a carefully directed diagnostic evaluation. The actual value of alarm features in distinguishing organic disease from IBS is limited. Whitehead and colleagues[21] performed a systematic chart review of 1434 patients diagnosed with IBS, abdominal pain, diarrhea, or constipation, with specific attention to the documentation of Rome II criteria and typical red-flag symptoms. Of 575 patients diagnosed with IBS using symptom-based criteria, organic disease was identified in 3% (1% gastrointestinal cancer, 1.2% IBD, 0.7% malabsorption). However, several of these diagnoses were already known to clinicians at the time

Table 2
Pretest probability and prevalence of frequently excluded organic diseases in patients with IBS and population norms

Disease	Prevalence Among Patients with IBS (%)	Prevalence Among General Population (%)
Colitis/IBD	0.51–0.98	0.3–1.2
Colorectal cancer	0–0.51	0–6
Thyroid dysfunction	4.2	5–9
Gastrointestinal infection	0–1.5	N/A
Lactose maldigestion	38	26
Celiac disease	0.4–4	0.7

Abbreviation: N/A, not applicable.
Data from Cash BD, Schoenfeld PS, Chey WD. The utility of diagnostic tests in irritable bowel syndrome patients: a systematic review. Am J Gastroenterol 2002;97:2812–9.

of the patient's initial visit, so the prevalence of organic disease in patients with IBS in this group is likely much smaller. Overall, 83% of patients reported at least 1 red-flag symptom, and the positive predictive value of 1 red flag for identifying organic disease was less than 10%. Despite this relatively low specificity for organic disease, identification of malignancy, IBD, or malabsorption is of sufficient importance that, alarm features, when reported, should be appropriately investigated.

Hammer and colleagues[22] also investigated the value of alarm features and their ability to predict organic disease in patients with suspected IBS who completed a validated symptom questionnaire and then underwent diagnostic evaluation. Age greater than 50 years at symptom onset (odds ratio [OR], 2.65; $P = .002$) and report of blood on the toilet paper (OR, 2.7; $P = .002$) discriminated IBS from organic disease in this series. Overall, however, the presence of alarm symptoms had a positive predictive value of only 31.8% for structural gastrointestinal disease. The real value of alarm features seemed to be in their negative predictive value. When symptom-based criteria (Manning) were combined with absent alarm features, a correct diagnosis of IBS was reached in 96% of cases. A recent analysis of more than 7500 patients undergoing colonoscopy identified abdominal pain, rectal bleeding, and change in bowel habits as independent predictors of CRC.[23] The risk was greatest in patients with less than 12 months of these symptoms, with the greatest risk associated with rectal bleeding (OR, 4.3; 95% confidence interval [CI], 2.89–6.36, $P<.001$). **Box 2** lists alarm symptoms that the ACG IBS Task Force considers important to consider in the evaluation of patients with possible IBS.[20]

YIELD OF DIAGNOSTIC TESTING IN PATIENTS WITH SUSPECTED IBS

The first systematic review of the English language medical literature regarding commonly used diagnostic tests for IBS was performed in conjunction with the ACG IBS Task Force statement in 2002.[19] This review included clinical trials that were published between 1980 and 2001, in which patients who fulfilled symptom-based criteria for IBS underwent diagnostic testing. After applying established criteria for the quality and validity of trials,[24,25] 6 studies fulfilled inclusion criteria.[26–31] Review of these studies suggested that the pretest probability of organic diseases such as colon cancer, IBD, thyroid disease, and lactose malabsorption was not different between patients with IBS and the general population. Based on the review of

---

Box 2
Classic alarm features to note in suspected IBS

Unintentional weight loss

Iron deficiency anemia

Family history of IBD

Family history of CRC

Family history of celiac disease

Rectal bleeding

Nocturnal diarrhea

Data from Brandt LJ, Chey WD, Foxx-Orenstein AE, et al. An evidence-based systematic review on the management of irritable bowel syndrome. Am J Gastroenterol 2009;104(Suppl 1):S1–35.

published data, when patients with suspected IBS fulfilled symptom-based criteria for the diagnosis of IBS, performance of commonly recommended tests, including colonic endoscopy, complete blood count (CBC), comprehensive metabolic panel (CMP), stool examination for ova and parasites, fecal occult blood testing, thyroid function test (TFT), and hydrogen breath test for lactose maldigestion, did not result in a significant increase in the diagnosis of organic gastrointestinal disease. The possible exception to this was celiac disease, which seemed to be more common in patients with suspected IBS in a single study conducted in a referral setting with a relatively homogeneous population.[30] However, during the ensuing decade, more evidence has been presented that both challenges and compliments these conclusions. The recently updated ACG IBS Task Force statement takes much of this evidence into account.[20]

Routine Blood Tests

Blood tests, such as CBC, CMP, TFT, and determination of inflammatory markers such as the erythrocyte sedimentation rate (ESR) and level of C-reactive protein (CRP), are often ordered on initial evaluation of patients with suspected IBS. These tests are relatively inexpensive, can be processed rapidly in a local laboratory, and are generally considered noninvasive. However, there is little evidence to suggest that their routine use enhances the diagnosis of organic disease or results in meaningful management changes in patients with suspected IBS. Tolliver and colleagues[27] found that evaluation with CBC, ESR, CMP, TFT, and urinalysis in patients with suspected IBS yielded no alternative diagnoses (other than IBS) to explain the patients' gastrointestinal symptoms. Sanders and colleagues evaluated 300 patients who fulfilled the Rome II criteria for IBS with a similar battery of blood tests and found 1 patient (0.3%) with an abnormal CBC, 2 (0.7%) with abnormal levels of liver-associated enzymes, and 1 (0.3%) with an elevated ESR.[30] Likewise, Cash and colleagues[32] found no differences in the results of routine blood tests (CBC, CMP, TFT, ESR, CRP) between a cohort of nearly 500 patients with IBS and 500 healthy controls. These results are consistent in that they confirm that the likelihood of identifying organic disease with routine laboratory tests seems to be no greater in patients with IBS (and absent alarm features) than in the general population. However, many of these studies arise from the clinical trial or tertiary care arenas and, therefore, may not be representative of the larger population of patients with suspected IBS who are encountered in community practice.

Testing for Celiac Disease

Patients with IBS often endorse specific food ingestion as a primary trigger of their gastrointestinal symptoms, and many identify gluten-containing foods as problematic, causing a concern of celiac disease in patients with suspected IBS. The symptoms of IBS and celiac disease may be indistinguishable. In a survey of 1032 members of the Celiac Disease Foundation, many respondents endorsed presenting symptoms characteristic of IBS and patients with celiac disease often have been diagnosed with IBS for some time before the formal diagnosis of celiac disease.[33] Celiac disease, a chronic enteropathy resulting from an immune-mediated response to deamidated gliadin, has a prevalence of about 0.7% to 1% in the United States.[34] Common symptoms of celiac disease include abdominal pain (77%), gas or bloating (73%), diarrhea (52%), constipation (7%), and fluctuation between diarrhea and constipation (24%). Untreated celiac disease can result in malnutrition, anemia, osteoporosis, infertility, and an increased risk of gastrointestinal lymphoma.[35–37] The diagnosis of celiac disease is typically based on the demonstration of elevated levels of antigliadin antibodies (AGAs), antiendomysial antibodies (anti-EMAs), or anti–tissue transglutami-nase antibodies, with the last 2 antibody tests preferred because of their higher sensi-tivity and specificity than AGA. The gold-standard diagnostic test for celiac disease is small intestinal biopsy demonstrating characteristic changes in the intestinal mucosa, including villous atrophy, crypt hyperplasia, and inflammation of the lamina propria.[38] Because of the invasiveness and expense of upper gastrointestinal endoscopy and biopsy, this diagnostic modality is typically reserved for confirmation of abnormal anti-body testing or evaluation of treatment effects after the diagnosis has been made.

Multiple case-control studies have demonstrated an increased prevalence of celiac disease among subjects with IBS compared with healthy controls. Sanders and colleagues[30] screened 300 consecutive new patients who met the Rome II IBS criteria and an age-and-gender–matched control group with anti-EMA and antigliadin IgG and IgA antibody tests and used duodenal biopsy to confirm celiac disease in serologically positive subjects. Celiac disease was identified in 14 (4.6%) patients with IBS but in only 2 (0.7%) of the controls (OR, 7.0; $P = .004$). A more recent prospective US study comparing the prevalence of celiac disease in patients with suspected IBS and in controls found that 7.3% of 492 patients with nonconstipated IBS (diagnosed by Rome II criteria) had elevated celiac disease antibodies. The prevalence of biopsy-confirmed celiac disease in this group was 0.4%, similar to that observed in 458 controls without IBS symptoms ($P = .28$) and US population prevalence estimates.[32] In a recent meta-analysis, the prevalence of celiac disease in individuals with sus-pected IBS was computed to be 4 times greater than in non-IBS controls when data from 14 studies comprising 4202 patients were included.[39]

In its revised statement, the ACG IBS Task Force recommended testing for celiac disease in patients presenting with nonconstipated IBS symptoms, based on studies such as those discussed earlier and analyses that suggest that serologic testing for celiac disease is cost-effective when the pretest probability exceeds 1%. Mein and Ladabaum[40] used decision analytic modeling to evaluate the cost-effectiveness of serologic screening for celiac disease in patients with IBS. They concluded that with a calculated cost per quality adjusted life-year gain of $4600 per case, testing patients with suspected celiac disease is cost-effective. Spiegel and colleagues[41] came to a similar conclusion in their cost-effectiveness study, even after biasing their model against testing by assuming low individual test characteristics and incomplete patient adherence to a gluten-free diet. Given the wide geographic variability in the prevalence of celiac disease among persons with IBS symptoms, it may be necessary to know local prevalence data to understand cost-effectiveness of serologic screening in a specific population.

Colonoscopy

Patients with typical IBS symptoms commonly undergo colonoscopy. For example, community-based surveys indicate that up to 50% of patients with IBS undergo colonoscopy in the course of their diagnostic evaluation.[42] Furthermore, available data suggest that 25% of all colonoscopies performed in the United States are for IBS-related symptoms and 10% of colonoscopies performed on patients younger than 50 years are conducted for the evaluation of IBS symptoms.[43] Despite such broad use of colonoscopy in the evaluation of IBS symptoms, data addressing the actual prevalence of colonic structural abnormalities in patients with IBS are limited.

In a post hoc analysis of data from 2 placebo-controlled IBS trials, Hamm and colleagues[26] examined the yield of flexible sigmoidoscopy in study participants younger than 50 years or colonoscopy/flexible sigmoidoscopy and barium enema in enrollees aged 50 years and older. Of 1452 study participants, 306 (21%) were included in this post hoc analysis. Colonic imaging identified important structural lesions in 4 patients (1.3%; 3 IBD, 1 colonic obstruction). Unfortunately, the results of this post hoc analysis are difficult to interpret, as the proportion of patients who underwent sigmoidoscopy versus colonoscopy was not reported, patients underwent colonic imaging only if they had not undergone such imaging within 2 years of study enrollment, and the proportion of patients with IBS who had undergone previous colonic imaging was not reported.

Tolliver and colleagues[27] evaluated the yield of sigmoidoscopy, barium enema, and/ or colonoscopy in an uncontrolled, prospective trial of 196 subjects with suspected IBS. Forty-three colonic structural abnormalities were found in 34 subjects. Most abnormalities found were thought to be incidental and not responsible for the patients' gastrointestinal symptoms (benign polyps, diverticulosis, hemorrhoids, lipomas, and melanosis coli). Two (1.0%) patients were found to have organic disease (1 IBD, 1 cancer) that could have explained their IBS symptoms. Again, there are several issues that complicate the interpretation of the results from this study, including the inclusion of patients with warning signs (family history of colon cancer and hemoccult positive stool), absence of a control group, and failure to report the percentage of patients with IBS who underwent each type of examination. In an uncontrolled study, Francis and colleagues[29] studied the yield of flexible sigmoidoscopy, barium enema, or colonoscopy in 125 patients who fulfilled the Rome I criteria for IBS. With the exception of diverticulosis that was judged to be an incidental finding, no structural lesions that changed the diagnosis of IBS were identified.

Vanner and colleagues[12] performed a prospective study in 95 patients referred to the general gastroenterology clinics over a 9-month period in 1995–1996 who met the Rome criteria and lacked warning signs. About 91% of patients older than 45 years underwent barium enema or colonoscopy. Aside from 1 patient with rectal bleeding who was found to have ulcerative proctitis, no colonic abnormalities were identified. In another study, investigators reviewed colonoscopy reports of 622 patients with suspected IBS and 642 patients without IBS.[44] All colonoscopies were performed to evaluate new gastrointestinal complaints. Colonoscopy results were normal in only 48.4% of the patients with IBS; however, the lesions identified, such as hemorrhoids (21.1%), polyps (20.3%), diverticulosis (19%), and angiodysplasia (12.1%), were just as frequent in the non-IBS group, and none of these findings were felt to be responsible for IBS symptoms.

In a prospective trial of colonoscopy in patients with suspected IBS, Chey and colleagues[45] performed colonoscopy on 466 patients with suspected IBS (IBS with diarrhea [IBS-D] or IBS with a mixed stool pattern [IBS-M]) and 451 healthy controls. Compared with the control group, the study group was younger and predominantly female. Colonoscopy revealed organic lesions in both groups, with the most common lesions being hemorrhoids, polyps, and diverticulosis. Polyps were more than 2 times as prevalent in the older control group (34.4% vs 14.6%, $P \leq .0001$) and were more likely to be adenomatous than in patients with suspected IBS (26.1% vs 7.7%, $P \leq .0001$). Two patients (0.4%) in the IBS group were diagnosed with IBD, and routine colonic mucosal biopsies yielded a diagnosis of microscopic colitis in an additional 7 patients (1.5%) with suspected IBS. The prevalence of microscopic colitis was higher in older patients with IBS-D. A retrospective review of patients with biopsy-proven microscopic colitis found that 56% met the diagnostic criteria for IBS (Rome II) and one-third had previously been diagnosed with IBS.[46] Routine biopsies in the sigmoid colon of patients with IBS older than 40 years undergoing colonoscopy revealed microscopic colitis in more than 5%. These findings provide the rationale for the recommendations of the ACG IBS Task Force to perform colonoscopy in patients with IBS older than 50 years (for colon cancer screening) and those with alarm features. According to the Task Force, when colonoscopy is performed in patients with suspected IBS-D, clinicians should consider performing random mucosal biopsies to rule out microscopic colitis.[20]

Breath Testing for Small Intestinal Bacterial Overgrowth or Carbohydrate Maldigestion

Bloating is one of the most common symptoms associated with IBS, occurring in more than 75% of patients with IBS.[47,48] The high prevalence of bloating and the increasing recognition of symptom improvement from antibiotic and probiotic therapy for IBS has prompted the consideration of breath testing of patients with IBS to detect small intestinal bacterial overgrowth (SIBO). Similarly, the frequent association of IBS-like symptoms with lactose or fructose ingestion suggests a rationale for the use of breath tests to detect carbohydrate maldigestion. Breath tests are performed by measuring expired hydrogen or methane levels after ingestion of a disaccharide load. Increased gas production resulting from fermentation of carbohydrates by bacteria, either because of an overabundance of fermenting bacteria in the small bowel or because of maldigestion of sugars serving as an additional substrate for these bacteria, is thought to be a possible organic cause for the bloating observed in patients with IBS symptoms.

Whether or not a correlation exists between IBS and SIBO remains controversial. Pimentel and colleagues[49] found that 84% of patients with IBS compared with 20% in a gender-matched control group (OR, 26.2; 95% CI, 4.7–103.9; $P<.00001$) had abnormal results in the lactulose breath test (LBT) indicative of SIBO. In their randomized, double-blind, placebo-controlled study of neomycin as a therapy for IBS, they found that patients with abnormal baseline LBTs were 10 times more likely to have a significant improvement in IBS symptoms after treatment with neomycin versus placebo. A recent systematic review and meta-analysis of pooled data from 12 case series and case-control studies examined the prevalence of abnormal breath testing in IBS.[50] Challenged by considerable heterogeneity between studies, including the use of 3 different types of breath tests (lactulose, glucose, or sucrose), these investigators concluded that the prevalence of SIBO among a total of nearly 2000 adults meeting the criteria for IBS ranged from 4% to 64%, depending on the type of test used and the criteria defining a positive test result. Even when comparing studies using the same substrate, a broad range of prevalence rates was evident. The ACG Task Force echoed this conclusion when they indicated that there was insufficient evidence to support the routine use of breath tests for SIBO in the evaluation of patients with suspected IBS.[20] Another study used jejunal aspirate and culture, considered to be a more accurate test for SIBO, and found that only 4% of patients with IBS had SIBO (defined as $>10^6$ colony-forming units/mL), similar to what was observed in non-IBS controls.[51] However, this study was considered supportive of a putative role of small bowel bacteria in the pathophysiology of IBS because it showed significantly higher concentrations of coliform bacteria (albeit at lower thresholds) in the small bowel of patients with IBS compared with those without IBS.

Maldigestion of lactose caused by lactase deficiency is common, with prevalence rates as high as 25% in the United States and 75% in other parts of the world.[52] Rates among certain ethnic populations within the United States can be as high as 90%.[53] In affected individuals, ingestion of significant quantities of lactose can result in a syndrome of diarrhea, abdominal pain, flatulence, and/or bloating. A study conducted by Vernia and colleagues[54] prospectively assessed the prevalence of lactose malabsorption among patients diagnosed with IBS. They compared the results of breath tests in 503 patients with IBS with those in 336 patients who subjectively identified themselves as lactose intolerant and found comparable rates of positive test results between the 2 groups, with 337 patients with IBS (66.9%) and 240 patients with reported lactose intolerance (71.4%) having greater than 20 ppm rise in hydrogen concentration in the expired breath after lactose ingestion. Choi and colleagues[55] identified fructose maldigestion in 33% of patients with Rome II IBS symptoms based on expired hydrogen and methane levels after the ingestion of 25 g of fructose. At 1-year follow-up evaluations, the 46% of patients with fructose maldigestion who adhered to a fructose-restricted diet reported significant improvement in 6 of 9 gastrointestinal symptoms ($P = .02$), whereas the fructose-tolerant group reported significant improvement in only 2 symptoms.

Although breath testing may objectively identify those patients who are unable to digest the particular sugar being tested, an optimal breath testing technique and results can be difficult to achieve, and many patients with troublesome gastrointestinal symptoms who have negative breath test results may still benefit from food avoidance or presumed manipulation of their intestinal microbiome with antibiotics or probiotics. Because of this and other concerns about the validity of breath test results in the diagnosis of carbohydrate maldigestion, some have questioned whether it should be used in the evaluation of this condition at all and suggested that patient report and response to a food challenge may be a more appropriate diagnostic tool.[56] Patient report alone is a poor predictor of SIBO or carbohydrate maldigestion. This fact was shown in a randomized, double-blind, cross-over trial of subjects reporting symptoms consistent with severe lactose intolerance in which they underwent blinded hydrogen breath testing and were then randomized to receive a daily 240-mL serving of milk (containing 12 g of lactose) or lactose-hydrolyzed milk (containing no lactose).[57] Subjects were instructed to avoid all other dairy products during the study period and maintain daily dietary records. After 1 week, the subjects were crossed-over to the other milk preparation. Of the 30 self-reported severe lactose-intolerant patients, nearly one-third had a negative result in the hydrogen breath test. Analysis of the symptoms reported during the study period revealed no significant difference in the amount of flatus episodes, abdominal pain, diarrhea, or bloating between the 2 milk preparations. Overall, symptoms experienced were minimal among those with normal and abnormal lactose breath test results. From a practical standpoint, whether food-related gastrointestinal symptoms result from actual enzyme deficiencies or simply food intolerance is of minimal clinical significance, because management is similar with either cause. Consequently, in patients reporting food-related symptoms, either by history or based on correlating symptoms with a food diary, trials of lactose- or fructose-restricted diets are a rational and pragmatic therapeutic approach. Similarly, it was recently reported that rifaximin at a dosage of 1650 mg/d for 14 days resulted in a statistically significant improvement in IBS symptoms and bloating in several large phase 3 trials of this therapy compared with placebo.[58,59] This approach may also be a realistic empiric therapeutic option in lieu of breath testing because breath testing for SIBO was not performed in patients enrolled in these trials.

Stool Studies

The ACG IBS Task Force does not recommend the routine use of stool studies to evaluate for infectious causes of IBS symptoms in the absence of a relevant travel history or specific alarm features (severe uncontrollable diarrhea, hematochezia, weight loss).[20] Studies by Hamm and colleagues[26] and Tolliver and colleagues[27] demonstrated a low prevalence of positive results of fecal ova and parasite tests in patients with IBS. Only 19 (2%) of Hamm's cohort of 1452 patients had evidence of intestinal parasites, with nearly half of those being from colonization with *Blastocystis hominis*, which has been implicated as a possible factor in IBS but is of questionable clinical significance.[60] Stool examinations for parasites in Tolliver's cohort of 196 patients with IBS had normal findings.

Several neutrophil-derived proteins excreted in the feces, such as lactoferrin and calprotectin, are highly sensitive and specific markers of inflammatory activity in the gut,[61] but their use in differentiating organic from functional disease has not been widely studied. Kane and colleagues[62] measured lactoferrin concentrations in outpatients with Crohn disease, ulcerative colitis, and IBS and in healthy controls. Lactoferrin concentrations were significantly higher in the 2 IBD groups than in the controls or in patients with IBS. An abnormal fecal lactoferrin level was 100% specific in ruling out IBS. Similarly, strong test characteristics were shown for both fecal calprotectin and lactoferrin in a prospective blinded study comparing 64 patients with IBD (all with endoscopically proven active disease) with 30 patients with IBS and 42 healthy controls.[63] Mean stool concentrations of both proteins were more than 10 times higher in the IBD groups than in the IBS group ($P \geq .0001$), whereas concentrations were similar in the IBS group and controls. A third study examined the ability of these 2 stool markers, as well as a third marker, polymorphonuclear elastase, to distinguish active IBD from inactive disease and IBS.[64] Concentrations of all of these proteins were significantly higher in active IBD than in quiescent disease or in IBS, but diagnostic accuracy of the 3 assays for differentiating IBS from IBD ranged from 69% to 87%. Because of the high negative predictive value of these tests in ruling out intestinal inflammation, many clinicians use them as a noninvasive screen for IBD in their patients with typical IBS symptoms.[65] Cost-effectiveness studies assessing this strategy are needed before this approach can be advocated.

Tests of Gut Hormones and Other Serologic Biomarkers

Numerous studies over the past several years have attempted to identify serum biomarkers correlating with the presence of IBS, based on many of the 600 different pathways implicated in the pathophysiology of IBS. Many of these tests have focused specifically on the suggestion that the clinical syndrome of IBS may be associated with alterations in the secretion of various gut hormones, neurotransmitters, and inflammatory mediators. Although no single serologic marker has been able to reliably diagnose IBS, the presumed multifactorial nature of IBS has prompted researchers to develop assays to measure plausible biomarkers to clarify the diagnosis of IBS.[66] The article by Spiller elsewhere in this issue discusses this exciting field of study and its implications for the management of IBS.

SUMMARY

The optimal diagnostic approach to IBS continues to evolve. Although there is no completely reliable biomarker that can objectively differentiate IBS from organic disease, the available evidence would support the application of validated symptom-based clinical criteria along with a judicious use of selected laboratory and endoscopic testing. In that sense, the diagnosis of IBS remains a diagnosis of exclusion. In a primary care setting or initial clinical encounter with a patient without previous diagnostic testing, clinicians must balance the lack of strong evidence supporting the value of diagnostic testing with their specific practice setting, individual patient characteristics, anecdotal experience, desire for reassurance, and medical-legal considerations when deciding what tests to obtain in patients with suspected

IBS. The absence of compelling evidence to pursue a detailed diagnostic evaluation in patients with suspected IBS does not address the potential reassurance value of a negative evaluation. Such a response has been demonstrated with other functional gastrointestinal conditions but not with IBS. It is possible that in some situations, diagnostic testing could prove counterproductive, with persistent negative results serving to increase patient anxiety or clinically unimportant test variances leading to more expensive and invasive testing.

In a referral setting, where basic blood tests such as CBC, CMP, and TFT are typically available to the specialist, it is reasonable to make a positive, symptom-based diagnosis and embark on empiric therapy for young patients with typical IBS symptoms and absent alarm features. Current evidence support the performance of celiac disease testing and colonoscopy with biopsies to exclude microscopic colitis in patients with a diarrhea-predominant IBS. Patients older than 50 years should undergo some form of CRC screening, preferably colonoscopy. Most alarm features are nonspecific and are not associated with reliable identification of organic gastrointestinal disease, but when endorsed by patients, alarm features mandate a directed and thoughtful diagnostic evaluation. As the understanding of the diverse pathophysiologic basis of IBS becomes clearer, it is possible that the diagnosis of this condition may eventually be made with more objective certainty. Whether or not increasing the certainty of the diagnosis of IBS translates into differences in important patient outcomes such as health care seeking behaviors or health-related quality of life will need to be evaluated in future studies.

REFERENCES

1. Longstreth GF, Wolde-Tsadik G. Irritable bowel-type symptoms in HMO examinees: prevalence, demographics and clinical correlates. Dig Dis Sci 1993;38: 1581–9.
2. Mitchell CM, Drossman DA. Survey of the AGA membership relating to patients with functional gastrointestinal disorders. Gastroenterology 1987;92:1282–4.
3. Sandler RS. Epidemiology of irritable bowel syndrome in the United States. Gastroenterology 1990;99:409–15.
4. Lacy BE, Rosemore J, Robertson D, et al. Physicians' attitudes and practices in the evaluation and treatment of irritable bowel syndrome. Scand J Gastroenterol 2006;41:892–902.
5. Spiegel BM, Farid M, Esrailian E, et al. Is irritable bowel syndrome a diagnosis of exclusion? A survey of primary care providers, gastroenterologists and IBS experts. Am J Gastroenterol 2010;105:848–58.
6. Manning AP, Thompson WG, Heaton KW, et al. Towards a positive diagnosis of the irritable bowel syndrome. Br Med J 1978;2:653–4.
7. Thompson WG, Dotewall G, Drossman DA, et al. Irritable bowel syndrome: guidelines for the diagnosis. Gastroenterol Int 1989;2:92–5.
8. Thompson WG, Longstreth GF, Drossman DA, et al. Functional bowel disorders and functional abdominal pain. Gut 1999;45(Suppl 2):II43–7.
9. Longstreth GF, Thompson WG, Chey WD, et al. Functional bowel disorders. Gastroenterology 2006;130(5):1480–91.
10. Brandt LJ, Locke R, Olden K, et al. An evidence based approach to the diagnosis of irritable bowel syndrome in North America. Am J Gastroenterol 2002;97(Suppl 11): S1–26.
11. Drossman DA, Camilleri M, Mayer EA, et al. AGA technical review on irritable bowel syndrome. Gastroenterology 2002;123:2108–31.

12. Vanner SJ, Depew WT, Paterson WG, et al. Predictive value of the Rome criteria for diagnosing the irritable bowel syndrome. Am J Gastroenterol 1999;94: 2912–7.

13. Whitehead WE, Drossman DA. Validation of symptom-based diagnostic criteria for IBS: a critical review. Am J Gastroenterol 2010;105:814–20.

14. Chey WD, Olden K, Carter E, et al. Utility of the Rome I and Rome II criteria for IBS in US women. Am J Gastroenterol 2002;97:2803–11.

15. Drossman DA. An integrated approach to the irritable bowel syndrome. Aliment Pharmacol Ther 1999;13(Suppl 2):3–14.

16. Camilleri M, Prather CM. The irritable bowel syndrome: mechanisms and a practical approach to management. Ann Intern Med 1992;116:1001–8.

17. American Gastroenterological Association. American Gastroenterological Association medical position statement: irritable bowel syndrome. Gastroenterology 2002;123:2105–7.

18. Spiller RC, Thompson WG. Bowel disorders. Am J Gastroenterol 2010;105:775–9.

19. Cash BD, Schoenfeld PS, Chey WD. The utility of diagnostic tests in irritable bowel syndrome patients: a systematic review. Am J Gastroenterol 2002;97: 2812–9.

20. Brandt LJ, Chey WD, Foxx-Orenstein AE, et al. An evidence-based systematic review on the management of irritable bowel syndrome. Am J Gastroenterol 2009;104(Suppl 1):S1–35.

21. Whitehead WE, Palsson OS, Feld AD, et al. Utility of red flag symptom exclusions in the diagnosis of irritable bowel syndrome. Aliment Pharmacol Ther 2006;24:137–46.

22. Hammer J, Eslick GD, Howell SC, et al. Diagnostic yield of alarm features in irritable bowel syndrome and functional dyspepsia. Gut 2004;53:666–72.

23. Adelstein BA, Irwig L, Macaskill P, et al. Who needs colonoscopy to identify colorectal cancer? Bowel symptoms do not add substantially to age and other medical history. Aliment Pharmacol Ther 2010;32:270–81.

24. Lijmer JG, Mol BW, Heisterkamp S, et al. Empirical evidence of design-related bias in studies of diagnostic tests. JAMA 1999;282:1061–6.

25. Irwig L, Tostetson AN, Gastonis C, et al. Guidelines for meta-analyses evaluating diagnostic tests. Ann Intern Med 1994;120:667–76.

26. Hamm LR, Sorrells SC, Harding JP, et al. Additional investigations fail to alter the diagnosis of irritable bowel syndrome in subjects fulfilling the Rome criteria. Am J Gastroenterol 1999;94:1279–82.

27. Tolliver BA, Herrera JL, DiPalma JA. Evaluation of patients who meet clinical criteria for irritable bowel syndrome. Am J Gastroenterol 1994;89:176–8.

28. MacIntosh DG, Thompson WG, Patel DG, et al. Is rectal biopsy necessary in irritable bowel syndrome? Am J Gastroenterol 1992;87:1407–9.

29. Francis CY, Duffy JN, Whorwell PJ, et al. Does routine ultrasound enhance diagnostic accuracy in irritable bowel syndrome? Am J Gastroenterol 1996;91: 1348–50.

30. Sanders DS, Carter MJ, Hurlstone DP, et al. Association of adult coeliac disease with irritable bowel syndrome: a case-control study in patients fulfilling the ROME II criteria referred to secondary care. Lancet 2001;358:1504–8.

31. Pimentel M, Chow EJ, Lin HC. Eradication of small intestinal bacterial overgrowth reduces symptoms of irritable bowel syndrome. Am J Gastroenterol 2000;95: 3503–6.

32. Cash BD, Lee D, Riddle M, et al. Yield of diagnostic testing in patients with suspected irritable bowel syndrome (IBS): a prospective, US multicenter trial [abstract 1184]. Am J Gastroenterol 2008;103(Suppl 1):S462.

33. Zipser RD, Patel S, Yahya KZ, et al. Presentations of adult celiac disease in a nationwide patient support group. Dig Dis Sci 2003;48:761–4.
34. Fasano A, Berti I, Gerarduzzi T, et al. Prevalence of celiac disease in at-risk and not at-risk groups in the United States. Arch Intern Med 2003;163:286–92.
35. McFarlane XA, Bhalla AK, Roberston DA. Effect of a gluten-free diet on osteopenia in adults with newly diagnosed coeliac disease. Gut 1996;39:180–4.
36. West J, Logan RF, Smith CJ, et al. Malignancy and mortality in people with celiac disease: population based cohort study. BMJ 2004;329:716–9.
37. Catassi C, Fabiani E, Corrao G, et al, Italian Working Group on Coeliac Disease and Non-Hodgkin's Lymphoma. Risk of non-Hodgkin lymphoma in celiac disease. JAMA 2002;287:1413–9.
38. Marsh MN. Gluten, major histocompatibility complex, and the small intestine: a molecular and immunobiologic approach to the spectrum of gluten sensitivity. Gastroenterology 1992;102:330.
39. Ford AC, Chey WD, Talley NJ, et al. Yield of diagnostic tests for celiac disease in individuals with symptoms suggestive of irritable bowel syndrome. Arch Intern Med 2009;169:651–8.
40. Mein SM, Ladabaum U. Serological testing for celiac disease in patients with symptoms of irritable bowel syndrome: a cost effectiveness analysis. Aliment Pharmacol Ther 2004;19:1199–210.
41. Spiegel BM, DeRosa VP, Gralnek IM, et al. Testing for celiac sprue in irritable bowel syndrome with predominant diarrhea: a cost-effectiveness analysis. Gastroenterology 2004;126:1721–32.
42. Talley NJ, Gabriel SE, Harmsen WS, et al. Medical costs in community subjects with irritable bowel syndrome. Gastroenterology 1995;109:1736–41.
43. Lieberman D, Holub J, Eisen G, et al. Utilization of colonoscopy in the United States: results from a national consortium. Gastrointest Endosc 2005;62: 875–83.
44. Akhtar AJ, Shaheen MA, Zha J. Organic lesions in patients with irritable bowel syndrome. Med Sci Monit 2006;12:363–7.
45. Chey WD, Nojkov B, Rubenstein JH, et al. The yield of colonoscopy in patients with non-constipated irritable bowel syndrome: results from a prospective controlled US trial. Am J Gastroenterol 2010;105:859–65.
46. Limsui D, Pardi DS, Camilleri M, et al. Symptomatic overlap between irritable bowel syndrome and microscopic colitis. Inflamm Bowel Dis 2007;13:175–81.
47. Chang L, Lee OY, Naliboff B, et al. Sensation of bloating and visible distension in patients with irritable bowel syndrome. Am J Gastroenterol 2001;96:3341–7.
48. Ringel Y, Williams RE, Kalliani L, et al. Prevalence, characteristics, and impact of bloating symptoms in patients with irritable bowel syndrome. Clin Gastroenterol Hepatol 2009;7:68–72.
49. Pimentel M, Chow EJ, Lin HC. Normalization of lactulose breath testing correlates with symptom improvement in irritable bowel syndrome: a double-blind, randomized, placebo-controlled study. Am J Gastroenterol 2003;98:412–9.
50. Ford AC, Spiegel BM, Talley NJ, et al. Small intestinal bacterial overgrowth in irritable bowel syndrome: systematic review and meta-analysis. Clin Gastroenterol Hepatol 2009;7:1279–86.
51. Posserud I, Stotzer PO, Bjornsson ES, et al. Small intestinal bacterial overgrowth in patients with irritable bowel syndrome. Gut 2007;56:802–8.
52. Scrimshaw NS, Murray AB. The acceptability of milk and milk products in populations with a high prevalence of lactose intolerance. Am J Clin Nutr 1988;48: 1079–159.

53. Jackson KA, Savaiano DA. Lactose maldigestion, calcium intake and osteoporosis in African-, Asian-, and Hispanic-Americans. J Am Coll Nutr 2001;20: 198s–207s.

54. Vernia P, Di Camillo M, Marinaro V. Lactose malabsorption, irritable bowel syndrome and self-reported milk intolerance. Dig Liver Dis 2001;33:234–9.

55. Choi YK, Kraft N, Zimmerman B, et al. Fructose intolerance in IBS and utility of fructose-restricted diet. J Clin Gastroenterol 2009;42:233–8.

56. Law D, Conklin J, Pimentel M. Lactose intolerance and the role of the lactose breath test. Am J Gastroenterol 2010;105:1726–8.

57. Suarez FL, Savaiano DA, Levitt MD. A comparison of symptoms after the consumption of milk or lactose-hydrolyzed milk by people with self-reported severe lactose intolerance. N Engl J Med 1995;333:1–4.

58. Chey W, Talley N, Lembo A, et al. Rifaximin significantly improves quality of life versus placebo in patients with diarrhea-predominant irritable bowel syndrome. Am J Gastroenterol 2008;103(Suppl 1):S461–2.

59. Pimentel M, Lembo A, Chey WD, et al. Rifaximin treatment for 2 weeks provides acute and sustained relief over 12 weeks of IBS symptoms in non-constipated irritable bowel syndrome: results from 2 North American phase 3 trials (Target 1 and Target 2) [abstract 475i]. Presented at Digestive Disease Week (DDW) 2010 in New Orleans (LA), 2010.

60. Stark D, van Hal S, Marriott D, et al. Irritable bowel syndrome: a review on the role of intestinal protozoa and the importance of their detection and management. Int J Parasitol 2007;37:11–20.

61. Sugi K, Saitoh O, Hirata I, et al. Fecal lactoferrin as a marker for disease activity in inflammatory bowel disease: comparison with other neutrophil-derived proteins. Am J Gastroenterol 1996;91:927–34.

62. Kane SV, Sandborn WJ, Rufo PA, et al. Fecal lactoferrin is a sensitive and specific marker in identifying intestinal inflammation. Am J Gastroenterol 2003;98: 1309–14.

63. Schoepfer AM, Trummler M, Seeholzer P, et al. Discriminating IBD from IBS: comparison of the test performance of fecal markers, blood leukocytes, CRP, and IBD antibodies. Inflamm Bowel Dis 2008;14:32–9.

64. Langhorst J, Elsenbruch S, Koelzer J, et al. Noninvasive markers in the assessment of intestinal inflammation in inflammatory bowel diseases: performance of fecal lactoferrin, calprotectin, and PMN-elastase, CRP and clinical indices. Am J Gastroenterol 2008;103:162–9.

65. Poullis A, Foster R, Mendall MA, et al. Emerging role of calprotectin in gastroenterology. J Gastroenterol Hepatol 2003;18:756–62.

66. Lembo AJ, Neri B, Tolley J, et al. Use of serum biomarkers in a diagnostic test for irritable bowel syndrome. Aliment Pharmacol Ther 2009;29:834–42.

Potential Biomarkers

Robin C. Spiller, MD

KEYWORDS

• Biomarkers • Irritable bowel syndrome • Diagnosis

WHAT IS A BIOMARKER?

A biomarker (biological marker) is an indicator of a physiological or pathological state that can be objectively measured and evaluated. It contrasts with subjective patient reported outcomes by usually having lower variability and therefore greater power to detect effect of treatments or differences between groups. A good example of a biomarker used in other fields is the forced expiratory volume in 1 second (FEV_1). This biomarker is an objective measure of respiratory function that assesses airway resistance, which is a critical feature of asthma. It is simple, inexpensive, and reproducible. The standard is to use the best of 3 to allow for learning of the technique. It has been widely used and shown to be reproducible, responsive to treatment, and also to indicate the state of the disease. In pulmonology other measures are also used to study asthma, including mucosal histology obtained from bronchial biopsy, sputum eosinophil counts and sputum culture. The advantages of the FEV_1 when compared with these other more invasive and technically demanding tests are its non-invasiveness, patient acceptability, and its responsiveness to many treatments. It is also apparent that the value of any particular biomarker will depend on the treatment being assessed; for example, if an antibiotic is being tested in infective exacerbation of asthma, then sputum culture might prove more valuable in predicting response.

Criteria for a Useful Biomarker in Irritable Bowel Syndrome

A useful biomarker for irritable bowel syndrome (IBS) would be simple and easy to use. It would be patient acceptable and reproducible (low intrasubject variability). Ideally it should also have low intersubject variability within defined groups. This variability is important because it reduces the number needed to test (NN test) to detect a minimally important difference with an acceptable power, which is particularly important when evaluating new treatments to allow a rapid decision on whether to pursue development or move on to another molecule. Because most studies are done in multiple centers, it is important that the technique of measurement should be readily transferable between

Financial disclosures: Professor Spiller had received research funding from McNeil, Lesaffre, Norgine and Johnson & Johnson. He has also acted on advisory boards for Norgine, McNeil, Albireo, and Takeda.
NIHR Biomedical Research Unit, Nottingham Digestive Diseases Centre, E Floor West Block, University Hospital, Nottingham, NG7 2UH, UK
E-mail address: robin.spiller@nottingham.ac.uk

centers and, therefore, should not need highly sophisticated equipment or require scarce expertise. Finally, all these things are of little value if the technique is too expensive.

Pathophysiology of IBS relevant to choosing a biomarker

IBS patients are a highly heterogeneous group because the symptoms are quite nonspecific and may reflect numerous pathophysiologies, including altered transit and sensitivity. For the purposes of this article, it is sufficient to say that most authors agree that in any one patient a range of factors, including stress, somatization, anxiety, neuroticism, diet, and prior infection, contribute to symptoms mediating both altered visceral sensitivity and disturbances of bowel transit. Biomarkers that could identify the main mechanism in each individual patient would be of undoubted value.

The other important consideration in using biomarkers to predict or evaluate response to a new therapy is that to be useful, the biomarker should relate to the mode of action of the drug being evaluated. Many recently introduced drugs have altered gastrointestinal (GI) transit, including prokinetics, such as tegaserod,[1,2] prucalopride,[3,4] and velusetrag[5]; and secretagogues aimed at treating constipation, including lubiprostone[6] and linaclotide.[7] Others delay transit, such as the 5HT3 receptor antagonists (alosetron[8] and ondansetron[9]), or reduce visceral hypersensitivity, such as amitriptyline[10–12] and the 2,3-benzodiazepine receptor agonist dextofisopam.[13] Although still in development, anti-inflammatory agents, such as mesalazine, have been shown to reduce mast cell numbers[14] or to inhibit release of mast cell mediators, such as ketotifen.[15] Since one of the main purposes of biomarkers is to identify subjects for which a specific treatment may be more appropriate, the majority of this article addresses measures of transit, visceral hypersensitivity, abnormal stress responsiveness, and inflammation. The author also considers newer proposed biomarkers that still require validation but might be useful in the future.

As **Table 1** shows, there are many potential biomarkers reflecting different aspects of the pathophysiology of IBS. These biomarkers focus on changes in gut function and the associated microbiota. Of course, it is well recognized that there are important influences of the brain on the gut in IBS but as yet apart from psychometric assessments based on patient reports, the complexity of the brain has defied the development of simple biomarkers. Although differences in brain activation in response to painful stimuli between subjects with IBS and controls can be demonstrated using positron emission tomography scanning or fMRI, the techniques are difficult and results variable between centers.[16] Furthermore, the equipment is extremely expensive, therefore, patterns of brain activation by peripheral stimuli do not meet our criteria for a good biomarker.

Link Between Biomarker and Clinical Response

Although in the end a treatment has to improve patients' quality of life and how they perceive their symptoms, such measures are always influenced by many factors other than the local GI ones. Thus, all stimuli coming from the gut have to be interpreted in light of previous experiences, current emotional state, and psychological stressors before they are converted to symptom reports. This means that an intervention or drug that alters gut function may have a weak effect on patient-reported outcomes and the size of the clinical trial needed to show the effect is likely to be large, on the order of many hundreds.

Biomarkers as Surrogate Endpoints

By restricting the end points to a biomarker closer to the gut function, variability should be less and hence standardized effect sizes should be larger and the number of

Table 1
Potential biomarkers and their relationship to possible mechanism of disease in IBS

Mechanism	Potential Biomarkers
Disordered motility/secretion leading to altered transit and altered stool form	Manometry/transit tests/stool charts
Visceral hypersensitivity	Rectal barostat/cutaneous stimulation
Abnormal autonomic reactivity	Heart rate variability/response to pain
Stress response	Cortisol/response to visceral stimulus
Mucosal inflammation	Mucosal biopsy
Evidence of immune activation	Serum/peripheral blood mononuclear cells cytokine production
Increase fecal proteases	Stool test
Altered gut flora	Stool DNA/culture/bacterial metabolite assessment
Food allergy	Skin prick test, serum antibodies
Genetic polymorphisms	Single-nucleotide polymorphism assays

individuals needed to test to show an effect much less. This is of considerable value in the development of new drugs. By being more focused and less holistic, these measures are much more likely to be culture independent and hence easier to translate across multiple centers and countries, again a value feature in drug development that is often multinational. A major use of biomarkers is therefore in mode of action or proof of concept studies during phase I and early phase II. Although on its own not acceptable as the only outcome measure in phase III studies, biomarkers might also be valuable as entry criteria to improve responder rates or as secondary end points.

Assessing gut motility

Motor patterns are important in determining transit and also because they may cause pain, a major symptom in IBS that substantially determines perceived severity.[17] The gut is insensitive to many stimuli, including thermal and chemical injury, but is responsive to distension and powerful contractions. Several studies have clearly linked powerful colonic contractions with abdominal pain (**Fig. 1**).[18,19]

Although these contractions are crucial to the pain, as a biomarker, manometry's major problem is the requirement for intestinal intubation. The original studies were done using naso-intestinal intubation, which is extremely arduous, taking several days to properly position the manometry catheter. These uncomfortable experiments have mainly been done with paid volunteers. The number of patient studies is limited and the subjects studied are likely to be a highly selected sample. Furthermore, the technique is expensive and technically demanding and hence impracticable for use as a biomarker. More recently, the technique of retrograde cannulation of the colon at colonoscopy allowing the positioning of probes, which are clipped to the mucosa, has been developed. This technique is much quicker and more patient acceptable but still highly invasive and expensive.[20] Although useful perhaps for the early stages of proof-of-principal concepts, such techniques are unlikely to win widespread use in clinical trials or in clinical practice.

Even if such techniques were patient-acceptable, measures such as the duodenal motility index, although reasonably reproducible, show substantial intersubject variability in normal subjects with a coefficient of variation (CoV) (standard deviation

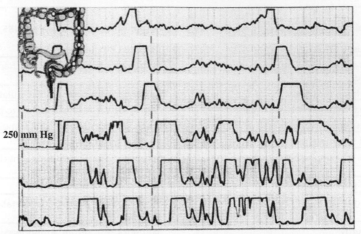

250 mm Hg

Fig. 1. Effect of cholecystokinin (CCK) on colonic motility. When CCK was infused intravenously, powerful abdominal contractions were seen, 90% of which were associated with abdominal cramps in IBS but none of which were associated with pain in healthy controls. (*From* Chey WY, Jin HO, Lee MH, et al. Colonic motility abnormality in patients with irritable bowel syndrome exhibiting abdominal pain and diarrhea. Am J Gastroenterol 2001;96:1499–506; with permission.)

divided by mean) of 13351/30708 (43%),[21] giving a total NN test of 96 (48 per group) to show a 25% change in mean index with a power of 80% in a random controlled trial (RCT) of drug against placebo.

Recordings in the colon show a highly erratic pattern requiring long-term recordings to give meaningful results, which has only been done in a few studies. However, Clemens studied 12 subjects with IBS and reported a CoV of sigmoid motility over 24 hours of just 7%, indicating this would require only 3 subjects per group in a parallel group design, a total of 6 to detect a 25% change with 80% power[22] if they could be persuaded to undergo 24-hour recordings. Almost identical figures were found by Rao[23] in healthy women with a CoV of 7% and just 5% in subjects who were constipated.[24] Alternative measures might be a frequency of specialized propagating pressure waves assessed over 24 hours with an indwelling rectal probe that gives a NN test of approximately 18.[23] Although attractive for proof-of-principle studies, 24-hour intubation is too demanding on subject and investigator to be practical for large clinical studies.

The barostat can be used to assess motility and also tone and compliance. The performance characteristics of colon in tone and motility indices have been recently reported.[25] The intersubject CoV was 22.8% for colonic compliance, 30.8% for fasting tone, and 35.9% for tone 30 minutes postprandially. This finding gave a NN test of 28, 25, and 28, respectively.

Wireless motility-pH capsule

Compared with manometry or a barostat study requiring intubation, this wireless pH, pressure and temperature sensitive capsule has obvious appeal. At 28.8 mm long by 11.7 mm in diameter, it is somewhat larger than a normal tablet but still readily swallowed by most patients. There is none of the pharyngeal discomfort associated with prolonged manometry and the patients are freely mobile. The temperature, pressure, and pH profile enable it to be tracked through the intestine with the sharp rise in pH that occurs on passing from the stomach to the duodenum and the sharp fall in temperature that occurs when the capsule is expelled readily identifying gastric, small bowel, and colonic transit. The rate of transit correlates well with the standard radio-opaque markers, although both show wide variability.[26] The pressure tracings can also be used to derive a motility index based on the area under the curve of the pressure versus time (**Fig. 2**) however, the clinical utility of this data has not been established. However, the intersubject CoV is high: 88% in constipated IBS and 127% in healthy volunteers.[27] With these values, the NN test to show a 25% change in motility using a parallel group design would be a prohibitive 195 subjects per group.

Transit as a surrogate for motility

In contrast to manometry, following the transit of a radioisotopically labeled meal through the gut is highly patient acceptable, can be done with low doses, and yields measures that have an acceptably low day-to-day variability while separating out important patient groups. The earliest techniques of measuring whole gut transit incorporated daily ingestion of radio opaque pellets on days 1 to 3 with a plain radiograph at day 4. Transit in hours through the colon was estimated to be 1.2 times the number remaining.[28] The normal range of such a measure is substantial with healthy individuals having transits that vary from 6 to 64 hours.[28] The coefficient of variance in women was 46%, giving a total NN test of 108 using a parallel group design, although this number falls to just 29 using a crossover design. Despite this variability, this method has been widely used and shown differences between patient groups, such as slow transit in those with constipated IBS.[29–31] Furthermore, colonic transit measured by this method is responsive to therapeutic interventions,[8,32] such as the prokinetic renzapride[33] or the effect of bowel cleansing in constipation,[34] although these studies used a crossover design that, by using each subject as their own control, reduces the numbers needed to test substantially. Mean colonic transit of markers measured in this way correlates well with geometric center of the pellets (r = 0.88) and with stool consistency (**Fig. 3**).[35]

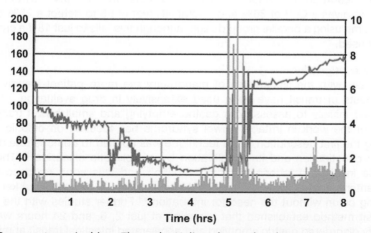

Time (hrs)

Fig. 2. Pressure trace in blue. The red pH line shows the sharp rise on entering the duodenum at around 5 hours. (*Data from* Chey WY, Jin HO, Lee MH, et al. Colonic motility abnormality in patients with irritable bowel syndrome exhibiting abdominal pain and diarrhea. Am J Gastroenterol 2001;96:1499–506, and Degen LP, Phillips SF. How well does stool form reflect colonic transit? Gut 1996;39:109–13.)

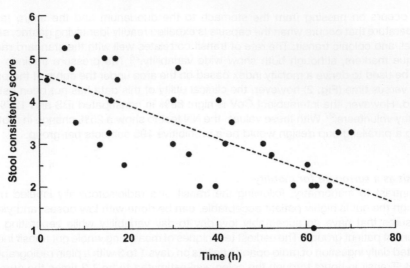

Fig. 3. Stool form score related to mean colonic transit time. Stool consistency as assessed by the Bristol Stool Form score correlated well with stool form, P<.001. (*From* Degen LP, Phillips SF. How well does stool form reflect colonic transit? Gut 1996;39:109–13; with permission.)

The reproducibility of median stool form in 2 28-day periods was tested by Degen and colleagues[35]and shown to have an intrasubject CoV of repeated measures of approximately 33%. Earlier studies have shown an intersubject CoV of 42% giving a NN test of 90 (45 per group).[28] However, it is easily assessed and in large clinical studies this measure shows the clinical efficacy of alosetron.[36]

The pressure-sensitive radio pill can also be used to measure transit, although it has high intersubject variability being a single estimate of transit of one particle rather than a weighted average of many, like scintigraphy or radio-opaque pellets.[28] In a recent study the mean transit time for constipated subjects was 46.7 (24.0–91.9) hours.[26] This finding gives a CoV of 36% and a total NN test of 68 to detect a 25% change in transit time using a parallel group design, although this falls to just 18 if a crossover design is used.

Transit by scintigraphy

By contrast, with the limited use of manometry the more patient-friendly scinti-graphic tests of transit have been used extensively in drug evaluation. Although being used initially to assess both gastric emptying and small bowel transit, the majority of the work in irritable bowel syndrome has focused on colonic transit. Following the first description,[37] the technique was applied to demonstrate delayed transit in constipation and its acceleration by a prokinetic cisapride.[38] The initial technique involved a laborious cecal intubation and was soon replaced by the use of enteric-coated pellets designed to release the radioactive marker in the ascending colon without the need for intubation.[39] Further studies with the whole-gut transit method established that scanning at just 2, 6, and 24 hours was able to identify disordered gastric emptying and accelerated intestinal transit at minimum cost.[40] Subsequent studies used this technique to demonstrate the efficacy of alosetron in subjects with carcinoid diarrhea,[41] the acceleration of oral cecal transit by tegaserod in constipation-predominant IBS,[2] and the effects of renzapride,[42] lubiprostone,[6] and linaclotide.[7]

Early studies suggested that the half clearance time of the ascending colon was an important predictor of stool form.[43] However, a recent study showed that the intersubject CoV was 40.9%, so the NN test would be 82 in a parallel group design.[7] The performance characteristics of the scintigraphic assessment of gut transit have been assessed looking at the reproducibility and intersubject variability in healthy volunteers (**Table 2**). The clinically important effect sizes based on previous studies were considered to be 25% different in gastric residual at 4 hours and a 1.5 difference in geometric center at 48 hours.[44] Certainly for the colonic transit measurement, the geometric center at 48 hours requires acceptably small NN test (14 per group) for the detection of a 25% difference with 80% power using the standard parallel group design.

However, abnormalities of transit are not a uniform feature of irritable bowel syndrome and in a recent, large study of 118 subjects with IBS, abnormal transit was only documented in 38 subjects, the remaining subjects showed a mixture of rectal hypersensitivity (25), hyposensitivity (20), and no abnormality in transit or sensitivity (39)[45]; therefore, it is apparent that other measures are needed.

Visceral sensitivity

Visceral hypersensitivity has been assessed over the last 15 years using the rectal barostat as a reproducible, ethically approved method of inducing abdominal pain without tissue injury. Although early studies suggested that 61% had an abnormally low pressure threshold for pain,[46] more recent studies have reported much lower incidence; the recent series from the Mayo Clinic reported only 7.6% having thresholds for pain sensation below the 10th percentile and 13% having thresholds above the 90th percentile.[47] Recent studies using decision theory analysis suggest that neurosensory sensitivity in IBS was no different from healthy controls and that the lower pain thresholds were a reflection of a greater tendency to report pain for any stimulus.[48] Although the reproducibility of the threshold for pain in the short term is reasonable, with intrasubject CoV being 23%, this is not true for other sensations, such as urgency and discomfort with CoV of 41% and 47%, respectively.[49] The same study showed that similar protocols performed at different centers produced similar results and that a 25% difference between 2 study groups could be demonstrated in a parallel group design for pain threshold using 14 individuals per group, a total of 28 in an RCT. Other endpoints, such as urgency and discomfort, would require much larger numbers, but a crossover design reduced the numbers substantially to just 6 per group.[49] By contrast, the more

Table 2
Performance characteristics of scintigraphic assessment of gut transit

	n	GE t1/2	Colon Filling 6 h	GC 24 h	GC 48 h
CoV intersubject	21	30.4	30	37	24
CoV intrasubject	21	14	19	28	14
NN test to detect a 25% difference	—	48	48	70	30
NN test[a]	—	82	96	46	28

Abbreviations: GC24h, geometric centre at 24 hours after marker ingestion; GEt1/2, time for 50% Gastric emptying in minutes.
[a] NN test is the number needed to test in an RCT of active versus placebo to detect clinically significant differences with 80% power.
Data from Cremonini F, Mullan BP, Camilleri M, et al. Performance characteristics of scintigraphic transit measurements for studies of experimental therapies. Aliment Pharmacol Ther 2002; 16:1781–90.

subjective sensory rating for pain at 36 mmHg distension gave a CoV of 56% and number needed to test of 80 per group.[25]

Despite reasonable reproducibility in the short term, the validity of pain thresholds as a measure of drug efficacy remains a problem for using this as a biomarker because the link between the reported thresholds and symptoms is weak. A longitudinal study performed over a period of 12 months with testing every 3 months showed that despite relative constant symptom severity the discomfort threshold in subjects with IBS moved into the normal range when the study was repeated, suggesting that part of the low thresholds in IBS relate to the stress of the first experience of the testing situation and that this may wear off with time.[50]

Although barostats have been developed for use in animals and widely used to screen drugs, the link between the animal data and subsequent success or failure in clinical trials has been poor. As **Table 3**[71] shows, drugs that increased barostat pain thresholds, such as asimadoline and fedotozine, failed in large clinical trials; whereas, drugs that do not alter the threshold, such as lubiprostone and citalopram, have been successful. There is also the striking example of the tachykinin antagonists that are effective in animal models[62,72] but that appear to have failed in clinical trials that have been completed some years ago but never published. Likewise, asimadoline, a kappa opioid agonist, was effective in decreasing sensation during rectal distension and decreased postprandial fullness during ingestion to maximum satiety of a liquid test meal.[63,64] However, in clinical trials it failed to achieve adequate relief of IBS pain compared to placebo and failed to improve symptoms in functional dyspepsia.[66] Subgroup analysis in the IBS trial showed that in diarrhea-predominant IBS with at least moderate pain at baseline, one of the 3 doses of asimadoline did produce improvement in the total number of months with adequate relief.[65] However, being an unplanned subgroup analysis, this may well represent a chance finding.

Clonidine stands out as being the exception in that it not only relaxes the rectum but also increases the threshold for pain and was effective in a small clinical trial, but unfortunately drowsiness limited its use.[70]

The conclusion of this experience must be that although the rectal barostat can be used to demonstrate changes in visceral hypersensitivity, the link between this observation and changes in clinical symptoms is weak and should not be used as a basis for decision to proceed with development of a new product. Furthermore, as already alluded to, the barostat technique is difficult to standardize and technically demanding. It is thus unsuitable for use as entry criteria for a clinical trial or indeed to use in clinical practice.

Autonomic reactivity
Many patients think that stress aggravates their symptoms and several recent studies have demonstrated enhanced hypothalamic-pituitary axis (HPA) response. Patients with IBS-D show increased cortisol response after a meal and an increase in the low-frequency/high-frequency band ratio of heart rate variability.[73] This ratio is thought to represent the balance between para sympathetic and sympathetic tone. Overall, women with IBS show no differences between controls and IBS, but when analysis is restricted to those with severe symptoms, parasympathetic tone appears lower in the constipated group compared with the diarrhea group.[74] Small studies have reported differences in other cardiovascular parameters including a higher resting heart rate in IBS.[75] Other measures, including cortisol response to the invasive procedure of sigmoidoscopy, did separate subjects with IBS from healthy controls and was higher in those with early life trauma regardless of whether they had IBS or

Table 3
Effectiveness of drugs in barostat test compared with effectiveness in clinical trial

Drug	Increase in Barostat Pain Threshold	Study	Effectiveness in Clinical Trial	Study/Meta-analysis
Ondansetron	No (compliance increased)	Zighelboim et al[51] 1995	Yes	—
Alosetron	No (compliance increased)	Delvaux et al[52] 1998	Yes	Cremonini[53]
Fedotozine	Yes	Delvaux et al[54] 1999	No	Lembo 2006[55]
Hypnosis	No	Palsson et al[56] 2002	Yes	Palsson et al[56] 2002
Fluoxetine	No	Kuiken 2003[57]	No	—
Citalopram	No	Tack et al[58] 2006	Yes	Tack et al[58] 2006
Talnetant	No	Houghton et al[59] 2007	No	Unpublished www.Clinicaltrials.gov, registered 2005
Lubiprostone	No	Sweetser et al[60] 2009	Yes	Drossman et al[61] 2009
Saredutant	Yes in animal models	Toulouse et al[62]	? No	Trials unpublished, 2006
Asimadoline	Yes	Delgard-Aros et al[63] Delvaux et al[64]	No in IBS or functional dyspepsia	Mangel et al[65] 2008 Talley et al[66] 2008
Amitriptyline	Yes	—	Yes	
Clonidine	Yes	Bharucha et al[67] 1997 Viramontes et al[68] 2001 Camilleri et al[69] 2009	Effective but drowsiness excessive	Camilleri et al[70] 2003

not.[76] The data from these trials suggests that salivary cortisol at baseline shows substantial variability and does not distinguish IBS from controls and would therefore not be a useful biomarker. Although the response to sigmoidoscopy showed clear-cut differences, it is not a practical test to be used in large numbers of subjects.

Markers of mucosal inflammation

The recognition that IBS can develop after a bout of gastroenteritis and the demonstration of evidence of immune activation in the mucosa[77] has stimulated examination of mucosal biopsies using a range of techniques, including quantitative histology, mRNA for cytokines, and assessment of mediators released into the supernatant of cultured biopsies. Although there are indeed differences in mean cell counts between healthy controls and subjects with IBS, there is also considerable overlap.[78] Furthermore, quantitative histology is demanding and highly dependent on technical expertise. Reproducibility has not been demonstrated, although recently evidence of responsiveness to treatment has been forthcoming. A recent randomized control trial of mesalazine against placebo did show a significant fall in mast cell numbers.[14] Thus, in mechanistic studies particularly using anti-inflammatory drugs, mast cell number could act as a biomarker both for entry into the study and as an endpoint. In that study, the placebo arm can be regarded as a reproducibility study with a CoV of approximately 20% and a number needed to test of 22, which is at least as good as other biomarkers. Further studies in this area would be valuable.

Several studies have reported on mediator release from incubated biopsies.[79–81] Although of great mechanistic interest, the variability in the biopsies is substantial and, without further standardization of the procedure, unsuitable as a biomarker. Whether this will change in the future with, for example, serotonin release correlating with response to serotonin antagonists remains to be established. In addition, there have also been several studies demonstrating increased cytokine production by peripheral blood mononuclear cells.[82,83] Again, the variability is substantial and these have not been shown to be responsive to treatments and do not seem ready to become biomarkers at present.

Stool markers of mucosal inflammation

Looking at markers released by neutrophils into the stool can assess inflammation in the gut. These markers are not a feature of irritable bowel syndrome where the mucosal changes are restricted to chronic inflammatory cells, such as lymphocytes and macrophages. The best-validated test is fecal calprotectin, a molecule resistant to bacterial degradation released by mucosal polymorphonuclear white blood cells with sensitivity for inflammatory bowel disease of 89% and a specificity of 79%. Therefore, a negative fecal calprotectin increases the risk of IBS but does not exclude inflammatory bowel disease because approximately 11% have normal values. Negative biomarkers are less useful than positive ones because they cannot be used to evaluate responses. In this respect, β defensin is interesting because, unlike calprotectin, it shows an increase in IBS.[84] However, variability is high and the intersubject CoV is substantial with a mean value of 76.0 ± 67.9, giving a CoV of 89% and requiring 400 subjects to detect a 25% difference with an 80% power.

Fecal proteases

Another potential biomarker recently described is the fecal protease. These functional assessments of enzyme activity detect serine proteases within the gut lumen, which are likely to be mainly of endogenous origin but also include possible bacterial enzymes. Recent reports indicate that these are elevated specifically in IBS-D.[85] The importance of this finding relates to the demonstration that there are protease activated receptors type 2 on epithelial cells and enteric nerves with activation that increases gut permeability and induces inflammation.[86] The fecal supernatants from subjects with IBS containing these serine protease were able to increase visceral hypersensitivity in a rat barostat model.[85] However, the values of trypsin units per milligram of protein were 2079 with a standard deviation of 1860, which gives a CoV of 89% and a number needed to test of 400 to detect a 25% difference with an 80% power in a parallel group design. Plainly, greater standardization of stool collection and assay methods will be needed before such a marker could be useful.

Assessment of gut flora

There has been a revolution in the approach to understanding the gut flora brought about by the development of new DNA-based assessments. These assessments reveal that nearly two-thirds of the bacteria cannot be cultured, indicating that the picture we have been obtaining so far has been incomplete. The new technologies include density gradient gel electrophoresis of DNA generated by polymerase chain reaction (PCR) of the 16S ribosomal RNA gene and the more sophisticated human intestinal tract chip (HITChip), a phylogenetic microarray which uses nanotechnology to PCR more than 5000 markers to characterize around 1000 bacterial species. These new techniques have revealed a previously unrecognized complexity. Studies so far in IBS have indicated important differences but also great variability.[87,88] Patterns are starting to emerge with evidence of imbalance in the different microbial communities, particularly in IBS-D.[89] One consistent feature appears to be a decrease in overall diversity and the number of aerobic bacteria with an increase in aerobes, including Proteobacteria. Similar features are seen after infection[90,91] and in inflammatory bowel disease.[92] These changes in gut microbiota may well prove to be useful biomarkers for studies of treatments likely to alter the flora, such as probiotics and antibiotics, but like some of the other more experimental techniques discussed, this will take a lot more work before it can be applied in clinical practice.

Serum antibodies

Reports of increased incidence of antibodies to common food antigens have been made for more than 2 decades but they lack consistency. A recent report showed an increase in antibodies to flagellin antigens A4Fla-2 and A4Fla-X in 29% and 25% of subjects with IBS versus 7% in controls.[93] However, similar increases were seen in Crohn disease, so this is not helpful diagnostically and antibodies rarely change rapidly in response to treatment, making this of little value on its own as a biomarker. There is already on the market the Prometheus serological panel, which combines several tests that detect the presence of inflammatory bowel disease anti-*Saccharomyces cerevisiae* antibody (ASCA), periplasmic antineutrophil cytoplasmic antibody (pANCA), and celiac disease (antihuman tissue transglutaminase [tTG]) together with some other antibodies in an unpublished algorithm to predict whether or not patients have IBS. Of the 10 antibodies examined, the ASCA, pANCA, and tTG are negative predictors[94]; whereas, the other antibodies, including antibodies against bacterial flagellin, tumor necrosis factor-α, and interleukin-1β, may be measures of previous infection and ongoing inflammation. Other proteins examined include Gro-α, a chemokine associated with chemotaxis, and a tissue inhibitor of metalloproteinase (TIMP-1), which may well be raised in inflammatory bowel disease. The sensitivity overall was only 50% with a specificity of 88%.[94] The positive-likelihood ratio of 4.2 is in fact rather similar to other clinical criteria, such as the Kruis criteria published in 1984.[95] Whether this can be improved on by adding different serum-based markers remains to be determined.

Skin prick tests and tests of food allergy

Although patients attending the immunology department with potential food allergy certainly share features in common with IBS, including abdominal pain and diarrhea, the true incidence of food allergy in patients attending IBS clinics seems fairly low with about 14.0% suspected and only 3.2% confirmed by objective testing.[96] Patients who present with classic food allergy, including diarrhea and urticaria, after ingesting offending food stuffs are rarely misdiagnosed as IBS and usually see immunologists rather than gastroenterologists. Those without these features rarely turn out to have true food allergy when assessed by the gold standard, which is a double blind, placebo-controlled food challenge. More careful attention to symptoms suggests that the presence of frequent lower abdominal pain relieved by defecation and associated with bloating can distinguish IBS from food allergy.[97] There are several poorly validated commercial tests that examine immunoglobulin G (IgG) antibodies for food that is extremely common within the normal population. One study showed IBS had significantly high IgG4 titres against wheat, beef, pork, and lamb compared with controls.[98] Unfortunately these are not consistent in other studies that report increased titres to mostly different protein, although wheat was positive in both studies.[99] One placebo-controlled trial did demonstrate a small benefit of a food-elimination diet based on IgG antibodies,[100] but the majority of individuals were treated by means of wheat and milk exclusion so it unclear to what extent the antibodies are useful in predicting the correct diet. One earlier study reported that the

Table 4
Total number of subjects needed to test (treatment and placebo group) to detect 25% difference with 80% power in an RCT of treatment versus placebo with a parallel group design using various biomarkers as endpoints

Biomarker	NN Test	References	Feasibility
Duodenal motility index	96	Penning et al[21]	-
24-h sigmoid motility index	6	Clemens et al [22]	-
Frequency of propagated pressure waves using 24-h sigmoid motility recording	18	Rao et al[23]	-
Radio pill manometry	390	Hasler et al[27]	-
Radio pill transit	68	Rao et al[26]	-
Colonic transit (radio-opaque pellets method)	108	Metcalf et al[28]	-
Geometric center at 48 h	30	Cremonini et al[44]	++
$T_{1/2}$ ascending colon	82	Andresen et al[7]	-
Bristol Stool form score	90	Metcalf et al[28]	-
Rectal compliance (barostat)	28	Odunsi et al[25]	+
Fasting rectal tone	50	Odunsi et al[25]	+
Pain threshold (rectal barostats)	27	Cremonini et al[49]	+
Subjective pain rating to 36 mm Hg distension	160	Odunsi et al[25]	-
Mast cell numbers	22	Barbara et al[14]	?
Fecal β-defensin	400	Langhorst et al[84]	-
Fecal protease	400	Gecse et al[85]	-

presence of a positive skin prick test to certain foods increased the chances of responding to sodium cromoglycate,[101] but this has never been repeated and in clinical practice skin prick testing in patients with IBS proves of little value.

Genetic polymorphisms

A genetic component of IBS is likely to be similar to that of many complex diseases with many genes providing small effects. The studies that have yielded information of the greatest value in gastroenterology have been performed in Crohn disease using more than 12,000 individuals to identify more than 30 genetic polymorphisms each associated with small (1.2) relative risks. By contrast, most IBS patient studies have less than 250 subjects and so it is not surprising that many of the findings are not reproducible. There are a small number of studies that suggest that genetic polymorphisms might predict drug responsiveness based on polymorphisms in drug metabolism enzymes and also the serotonin transporters gene. Thus, the homozygote *ll* for the SERT promoter polymorphism was associated with greater response to the 5HT3 receptor antagonist than the heterozygote *sl*.[102] Likewise, the homozygote *ll* responded less well to the prokinetic 5HT4 receptor agonist, tegaserod.[103] However, these studies were small and require replication in larger studies before they can be considered potential biomarkers of drug responsiveness.

SUMMARY

A wide range of possible biomarkers has been considered, but at present only transit measures using radioisotope markers meet the criteria of reproducibility and availability with a low NN test. Although barostats studies give reasonable NN test (**Table 4**), reproducibility requires considerable effort and standardization because the precise wording used in the questions and instructions to subjects can make a critical difference in the outcome, which makes them less suitable for widespread use. However, radioisotope tests are expensive and are only of value with drugs that alter transit, so the search for other more convenient markers, including blood and stool tests, is still an important research goal for the future.

REFERENCES

1. Harish K, Hazeena K, Thomas V, et al. Effect of tegaserod on colonic transit time in male patients with constipation-predominant irritable bowel syndrome. J Gastroenterol Hepatol 2007;22:1183–9.
2. Prather CM, Camilleri M, Zinsmeister AR, et al. Tegaserod accelerates orocecal transit in patients with constipation-predominant irritable bowel syndrome. Gastroenterology 2000;118:463–8.
3. Bouras EP, Camilleri M, Burton DD, et al. Prucalopride accelerates gastrointestinal and colonic transit in patients with constipation without a rectal evacuation disorder. Gastroenterology 2001;120:354–60.
4. Sloots CE, Poen AC, Kerstens R, et al. Effects of prucalopride on colonic transit, anorectal function and bowel habits in patients with chronic constipation. Aliment Pharmacol Ther 2002;16:759–67.
5. Manini ML, Camilleri M, Goldberg M, et al. Effects of velusetrag (TD-5108) on gastrointestinal transit and bowel function in health and pharmacokinetics in health and constipation. Neurogastroenterol Motil 2010;22:42–8.
6. Camilleri M, Bharucha AE, Ueno R, et al. Effect of a selective chloride channel activator, lubiprostone, on gastrointestinal transit, gastric sensory, and motor

functions in healthy volunteers. Am J Physiol Gastrointest Liver Physiol 2006; 290:G942–7.

7. Andresen V, Camilleri M, Busciglio IA, et al. Effect of 5 days linaclotide on transit and bowel function in females with constipation-predominant irritable bowel syndrome. Gastroenterology 2007;133:761–8.

8. Houghton LA, Foster JM, Whorwell PJ. Alosetron, a 5-HT3 receptor antagonist, delays colonic transit in patients with irritable bowel syndrome and healthy volunteers. Aliment Pharmacol Ther 2000;14:775–82.

9. Gore S, Gilmore IT, Haigh CG, et al. Colonic transit in man is slowed by ondansetron (GR38032F), a selective 5-hydroxytryptamine receptor (type 3) antagonist. Aliment Pharmacol Ther 1990;4:139–44.

10. Poitras P, Riberdy PM, Plourde V, et al. Evolution of visceral sensitivity in patients with irritable bowel syndrome. Dig Dis Sci 2002;47:914–20.

11. Thoua NM, Murray CD, Winchester WJ, et al. Amitriptyline modifies the visceral hypersensitivity response to acute stress in the irritable bowel syndrome. Aliment Pharmacol Ther 2009;29:552–60.

12. Morgan V, Pickens D, Gautam S, et al. Amitriptyline reduces rectal pain related activation of the anterior cingulate cortex in patients with irritable bowel syndrome. Gut 2005;54:601–7.

13. Leventer SM, Raudibaugh K, Frissora CL, et al. Clinical trial: dextofisopam in the treatment of patients with diarrhoea-predominant or alternating irritable bowel syndrome. Aliment Pharmacol Ther 2008;27:197–206.

14. Barbara G, Cremon C, Gargano L, et al. Mesalazine treatment for intestinal immune activation in patient with irritable bowel syndrome: a randomized controlled pilot. Gastroenterology 2008;134:A546.

15. Klooker TK, Koopman KE, Heide SV, et al. Treatment with the mast cell stabilizer ketotifen decreases visceral hypersensitivity and improves intestinal symptoms in IBS patients. Gut 2009;57:A86.

16. Derbyshire SW. Visceral Afferent Pathways and Functional Brain Imaging. ScientificWorldJournal 2003;3:1065–80.

17. Spiegel B, Bolus R, Harris LA, et al. Measuring IBS patient reported outcomes with an abdominal pain numeric rating scale: results from the proof cohort. Aliment Pharmacol Ther 2009;30:1159–70.

18. Kellow JE, Miller LJ, Phillips SF, et al. Altered sensitivity of the gallbladder to cholecystokinin octapeptide in the irritable bowel syndrome. Am J Physiol 1987;253:G650–5.

19. Spiller RC, Brown ML, Phillips SF. Decreased fluid tolerance, accelerated transit, and abnormal motility of the human colon induced by oleic acid. Gastroenterology 1986;91:100–7.

20. Dinning PG, Arkwright JW, Gregersen H, et al. Technical advances in monitoring human motility patterns. Neurogastroenterol Motil 2010;22:366–80.

21. Penning C, Gielkens HA, Hemelaar M, et al. Reproducibility of antroduodenal motility during prolonged ambulatory recording. Neurogastroenterol Motil 2001;13:133–41.

22. Clemens CH, Samsom M, Berge Henegouwen GP, et al. Abnormalities of left colonic motility in ambulant nonconstipated patients with irritable bowel syndrome. Dig Dis Sci 2003;48:74–82.

23. Rao SS, Sadeghi P, Beaty J, et al. Ambulatory 24-h colonic manometry in healthy humans. Am J Physiol Gastrointest Liver Physiol 2001;280:G629–39.

24. Rao SS, Sadeghi P, Beaty J, et al. Ambulatory 24-hour colonic manometry in slow-transit constipation. Am J Gastroenterol 2004;99:2405–16.

25. Odunsi ST, Camilleri M, Bharucha AE, et al. Reproducibility and performance characteristics of colonic compliance, tone, and sensory tests in healthy humans. Dig Dis Sci 2010;55:709–15.
26. Rao SS, Kuo B, McCallum RW, et al. Investigation of colonic and whole gut transit with wireless motility capsule and radio-opaque markers in constipation. Clin Gastroenterol Hepatol 2009. [Epub ahead of print].
27. Hasler WL, Saad RJ, Rao SS, et al. Heightened colon motor activity measured by a wireless capsule in patients with constipation: relation to colon transit and IBS. Am J Physiol Gastrointest Liver Physiol 2009;297:G1107–14.
28. Metcalf AM, Phillips SF, Zinsmeister AR, et al. Simplified assessment of segmental colonic transit. Gastroenterology 1987;92:40–7.
29. Dunlop SP, Coleman NS, Blackshaw E, et al. Abnormalities of 5-hydroxytryptamine metabolism in irritable bowel syndrome. Clin Gastroenterol Hepatol 2005; 3:349–57.
30. Evans JM, Fleming KC, Talley NJ, et al. Relation of colonic transit to functional bowel disease in older people: a population-based study. J Am Geriatr Soc 1998;46:83–7.
31. Gorard DA, Libby GW, Farthing MJ. Influence of antidepressants on whole gut and orocaecal transit times in health and irritable bowel syndrome. Aliment Pharmacol Ther 1994;8:159–66.
32. Emmanuel AV, Kamm MA, Roy AJ, et al. Effect of a novel prokinetic drug, R093877, on gastrointestinal transit in healthy volunteers. Gut 1998;42:511–6.
33. Tack J, Middleton SJ, Horne MC, et al. Pilot study of the efficacy of renzapride on gastrointestinal motility and symptoms in patients with constipation-predominant irritable bowel syndrome. Aliment Pharmacol Ther 2006;23: 1655–65.
34. Sloots CE, Felt-Bersma RJ. Effect of bowel cleansing on colonic transit in constipation due to slow transit or evacuation disorder. Neurogastroenterol Motil 2002;14:55–61.
35. Degen LP, Phillips SF. How well does stool form reflect colonic transit? Gut 1996; 39:109–13.
36. Camilleri M, Chey WY, Mayer EA, et al. A randomized controlled clinical trial of the serotonin type 3 receptor antagonist alosetron in women with diarrhea-predominant irritable bowel syndrome. Arch Intern Med 2001;161:1733–40.
37. Krevsky B, Malmud LS, D'Ercole F, et al. Colonic transit scintigraphy. A physiologic approach to the quantitative measurement of colonic transit in humans. Gastroenterology 1986;91:1102–12.
38. Krevsky B, Maurer AH, Malmud LS, et al. Cisapride accelerates colonic transit in constipated patients with colonic inertia [see comments]. Am J Gastroenterol 1989;84:882–7.
39. Stivland T, Camilleri M, Vassallo M, et al. Scintigraphic measurement of regional gut transit in idiopathic constipation. Gastroenterology 1991;101:107–15.
40. Charles F, Camilleri M, Phillips SF, et al. Scintigraphy of the whole gut: clinical evaluation of transit disorders. Mayo Clin Proc 1995;70:113–8.
41. Saslow SB, Scolapio JS, Camilleri M, et al. Medium-term effects of a new 5HT3 antagonist, alosetron, in patients with carcinoid diarrhoea. Gut 1998;42:628–34.
42. Camilleri M, McKinzie S, Fox J, et al. Effect of renzapride on transit in constipation-predominant irritable bowel syndrome. Clin Gastroenterol Hepatol 2004;2:895–904.
43. Vassallo M, Camilleri M, Phillips SF, et al. Transit through the proximal colon influences stool weight in the irritable bowel syndrome. Gastroenterology 1992;102:102–8.

44. Cremonini F, Mullan BP, Camilleri M, et al. Performance characteristics of scintigraphic transit measurements for studies of experimental therapies. Aliment Pharmacol Ther 2002;16:1781–90.
45. Camilleri M, Bharucha AE, Di LC, et al. American Neurogastroenterology and Motility Society consensus statement on intraluminal measurement of gastrointestinal and colonic motility in clinical practice. Neurogastroenterol Motil 2008; 20:1269–82.
46. Mertz H, Naliboff B, Munakata J, et al. Altered rectal perception is a biological marker of patients with irritable bowel syndrome. Gastroenterology 1995;109:40–52.
47. Camilleri M, McKinzie S, Busciglio I, et al. Prospective study of motor, sensory, psychologic, and autonomic functions in patients with irritable bowel syndrome. Clin Gastroenterol Hepatol 2008;6:772–81.
48. Dorn SD, Palsson OS, Thiwan SI, et al. Increased colonic pain sensitivity in irritable bowel syndrome is the result of an increased tendency to report pain rather than increased neurosensory sensitivity. Gut 2007;56:1202–9.
49. Cremonini F, Houghton LA, Camilleri M, et al. Barostat testing of rectal sensation and compliance in humans: comparison of results across two centres and overall reproducibility. Neurogastroenterol Motil 2005;17:810–20.
50. Naliboff BD, Berman S, Suyenobu B, et al. Longitudinal change in perceptual and brain activation response to visceral stimuli in irritable bowel syndrome patients. Gastroenterology 2006;131:352–65.
51. Zighelboim J, Talley NJ, Phillips SF, et al. Visceral perception in irritable bowel syndrome. Rectal and gastric responses to distension and serotonin type 3 antagonism. Dig Dis Sci 1995;40:819–27.
52. Delvaux M, Louvel D, Mamet JP, et al. Effect of alosetron on responses to colonic distension in patients with irritable bowel syndrome. Aliment Pharmacol Ther 1998;12:849–55.
53. Cremonini F, Delgado-Aros S, Camilleri M. Efficacy of alosetron in irritable bowel syndrome: a meta-analysis of randomized controlled trials. Neurogastroenterol Motil 2003;15:79–86.
54. Delvaux M, Louvel D, Lagier E, et al. The kappa agonist fedotozine relieves hypersensitivity to colonic distention in patients with irritable bowel syndrome. Gastroenterology 1999;116:38–45.
55. Lembo A. Peripheral opioids for functional GI disease: a reappraisal. Dig Dis 2006;24:91–8.
56. Palsson OS, Turner MJ, Johnson DA, et al. Hypnosis treatment for severe irritable bowel syndrome: investigation of mechanism and effects on symptoms. Dig Dis Sci 2002;47:2605–14.
57. Kuiken SD, Tytgat GN, Boeckxstaens GE. The selective serotonin reuptake inhibitor fluoxetine does not change rectal sensitivity and symptoms in patients with irritable bowel syndrome: a double blind, randomized, placebo-controlled study. Clin Gastroenterol Hepatol 2003;1:219–28.
58. Tack J, Broekaert D, Fischler B, et al. A controlled cross-over study of the selective serotonin reuptake inhibitor citalopram in irritable bowel syndrome. Gut 2006;55(8):1095–103.
59. Houghton LA, Cremonini F, Camilleri M, et al. Effect of the NK(3) receptor antagonist, talnetant, on rectal sensory function and compliance in healthy humans. Neurogastroenterol Motil 2007;19:732–43.
60. Sweetser S, Busciglio IA, Camilleri M, et al. Effect of a chloride channel activator, lubiprostone, on colonic sensory and motor functions in healthy subjects. Am J Physiol Gastrointest Liver Physiol 2009;296:G295–301.

61. Drossman DA, Chey WD, Johanson JF, et al. Clinical trial: lubiprostone in patients with constipation-associated irritable bowel syndrome–results of two randomized, placebo-controlled studies. Aliment Pharmacol Ther 2009;29:329–41.

62. Toulouse M, Coelho AM, Fioramonti J, et al. Role of tachykinin NK2 receptors in normal and altered rectal sensitivity in rats. Br J Pharmacol 2000;129:193–9.

63. Delgado-Aros S, Chial HJ, Camilleri M, et al. Effects of a kappa-opioid agonist, asimadoline, on satiation and GI motor and sensory functions in humans. Am J Physiol Gastrointest Liver Physiol 2003;284:G558–66.

64. Delvaux M, Beck A, Jacob J, et al. Effect of asimadoline, a kappa opioid agonist, on pain induced by colonic distension in patients with irritable bowel syndrome. Aliment Pharmacol Ther 2004;20:237–46.

65. Mangel AW, Bornstein JD, Hamm LR, et al. Clinical trial: asimadoline in the treatment of patients with irritable bowel syndrome. Aliment Pharmacol Ther 2008; 28:239–49.

66. Talley NJ, Choung RS, Camilleri M, et al. Asimadoline, a kappa-opioid agonist, and satiation in functional dyspepsia. Aliment Pharmacol Ther 2008;27: 1122–31.

67. Bharucha AE, Camilleri M, Zinsmeister AR, et al. Adrenergic modulation of human colonic motor and sensory function. Am J Physiol 1997;273:G997–1006.

68. Viramontes BE, Malcolm A, Camilleri M, et al. Effects of an alpha(2)-adrenergic agonist on gastrointestinal transit, colonic motility, and sensation in humans. Am J Physiol Gastrointest Liver Physiol 2001;281:G1468–76.

69. Camilleri M, Busciglio I, Carlson P, et al. Pharmacogenetics of low dose clonidine in irritable bowel syndrome. Neurogastroenterol Motil 2009;21:399–410.

70. Camilleri M, Kim DY, McKinzie S, et al. A randomized, controlled exploratory study of clonidine in diarrhea-predominant irritable bowel syndrome. Clin Gastroenterol Hepatol 2003;1:111–21.

71. Mayer EA, Bradesi S, Chang L, et al. Functional GI disorders: from animal models to drug development. Gut 2008;57:384–404.

72. Laird JM, Olivar T, Lopez-Garcia JA, et al. Responses of rat spinal neurons to distension of inflamed colon: role of tachykinin NK2 receptors. Neuropharmacology 2001;40:696–701.

73. Elsenbruch S, Lovallo WR, Orr WC. Psychological and physiological responses to postprandial mental stress in women with the irritable bowel syndrome. Psychosom Med 2001;63:805–13.

74. Heitkemper M, Jarrett M, Cain KC, et al. Autonomic nervous system function in women with irritable bowel syndrome. Dig Dis Sci 2001;46:1276–84.

75. Gupta V, Sheffield D, Verne GN. Evidence for autonomic dysregulation in the irritable bowel syndrome. Dig Dis Sci 2002;47:1716–22.

76. Videlock EJ, Adeyemo M, Licudine A, et al. Childhood trauma is associated with hypothalamic-pituitary-adrenal axis responsiveness in irritable bowel syndrome. Gastroenterology 2009;137(6):1954–62.

77. Dunlop SP, Jenkins D, Neal KR, et al. Relative importance of enterochromaffin cell hyperplasia, anxiety, and depression in postinfectious IBS. Gastroenterology 2003;125:1651–9.

78. Cremon C, Gargano L, Morselli-Labate AM, et al. Mucosal immune activation in irritable bowel syndrome: gender-dependence and association with digestive symptoms. Am J Gastroenterol 2009;104:392–400.

79. Barbara G, Cremon C, Vicini R, et al. Excitatory effects of colonic mast cell mediators of irritable bowel syndrome patients on enteric cholinergic motor neurones. 2005:49.

80. Buhner S, Li Q, Vignali S, et al. Activation of human enteric neurons by supernatants of colonic biopsies from patients with irritable bowel syndrome. Gastroenterology 2009;137(4):1425–34.

81. Corinaldesi R, Stanghellini V, Cremon C, et al. Effect of mesalazine on mucosal immune biomarkers in irritable bowel syndrome: a randomized controlled proof of concept study. Aliment Pharmacol Ther 2009;30(3):245–52.

82. Liebregts T, Adam B, Bredack C, et al. Immune activation in patients with irritable bowel syndrome. Gastroenterology 2007;132:913–20.

83. Ohman L, Isaksson S, Lindmark AC, et al. T-cell activation in patients with irritable bowel syndrome. Am J Gastroenterol 2009;104:1205–12.

84. Langhorst J, Junge A, Rueffer A, et al. Elevated human beta-defensin-2 levels indicate an activation of the innate immune system in patients with irritable bowel syndrome. Am J Gastroenterol 2009;104:404–10.

85. Gecse K, Roka R, Ferrier L, et al. Increased faecal serine protease activity in diarrhoeic IBS patients: a colonic lumenal factor impairing colonic permeability and sensitivity. Gut 2008;57:591–9.

86. Hyun E, Andrade-Gordon P, Steinhoff M, et al. Protease-activated receptor-2 activation: a major actor in intestinal inflammation. Gut 2008;57:1222–9.

87. Malinen E, Rinttila T, Kajander K, et al. Analysis of the fecal microbiota of irritable bowel syndrome patients and healthy controls with real-time PCR. Am J Gastroenterol 2005;100:373–82.

88. Matto J, Maunuksela L, Kajander K, et al. Composition and temporal stability of gastrointestinal microbiota in irritable bowel syndrome–a longitudinal study in IBS and control subjects. FEMS Immunol Med Microbiol 2005;43:213–22.

89. Krogius-Kurikka L, Lyra A, Malinen E, et al. Microbial community analysis reveals high level phylogenetic alterations in the overall gastrointestinal microbiota of diarrhoea-predominant irritable bowel syndrome sufferers. BMC Gastroenterol 2009;9:95.

90. Balamurugan R, Janardhan HP, George S, et al. Molecular studies of fecal anaerobic commensal bacteria in acute diarrhea in children. J Pediatr Gastroenterol Nutr 2008;46:514–9.

91. Lupp C, Robertson ML, Wickham ME, et al. Host-mediated inflammation disrupts the intestinal microbiota and promotes the overgrowth of Enterobacteriaceae. Cell Host Microbe 2007;2:204.

92. Cucchiara S, Iebba V, Conte MP, et al. The microbiota in inflammatory bowel disease in different age groups. Dig Dis 2009;27:252–8.

93. Schoepfer AM, Schaffer T, Seibold-Schmid B, et al. Antibodies to flagellin indicate reactivity to bacterial antigens in IBS patients. Neurogastroenterol Motil 2008;20(10):1110–8.

94. Lembo AJ, Neri B, Tolley J, et al. Use of serum biomarkers in a diagnostic test for irritable bowel syndrome. Aliment Pharmacol Ther 2009;29(8):834–42.

95. Spiller R, Camilleri M, Longstreth GF. Do the symptom-based, Rome criteria of irritable bowel syndrome lead to better diagnosis and treatment outcomes? Clin Gastroenterol Hepatol 2010;8:125–9.

96. Bischoff SC, Herrmann A, Manns MP. Prevalence of adverse reactions to food in patients with gastrointestinal disease. Allergy 1996;51:811–8.

97. Neri M, Laterza F, Howell S, et al. Symptoms discriminate irritable bowel syndrome from organic gastrointestinal diseases and food allergy. Eur J Gastroenterol Hepatol 2000;12:981–8.

98. Zar S, Benson MJ, Kumar D. Food-specific serum IgG4 and IgE titers to common food antigens in irritable bowel syndrome. Am J Gastroenterol 2005;100:1550–7.

99. Zuo XL, Li YQ, Li WJ, et al. Alterations of food antigen-specific serum immuno-globulins G and E antibodies in patients with irritable bowel syndrome and functional dyspepsia. Clin Exp Allergy 2007;37:823–30.
100. Atkinson W, Sheldon TA, Shaath N, et al. Food elimination based on IgG antibodies in irritable bowel syndrome: a randomised controlled trial. Gut 2004; 53:1459–64.
101. Paganelli R, Fagiolo U, Cancian M, et al. Intestinal permeability in irritable bowel syndrome. Effect of diet and sodium cromoglycate administration. Ann Allergy 1990;64:377–80.
102. Camilleri M, Atanasova E, Carlson PJ, et al. Serotonin-transporter polymorphism pharmacogenetics in diarrhea-predominant irritable bowel syndrome. Gastroenterology 2002;123:425–32.
103. Li YY, Nie YQ, Xie J, et al. [Serotonin transporter gene polymorphisms in irritable bowel syndrome and their impact on tegaserod treatment]. Zhonghua Nei Ke Za Zhi 2006;45:552–5 [in Chinese].

Food: The Forgotten Factor in the Irritable Bowel Syndrome

Shanti Eswaran, MD[a], Jan Tack, MD, PhD[b],
William D. Chey, MD, AGAF[a],*

KEYWORDS

- Carbohydrate • Lactose • Fructose • FODMAP
- Gluten • Lipid • Diet

Between 7% and 20% of adults experience symptoms compatible with the irritable bowel syndrome (IBS), a disorder defined by the presence of recurring episodes of abdominal pain in association with altered bowel habits and no evidence of a structural or easily identifiable biochemical abnormality that might explain these symptoms.[1,2] Several factors have been suggested as playing a role in the pathogenesis of IBS, including disturbed motility, the brain-gut axis, genetic factors, impaired gut barrier function, immunologic dysregulation, the gut microbiome, and psychosocial factors. More recently, there has been increasing attention on the role of food in IBS. Patients have long associated their IBS symptoms with the ingestion of certain foods, combinations of foods, or a meal itself. More than 60% of IBS patients report worsening of symptoms after meals, 28% of these within 15 minutes after eating and 93% within 3 hours.[1] Unfortunately, the lack of empiric data proving a causal link or consistently documenting symptom improvement has caused health care providers to view dietary interventions with skepticism. Furthermore, even to this day, gastroenterologists and primary care providers receive virtually no structured training in dietary interventions for IBS. This lack of enthusiasm for dietary counseling has increasingly caused providers to be misaligned with their patients who are increasingly seeking more holistic solutions for their IBS symptoms. Out of desperation, many providers recommend or passively stand by as their patients empirically attempt various dietary manipulations, such as the elimination of fatty foods, fruits, gluten, or milk/dairy products or modifying dietary fiber content. This haphazard approach not surprisingly leads to inconsistent results, which can be frustrating to both patients and providers.

Conflicts of Interest: The authors declare no conflict of interest and have nothing to disclose.
[a] Division of Gastroenterology, University of Michigan Health System, 3912 Taubman Center, SPC 5362, Ann Arbor, MI 48109-5362, USA
[b] Department of Gastroenterology, University Hospital Gasthuisberg, University of Leuven, Herestraat 49, B-3000 Leuven, Belgium
* Corresponding author.
E-mail address: wchey@med.umich.edu

Gastroenterol Clin N Am 40 (2011) 141–162
doi:10.1016/j.gtc.2010.12.012
0889-8553/11/$ – see front matter © 2011 Elsevier Inc. All rights reserved.

Several disorders and diseases can masquerade as or exacerbate the symptoms of IBS. For example, few clinicians would dispute that celiac disease and lactose intolerance are important considerations in patients presenting with IBS symptoms. These two well-defined disorders likely represent the tip of the iceberg, however, pertaining to the role of food in IBS. This article reviews the literature supporting a causal link between food and the symptoms of IBS as well as the evidence supporting dietary intervention as a means of treating IBS.

THE SCOPE OF THE PROBLEM

Adverse reactions to food are acknowledged by 5% to 45% of the general population,[3–5] and GI complaints are predominant in approximately one-third to one-half of those affected.[1,6] Offending foods are often referred to as trigger foods, dietary triggers, or culprit foods,[7] sometimes leading to a nutritionally inadequate diet.[3] Although food intolerance is a common perception among the general population, it can be demonstrated in only a relatively small proportion of the population when double-blind food elimination and challenge studies are employed. In a population study of food intolerance of 20,000 patients, 20.4% complained of food intolerance. Of the 93 subjects who entered the double-blind, placebo-controlled food challenge, 11.4%–27.4% had a positive reaction, with estimated prevalence of reactions to the 8 foods tested varying from 1.4% to 1.8% depending on the method of testing used. Women perceived food intolerance more frequently and showed a higher rate of positive results to food challenge.

Among individuals with IBS,[3,5,8–12] 20% to 67% complain of subjective food intolerance, which is more prevalent than similar reports in matched controls.[5,9,13] One population-based study reported a prevalence rate of perceived food intolerance of greater than 50% among subjects with IBS, a rate that was 2-fold greater than that reported by those without IBS.[5] Another found that patients in a GI clinic with a final diagnosis of a functional disorder were four times more likely to report food allergies (FAs) or adverse reaction to food.[13] The likelihood of a patient's symptoms being functional increased even further if adverse reactions to both drugs and foods were reported. Such complaints seem to correlate with female gender and anxiety level in those with functional GI disorders.[14]

Many patients suffering from IBS report an association of symptoms with specific foods. Although the foods that induce symptoms may be specific, the associated symptoms are often nonspecific and consistent with functional disorders, such as IBS. Many patients identify specific trigger foods (most commonly dairy, fructose, wheat products, and caffeine), but there is little evidence that IBS patients with food-related complaints are suffering from a true FA.[15] Although there are undoubtedly some patients with IBS symptoms who suffer from an FA, the proportion of the total population of IBS sufferers with a true FA is small.[16–21] Alternatively, there is likely to be substantial overlap between food intolerances/sensitivities and IBS, because these syndromes often have similar clinical presentations.

It is not uncommon for IBS patients to experiment with their diet or limit their diet before seeking medical attention.[3] The foodstuffs most commonly implicated are wheat, corn, dairy products, coffee, tea, and citrus fruits. In a 2005 population-based sample comparing dietary consumption of specific food items and nutrients between individuals with IBS or dyspeptic symptoms and those without symptoms, no differences were seen in the consumption of frequently suspected culprit foods.[22] In a survey of more than 1200 individuals with IBS, 63% were interested in knowing which foods to avoid. The lifestyle changes they had made or considered for treatment of IBS included small meals (69%); avoiding fatty foods (64%); higher fiber intake (58%); and avoiding milk products (54%), carbohydrates (43%), caffeine (41%), alcohol (27%), and high-protein foods, such as meats (21%).[23]

HOW DOES FOOD CAUSE IBS SYMPTOMS?

Food processing is the primary function of the gastrointestinal (GI) tract, and food ingestion, through mechanosensation and nutrient sensing, causes major changes in GI sensorimotor and secretory function, which may contribute to symptom generation in IBS. On ingestion of nutrients, the proximal stomach relaxes and upper GI motility switches from interdigestive to fed state motility, characterized by phasic contractions in the antrum and the small bowel.[24] In addition, food ingestion stimulates gastric and pancreatic secretion and is associated with the release of several anorexigenic hormones, such as cholecystokinin (CCK) and glucagon-like peptide-1 (GLP-1).[24,25] Hence, food can influence symptom generation from the GI tract by stimulation of mechano- or chemoreceptors, activation of motor reflexes pathways, by altered secretion, and by (colonic) fermentation.

Most investigators agree that the stomach does not meaningfully detect the nutrient or caloric composition of a meal and that mechanical distention by the meal is the major gastric sensory signal upon food intake.[26] Tension-sensitive mechanoreceptors in the stomach are involved in detecting the ingested nutrient volume and in triggering relaxation of the proximal stomach, which enables storage of the meal without a rise in intragastric pressure.[27,28] Probably through similar mechanisms, the volume of the meal in the stomach is a trigger for the initial phase of the gastrocolonic reflex, a meal-induced increase in tone, and phasic contractility of the colon.[29,30] The early (gastric) phase of colonic contractile activity in response food intake is mediated by activation of gastric mechanoreceptors and can be reproduced by distention of a gastric balloon, and suppressed by atropine. A later (intestinal) phase depends on duodenal delivery of nutrients.[29]

Passage of nutrients to the small intestine activates a different set of neural and hormonal responses.[24] The small intestine is well equipped to sense the presence of nutrients and their composition. Specialized receptors on enteroendocrine cells detect the presence of specific food constituents, pH, and osmolarity of small intestinal contents, and through altered release of peptides and other signaling molecules, neural and hormonal pathways are activated that may influence GI sensorimotor function and afferent signaling. In general, the presence of nutrients, gastric acid, or hyperosmolar fluids in the duodenum activates neurohormonal pathways that slow further delivery of gastric contents to the small intestine through inhibition of gastric tonic and phasic contractions and through closure of the pylorus.[24,31] For instance, lipids in the duodenum activate long-chain free fatty acid receptors GPR120 and possibly GPR40 and release CCK from I-cells.[32] CCK is a potent enhancer of colonic motility and of GI motility and has been implicated in the intestinal phase of the gastrocolonic reflex, based on observations in a dog model.[33] The gastrocolonic reflex is exaggerated in IBS patients as a group, and this reflex has been implicated in the early postprandial increase in IBS symptoms that is present in the majority of patients.[34,35] In humans, however, the colonic response to food ingestion was not inhibited by the CCK-A receptor antagonist loxiglumide.[34] Recent studies have shown an exaggerated increase in rectal sensitivity to distention after ingestion of a meal in IBS.[35,36] Because lipids were the strongest stimulus in these studies, it has been suggested that CCK might be involved, and exogenously administered CCK was shown to enhance rectal sensitivity in health.[36,37]

Intestinal nutrient sensing is extensive, and several nutrient-related components have the ability to activate afferent pathways, alter GI reflex activity, or change the release of GI peptides. The presence of glucose in the lumen induces release of GLP-1 and serotonin, among other gut hormones, from enteroendocrine cells, through the sodium-glucose cotransporters, SGLT1 and SGLT3.[38] These peptides may alter visceral sensorimotor function and could contribute to food-induced symptom aggravation.[9,39] More recently, it has been shown that the small intestine also expresses the T1R and T2R G-protein–coupled taste receptors families.[40] Taste receptors interact with specific Gα subunits, including α-gustducin, a taste-specific signaling protein. Because immuno-histochemical studies have shown expression of α-gustducin in several types of enteroendocrine cells, it has been hypothesized that activation of taste receptor signaling molecules may alter the release of GI peptides, such as PYY, GLP1, or CCK.[40] In turn, these hormones may alter endocrine secretions and appetite, but they may also affect motor behavior and sensory signaling, thereby contributing to changes in symptoms induced by ingestion of a meal.[39] Finally, the gut also expresses members of the superfamily of transient receptor potential cation channels on enteroendocrine cells and afferent nerves.[41] These may sense aspects of luminal contents, such as acidity, or the presence of food components, such as menthol or capsaicin, which may alter GI sensorimotor function through activation of neural or humoral pathways.[41] The presence of taste receptors and transient receptor potential channels and their coupling to release of functionally relevant GI signaling molecules or activation or neural pathways could potentially help explain some of the intolerances to specific foods or tastes that IBS patients report and which cannot be explained by food allergies.[9,39]

The physical properties of nutrients may also contribute to meal-related symptom aggravation, without involvement of sensing of nutrient composition. Nonabsorbable components of ingested food may also contribute to symptom generation and perception in IBS, either through changes in motility and transit that they induce or through fermentation by bacterial flora in the colon. Osmotically active substances in the small intestine, such as nonabsorbable sugars, attract fluids and this may lead to increased intestinal contractility, accelerated colonic transit, increased flatulence, and diarrhea.[42–44] It is conceivable that such responses may be aggravated in IBS patients, where small intestinal transit and water content may already differ from health.[45] Fiber, especially insoluble, may promote bacterial fermentation in the large intestine and symptoms of bloating and distention.[46] Because the colonic flora may differ in IBS from health, these processes could potentially be altered in IBS, but additional studies are needed.[47]

In summary, food can influence symptom generation from the GI tract through many pathways. These include activation of mechanoreceptors by the volume and physical properties of the meal and activation of chemoreceptor-activated pathways through a multitude of nutrient-sensing mechanisms. Nonabsorbable components may influence GI function and sensations through osmotic actions and colonic fermentation. There is emerging evidence of some altered nutrient-related GI functions in IBS, which include an exaggerated gastrocolonic reflex, enhanced sensitization to rectal distention after lipid ingestion, and changes in colonic bacterial flora that may be relevant for fermentation of nonabsorbable remnants. Detailed studies investigating potentially altered nutrient sensing in IBS are still lacking.

FOOD ALLERGY VERSUS FOOD INTOLERANCE

Up to 25% of the general US population believes they have an FA.[48] True FA, however, occurs in approximately 4% to 8% of children and 1% to 4% of adults in the United

States. Although controversial, there are data to suggest that the prevalence of FA is increasing.[49–53] Few children retain their FA into adulthood, which accounts for the decrease in prevalence between children and adults. Many studies demonstrate that 50% to 90% of presumed food allergies are not actually allergies but rather a food intolerance (some adverse reaction to food) or food aversion (refusal to eat a food because it is potentially hazardous, socially inappropriate, or distasteful).

True FA is an immunologically mediated, adverse reaction that occurs reproducibly after a susceptible individual ingests a specific food. Although nonfood allergies can be diagnosed by well-defined criteria, the diagnosis of FA is far more difficult. This is particularly true for the clinical spectrum of food-related allergic manifestations that occur in the digestive tract, because many symptoms, such as oral/throat itching, nausea, vomiting, abdominal pain, diarrhea, and constipation, are vague and can be mistaken for other conditions. The best-established food reactions are IgE-mediated (considered type I hypersensitivity) and non–IgE-mediated reactions (including type III hypersensitivity [IgG or IgM immune complex reactions] and type IV hypersensitivity [delayed-type or cell-mediated reactions]). (See **Table 1** for a classification of pathophysiologic reactions to foods.)

The best-established mechanism in FA is due to the development of IgE antibodies against the offending food (most commonly cow milk, eggs, peanuts, tree nuts, seafood, and shellfish). The diagnosis of an IgE-mediated FA is made by a carefully taken case history, supported by the demonstration of IgE sensitization either by skin prick tests or in vitro tests, and confirmed by positive food challenge. If the reaction is not IgE mediated (as in some children with cow milk allergy), however, these tests are often unrevealing. A helper T cells type 2 cytokine pattern is prevalent in allergic individuals at the site of the gut-associated lymphoid and mucosal system. Because individuals can develop immunologic sensitization (as evidenced by the presence of allergen-specific IgE) to food allergens without having clinical symptoms on exposure to those foods, an IgE-mediated FA requires both the presence of sensitization and the development of specific signs and symptoms on exposure to that food. Sensitization alone is not sufficient to define FA.[54] The formation of IgE antibodies on antigen exposure may not necessarily induce clinical manifestations and vice versa (the

Table 1
Pathophysiologic classification of adverse reactions to food

	Immunopathology	Disorder
Allergic	IgE dependent (acute onset)	Urticaria/angioedema Oral-allergy syndrome (pollen-food related) Asthma, rhinitis Anaphylaxis
	IgE antibody associated/cell mediated (delayed onset/chronic)	Atopic dermatitis Eosinophillic gastroenteropathies
	Cell mediated (delayed onset/chronic)	Dietary protein enterocolitis Dietary protein proctitis Celiac disease
Nonimmunologic	Toxic	Infection/food poisioning
	Pharmacologic	Caffeine, histamine, tyramine, monosodium glutamate
	Metabolic	Galactosemia, alcohol intolerance, lactose intolerance

quiescence of atopic disease does not necessarily correlate with a decrease in antibodies). Clinicians, however, may use the detection of these antibodies to identify potential offending antigens, the clinical significance of which can only be confirmed by reproduction of symptoms after oral food challenge. Furthermore, the absence of such antibodies helps exclude the presence of IgE-mediated FA. A double-blind placebo-controlled food challenge is the gold standard for establishing the presence of FA. Reproduction of GI symptoms with a single-blind or open food challenge is suggestive but subject to a higher likelihood of placebo response.

The spectrum of food allergies also includes delayed-onset or cell-mediated diseases, such as eosinophilic GI diseases (esophagitis, gastroenteritis, and colitis), food protein–induced enterocolitis syndromes (occurring in young children), and food-induced atopic dermatitis. These may be T-cell or IgE mediated. Two specific presentations that also fall within the FA category are the pollen food syndrome and the latex-FA syndrome, which both present with cutaneous and GI complaints and may include bronchospasm and anaphylaxis.

Food intolerances are non–immune-mediated adverse reactions to food and may be due to factors within foods, such as pharmacologic agents (histamine, sulfites, and caffeine), enzyme deficiency of the host (lactase deficiency), host-specific metabolic disorders (galactosemia and alcohol intolerance), or idiosyncratic responses induced by an unknown mechanism. To date, there has been no widely accepted definition put forth by an internationally sanctioned organization. Symptoms may cover a wide spectrum, but are usually minor complaints, such as headaches. Pharmacologic reactions to food and food additives may be caused by vasoactive amines (dopamine, histamine, serotonin, phenylethylamine, and tryamine) in selected foods, and food additives, such as sulfites, tartrazine, and monosodium glutamate. Symptoms of this type of reaction usually manifest outside of the GI tract in the form of headache, asthma, and urticaria.

FOOD ALLERGY AND FOOD INTOLERANCE IN IBS

Many studies have tried to examine the prevalence of FA in patients with GI symptoms. In one study of patients with IBS and inflammatory bowel disease (IBD), 32% complained of adverse reactions to food as a cause of their GI symptoms.[8] FA was suspected, however, according to several criteria in only 14% and could be confirmed by endoscopic allergen provocation and/or elimination diet and rechallenge in only 3.2% of patients. Similar results were reported by Dainese and colleagues[10] who found no difference in the frequency of positive skin prick tests in IBS patients when comparing those with and without self-reported adverse reactions to food. Similarly, there was little consistency between the specific foods reported to cause intolerance and those resulting from the tests (11 of 80 patients, 13.7%).

The prevalence of IBS-like symptoms is increased in patients with allergic symptoms, such as rhinitis and asthma, when compared with nonallergic patients.[55–57] Another study showed that patients with asthma have an increased prevalence of IBS relative to patients with other pulmonary disorders and healthy subjects.[58] Minor histologic abnormalities in the GI tract of patients with atopic diseases have been documented.[59–62] Likewise, the presence of atopic conditions is increased in patients with diarrhea-predominant IBS.[17,63] This higher prevalence of allergic symptoms in unselected gastroenterology patients and the higher prevalence of IBS-like symptoms in allergic patients both suggest that atopic disease and GI complaints may be associated, independently of whether or not patients suspect food hypersensitivity as the main cause of their symptoms.[55,57]

Some authors have posited that patients with atopic diseases have impaired gut barrier function as indicated by increased intestinal permeability.[64–66] The potential association between atopic disease, mild intestinal mucosal inflammation, and IBS symptoms in patients with self-reported food hypersensitivity was recently explored by Lillestol and colleagues.[67] Symptoms, skin prick tests, serum markers of allergy, and intestinal permeability were recorded in 71 adult patients with self-reported FH. Patients with self-reported food hypersensitivity had a high prevalence of IBS and atopic disease (93% and 61%, respectively). Atopic patients had increased intestinal permeability and density of IgE-bearing cells compared with nonatopic patients, but GI symptoms did not differ between groups. Some investigators have suggested atopic IBS as a new subgroup of IBS, with the intestinal mucosal mast cell as a possible pivotal pathophysiologic factor.[57] For further discussion on the link between immune response and functional bowel disease, readers are directed to a recent comprehensive review.[68]

Elevated levels of both food-specific serum IgE and IgG4 antibodies have been associated with food hypersensitivity–induced atopic conditions also, although the significance of elevated IgG4 antibody has been questioned. There is emerging evidence that these antibodies are pathophysiologically relevant in IBS.[20,69] Zar and colleagues[20] tested 108 IBS patients with IgG4 titers, skin prick tests, and IgE titers and compared with controls. Of 16 common food articles, there were significantly higher titers in the IBS group to wheat, soy, beef, pork, and lamb compared with controls but no difference in IgE titers or skin prick tests. No correlation was seen between the pattern of elevated IgG4 antibody titers and patient symptoms (ie, no difference among IBS subtypes).

The identification of patients with FH and IBS symptoms can be challenging, and a newer application of the basophil activation assay has been used in attempt to further characterize these patients. A recent report by Carroccio and colleagues[70] evaluated the prevalence of food hypersensitivity to milk or wheat and the performance of this in vitro basophil activation assay for FH in patients with IBS symptoms. This test has previously been applied to allergy diagnoses, but the investigators used this technique to identify FH in a group of IBS patients. One hundred and twenty patients with IBS based on Rome II criteria completed questionnaires addressing their symptoms and any possible self-perceived FH. Patients underwent a 4-week diet that strictly eliminated milk, wheat, egg, tomato, and chocolate. Responders subsequently underwent a series of double-blind, placebo-controlled, 2-week oral food challenges with milk and wheat. Ultimately, 24 (20%) of the IBS patients had a positive food challenge to milk and/or wheat (16% both, 3% milk, and 2% wheat) and were diagnosed with FH. Patients with FH developed symptoms after a median of 3 days of food challenge and 50% had to discontinue the food challenge because of recurrent symptoms. The FH patients tended to carry a longer diagnosis of IBS and showed a higher frequency of self-perceived food intolerance. Still, the majority of patients with self-perceived food intolerance had a negative response to double-blind food challenge. A small subset of patients who denied a relationship between food and their symptoms had a positive response to double-blind food challenge. The in vitro basophil activation assay was more often abnormal than were the serum measurements of total IgE and serum food-specific IgE. Using double-blind food challenge as a gold standard, specificity of the in vitro basophil activation assay was 86% in the IBS subjects with no false-positive results identified in the healthy controls. There was a high frequency of false-positive results when patients with other chronic intestinal inflammatory diseases were tested. More work is needed to validate the accuracy of the basophil activation assay used in this study.

Useful information on the role of foods in GI immunoallergic reactions could come from the colonoscopic allergen provocation test developed by Bischoff and colleagues.[71] Briefly, during colonoscopy, specific food allergens were found to trigger mucosal weal and flare reactions in 54 of 70 (77%) patients with abdominal symptoms suspected of being food related, whereas no reaction was observed in healthy volunteers. The clinical relevance of these findings, however, requires further study.

ELIMINATION DIETS

Many investigators have investigated dietary manipulation as a potential treatment strategy for patients with IBS. In 1982, Jones and colleagues[12] were among the first to demonstrate symptom improvement after an elimination diet in two-thirds of their IBS patients. Based on such results, they and others hypothesized that food intolerance was the major factor underlying the pathogenesis of IBS and that a therapy based on a diet that excluded certain foods could be effective in IBS patients[11] Subsequent studies, however, failed to conclusively confirm this hypothesis, with some groups demonstrating food hypersensitivity in only IBS patients with associated atopic disease or IBS-D and still others finding little benefit from exclusion diets.[72–74] Overall, response rates to exclusion diets have ranged from 15% to 71%,[11,12,18,72–75] with dairy products, wheat, and eggs the most commonly implicated food items. Foods high in salicylates or amines may also be problematic for IBS patients.

The reasons that underlie the widely variable response rates with exclusion diets are unknown but may include the lack of standardized protocols among the studies, varying inclusion/exclusion criteria, and inconsistent definitions of food intolerance and positive food challenge. Furthermore, a placebo diet is difficult to incorporate in clinical trials and the high placebo response in such trials necessitates large sample sizes to achieve appropriate power. Well-designed studies are needed to evaluate the role of exclusion diets in patients with IBS symptoms.

SPECIFIC DIETS
Fiber Supplements

Although increasing dietary fiber continues to be a standard recommendation for patients with IBS, the efficacy of fiber for IBS is more nuanced than appreciated by most clinicians. A recent systematic review and meta-analysis, which evaluated the efficacy of fiber as a treatment for IBS, included 12 trials and 591 patients.[76] Included studies compared various forms of fiber with placebo or, in one study, a low-fiber diet. Two of the studies included only IBS-C patients and another had 49% IBS-C patients. Overall, 52% patients assigned to fiber had persistent symptoms or no improvement in symptoms after treatment compared with 57% assigned to placebo or a low-fiber diet (relative risk [RR] 0.87; 95% CI, 0.76 to 1.00; $P = .05$). There was no statistically significant heterogeneity detected between studies ($I2 = 14.2\%$, $P = .31$). The number needed to treat (NNT) with fiber to prevent one patient with persistent symptoms was 11 (95% CI, 5 to 100). There was no evidence of funnel plot asymmetry, suggesting no publication bias. Only 7 of the 12 studies, however, scored 4 or more on the Jadad scale. When only these 7 higher-quality studies were included in the analysis, the borderline treatment benefit for fiber was no longer evident (RR of persistent symptoms 0.90; 95% CI, 0.75 to 1.08).

The data suggest that not all types of fiber supplementation are created equally, at least not as pertaining to the treatment of IBS. In 5 studies (221 patients) that compared insoluble bran with placebo or a low-fiber diet, bran failed to improve overall

IBS symptoms (RR of persistent or unimproved symptoms 1.02; 95% CI, 0.82 to 1.27).[76] In one study that evaluated bran in IBS patients, 55% of patients were actually made worse by bran whereas only 10% found it helpful.[77] All symptoms of IBS were exacerbated by bran, with bowel disturbance most often adversely affected, followed by abdominal distension and pain. Alternatively, 6 studies (321 patients) evaluated soluble ispaghula/psyllium versus placebo. Ispaghula was effective at improving overall IBS symptoms (RR of persistent or unimproved symptoms 0.78; 95% CI, 0.63 to 0.96). The NNT with ispaghula to prevent one patient from experiencing persistent symptoms was 6 (CI, 3 to 50). There was no evidence of funnel plot asymmetry and 5 of 6 studies scored 4 or more on the Jadad scale. A recent comparative effectiveness trial evaluated the relative efficacy of psyllium, 10 g (n = 85); bran, 10 g (n = 97); or rice flour (placebo) (n = 93), twice daily (mixed with food, preferably yogurt) for 12 weeks.[78] At 1 month, 57% of patients taking psyllium experienced adequate symptom relief for 2 of 4 weeks of treatment compared with 40% with bran (NNT = 6; 95% CI, 4–104) and 35% with placebo (NNT = 5; 95% CI, 3–15). Although psyllium yielded significant benefits after the second month, treatment benefits were no longer significant after 3 months. Bran offered significant benefits only after 3 months of treatment. More than 60% of subjects randomized to psyllium or bran reported moderate adverse events, the most common of which were constipation and diarrhea.

When fiber is recommended, use of a soluble supplement, such as ispaghula or psyllium, is best supported by the available evidence. Fiber should be started at a nominal dose and slowly titrated up over the course of weeks to a target dose of 20 to 30 g of total dietary fiber per day. Even when used judiciously, fiber can exacerbate problems with abdominal distension, flatulence, constipation, and diarrhea.[11,76–79]

Gluten Restriction

Celiac disease is an immune-mediated disease that occurs as a consequence of exposure to gluten, a storage protein in wheat, barley, and rye. In patients with celiac disease, dietary gluten induces an abnormal mucosal immune response in genetically susceptible individuals associated with the markers HLA-DQ2 and HLA-DQ8. Patients with classic celiac disease suffer a variety of GI symptoms, such as bloating, abdominal pain, and diarrhea, and have villous atrophy on small bowel mucosal biopsies.[80] Patients with celiac disease typically experience rapid clinical and more gradual histologic improvements on a gluten-free diet.[81] Recent literature from around the world suggests that approximately 4% of patients with IBS symptoms actually have celiac disease.[82] Studies from the United States suggest that a smaller proportion, approximately 1%, of patients with typical IBS symptoms turn out to have biopsy-proved celiac disease.[83,84] There are data to suggest that a larger proportion of patients with IBS symptoms, although not meeting criteria for the diagnosis of celiac disease, are gluten sensitive.[85,86] Gluten sensitivity is a term used to refer to a heterogeneous group of conditions in which gluten leads to some adverse clinical, serologic, or histologic reaction, which improves with dietary gluten restriction. Such patients often experience GI symptoms that can be clinically indistinguishable from patients with celiac disease or IBS.[87–89]

Gluten sensitivity encompasses a broad array of disorders ranging from latent celiac disease to FA/hypersensitivity to simple intolerance. There is some acceptance that persistent low-grade inflammation may be present in a subset of patients with IBS, and multiple driving factors have been proposed, including small bowel bacterial overgrowth, postinfectious causes, and immune-mediated responses to specific dietary constituents, such as gluten.[90–94] Several proposed mechanisms for gluten sensitivity without celiac disease exist, including increasing intestinal permeability of tight junctions or stimulating lamina propria macrophages and leading to a proinflammatory cytokine milieu.[86] Nonceliac disease subjects who are +HLA-DQ2 may possess innate cells in a state of heightened activation compared with subjects who are DQ2−.

It has been argued that some patients with positive celiac antibody tests and evidence of genetic predisposition (+HLA-DQ2 or -DQ8) but only subtle abnormalities or entirely normal small bowel histology eventually develop villous atrophy and, thus, belong to the spectrum of celiac disease.[86,95] Wahnschaffe and colleagues[87] described a group of patients reporting IBS-D symptoms with +HLA-DQ2, minimal immunopathologic changes on duodenal biopsies (increased intraepithelial lymphocytes [IELs]), elevated celiac disease–associated antibodies in duodenal aspirate, and increased IgA deposition in the intestinal villi. Such IBS-D patients experienced significant reductions in symptoms with a gluten-free diet. Subsequent studies have shown a high likelihood of response to GFD in patients with GI symptoms, abnormal celiac disease antibody testing and genetic markers DQ2/DQ8, but normal or minimal small intestinal mucosal lesions.[87,95–97] In a follow-up study, Wahnschaffe and colleagues enrolled 41 patients with IBS-D, +HLA-DQ2/DQ8, and positive IgA and IgG antibodies to tissue tranglutaminase and/or gliadin. GI symptoms and antibody levels were followed after 6 months of a gluten-free diet.[85] In IBS-D patients, celiac disease–associated serum IgG antibodies (37%) and HLA-DQ2 expression (39%) were significantly more frequent than in a control group of IBD patients (18% and 23%, respectively). After 6 months of a gluten-free diet, stool frequency and GI symptom score returned to normal values in 60% of IBS-D patients who were positive and in 12% who were negative for HLA-DQ2 and celiac disease–associated serum IgG ($P<.05$). The investigators concluded that celiac disease–associated serum IgG and HLA-DQ2 expression may identify a subset of IBS-D patients who respond to a gluten-free diet.

It is also important to emphasize that the finding of increased IELs on small bowel biopsy is not specific for celiac disease. A variety of other conditions, including *Helicobacter pylori* infection, small intestinal bacterial overgrowth, IBS, diabetes mellitus, microscopic colitis, and the use of various medications, have been associated with this histologic finding.[98] Thus, in the absence of abnormal celiac antibodies or HLA-DQ2/8, other causes for duodenal lymphocytosis should be sought. That being said, the proportion of IBS patients with the isolated finding of increased IELs on small bowel biopsy who respond to a gluten-free diet remains to be clearly defined. Similarly, the proportion of IBS patients with isolated abnormal celiac antibody test results who will improve on a gluten-free diet is also unknown. **Table 2** may serve as a useful

Table 2
Proposed management of patients with IBS symptoms and testing for celiac disease

Symptom	LD	HLA-DQ2/8	Serology	Treatment
IBS	+	+	+	Trial of GFD
IBS	+	−	−	Consider other cause
IBS	−	+	+	GFD or follow
IBS	−	−	−	Treat IBS

Abbreviations: GFD, gluten-free diet; LD, lymphocytic duodenosis.
Data from Verdu EF, Armstrong D, Murray JA. Between celiac disease and irritable bowel syndrome: the "no man's land" of gluten sensitivity. Am J Gastroenterol 2009;104(6):1587–94.

guide for identifying patients who may benefit from a trial of a gluten-free diet, depending on their symptoms, biopsies, genotype, and serologies.

Sugar/Carbohydrate Restriction

Carbohydrate malabsorption is a potential cause of symptoms in patients with IBS. Of the various sugars that have been suggested as playing a role in IBS, lactose has been most extensively studied. Lactose is a disaccharide that is cleaved to its constituent monosaccharides, glucose and galactose, by the intestinal brush border enzyme lactase. In the face of lactase deficiency, lactose is presented to colonic bacteria, leading to fermentation and the production of short chain fatty acids as well as various gases, including hydrogen, methane, and/or carbon dioxide.[99] Lactose malabsorption does not universally lead to symptoms in persons with lactase deficiency.[100,101] When individuals with lactose malabsorption develop GI symptoms, such as abdominal cramping, bloating, flatulence, and diarrhea, they are said to suffer with lactose intolerance. Many patients who associate their GI symptoms with the ingestion of dairy products have no evidence of lactose malabsorption.[102] On the basis of data from 7 studies using lactose hydrogen breath testing, a recent systematic review found that more than a third of IBS patients have lactose malabsorption and that lactose intolerance is more common in IBS patients than controls.[103] From a pragmatic standpoint, this should not be surprising because the clinical consequences of lactose malabsorption are likely to be exaggerated in patients with IBS who often have underlying abnormalities in motility and visceral sensation. Patients who are thought to have lactose intolerance are typically treated with a lactose-restricted diet. Data from largely uncontrolled studies suggest that 40% to 85% of IBS patients with lactose malabsorption improve on a lactose-restricted diet.[39,104,105] A recent systematic review found that there were insufficient data to support the efficacy of lactose-reduced solutions, milk with reduced lactose content, probiotics, or incremental lactose administration in the hopes of inducing colonic adaptation for lactose intolerance.[106]

Fructose is another sugar that has been implicated as a potential trigger for symptoms in patients with IBS. Fructose is naturally found in honey, fruits, and table sugar. In the modern Western diet, one of the largest sources of fructose is high-fructose corn syrup, which is the primary sweetener in soft drinks and many prepared foods. The human intestine does not have a specific enzyme for digestion or transport of fructose; absorption of fructose primarily relies on facilitation by glucose transporters (GLUT 5 and GLUT 2), which can be overwhelmed after the ingestion of large amounts of fructose.[107–109] Fructose absorption is much more efficient in the presence of glucose; in fact, fructose malabsorption (FM) is more likely to occur when fructose is taken alone as opposed to in combination with glucose. This provides an explanation for why most persons tolerate high-fructose corn syrup, which contains near equimolar amounts of fructose and glucose. Delivery of the free fructose to the lumen of the distal small intestine and proximal large bowel may exert an osmotic effect and result in more luminal water, increasing the liquidity of intestinal contents and increasing transit. Malabsorbed fructose and nonabsorbed fructans (long chains of fructose molecules) are, like malabsorbed lactose, fermented by colonic bacteria, leading to the development of GI symptoms in some individuals.[108]

The literature suggests that the prevalence of FM is similar between healthy volunteers and patients with functional disorders, but there is some literature to suggest that FM is associated with the development of GI symptoms in a subset of individuals.[107,108,110,111] In a study by Shepherd and Gibson,[112] nearly 30% of IBS patients were unable to tolerate a large load of fructose or fructans, and no such problem occurred in non-IBS patients with or without FM. This reinforces the notion that in IBS patients, any form of carbohydrate malabsorption is likely to result in the development of symptoms. Restricting dietary intake of fructose may lead to symptomatic benefits in patients with IBS, but high-quality evidence is lacking. In particular, the methodology and clinical value of the fructose hydrogen breath test has been questioned.[109]

Acknowledging the limitations of the fructose hydrogen breath test, the prevalence of a positive result has been reported to be 11% to 70% in healthy individuals[108] and 40% to 80% in individuals with functional gastrointestinal disorders, such as IBS. As both natural and processed dietary sources of fructose usually contain glucose, including high-fructose corn syrup, breath testing with pure fructose may not reflect fructose ingestion under normal circumstances. Fructose breath testing alone may overestimate the true prevalence of FM in controls and IBS. When breath testing was performed with both fructose alone and with high-fructose corn syrup in IBS patients and healthy controls, FM was more prevalent with fructose alone than with high-fructose corn syrup, but this did not vary significantly between healthy patients and those with IBS.[110]

Other symptoms linked with FM, in particular mood disorders and depression, have also been improved with dietary restriction of fructose.[113]

In patients with functional abdominal bloating and evidence of fructose or lactose malabsorption, 67% of patients who were educated in dietary restriction had 50% symptom resolution.[114] The specificity of this response is questioned by the fact that only patients with positive HBTs were offered the fructose-restricted diet.

The concepts put forth in the preceding paragraphs addressing lactose and fructose malabsorption/intolerance can almost certainly be extended to any of a number of other carbohydrates when ingested in sufficient quantities. The excessive ingestion of sorbitol or mannitol can result in a similar spectrum of GI symptoms as lactose malabsorption or FM and can exacerbate the symptoms of IBS. A recent prospective, randomized, controlled pilot study tested the hypothesis that a very low carbohydrate diet might provide benefit to the symptoms of IBS. Austin and colleagues[115] reported that 10 of 13 patients with IBS (77%) experienced adequate relief for 4 of 4 weeks of a very low carbohydrate diet. Another study of 239 individuals with either IBS or nonspecific functional bowel complaints showed an improvement in symptoms after elimination of some combination of sorbitol, lactose, or fructose for 1 month.[116] Also, a very low carbohydrate diet based on animal sources of fat and protein is associated with an increased all-cause, cardiovascular, and cancer-related mortality compared with a very low carbohydrate diet based on plant sources of fat and protein.[117]

FODMAP Restriction

An extension of the concept of sugar/carbohydrate restriction as a treatment for IBS is offered by the restricted Fermentable Oligo-, Di-, and Mono-saccharides And Polyols (FODMAP) diet. FODMAPs represent a family of poorly absorbed, short-chain carbohydrates, which are highly fermentable in the presence of gut bacteria. Taking into consideration comments regarding gluten sensitivity as well as sugar/carbohydrate malabsorption (discussed previously), the major FODMAPs in the Western diet include fructose, linear or branched fructose polymers called fructans, and lactose. **Table 3** provides information regarding the FODMAP food groups and examples of specific foods within each group. Fermentation of these substrates results in gas production and an increased fluid load with secondary luminal distension and resultant peristalsis involving the distal small bowel and proximal colon.

Table 3
Foods rich in FODMAPs by category

FODMAP	Fructose	Polyols	Lactose	Fructans and Galactans
High FODMAP food sources	Apples, pears, watermelon, honey, fruit juices, dried fruits, high-fructose corn syrup	Sugar alcohols (sorbitol, maltitol, mannitol, xylitol, and isomalt), stone fruits, avocado, mushrooms, cauliflower	Milk (cow, goat, sheep), yogurt, soft cheeses (ricotta, cottage)	Wheat, rye, garlic, onions, artichokes, asparagus, inulin, soy, leeks, legumes, lentils, cabbage, Brussels sprouts, broccoli
Alternative lower FODMAP food sources	Citrus, berries, bananas, grapes, honeydew, cantaloupe, kiwifruit	Sweeteners, such as sugar, glucose, other artificial sweeteners not ending in "-ol" (sucralose, aspartame)	Lactose-free dairy products, rice milk, hard cheeses	Starches, such as rice, corn, potato, quinoa. Vegetables, such as winter squash, lettuce, spinach, cucumbers, bell peppers, green beans, tomato, eggplant

All nonprocessed meats are generally low in FODMAPs.

It is not difficult to imagine how these physiologic events could lead to the development of symptoms, such as bloating, distension, abdominal pain/cramping, or diarrhea, in particular in patients with underlying IBS.[118] The effect of dietary FODMAP content on the production of hydrogen and methane gases and the induction of functional symptoms was recently studied by Ong and colleagues,[119] who performed a randomized, single-blind, crossover trial in 15 healthy controls and 15 patients with IBS by Rome III criteria. Each group consumed a high or low FODMAP diet for 2 days. Higher levels of breath hydrogen excretion were seen with the high-FODMAP diet in both healthy volunteers and IBS patients. Breath hydrogen but not methane levels were higher in the IBS patients than controls. The investigators concluded that dietary FODMAPs were associated with prolonged hydrogen production and led to a greater degree of GI symptoms in IBS patients than controls. In addition to simply reducing exposure to fermentable substrates, it is also conceivable that elimination of dietary FODMAPs might alter the gut microbiome through prebiotic effects, reduce or change the products of fermentation, improve intestinal barrier function, or affect function of smooth muscle or the enteric nervous system.[120,121] The effects of FODMAPs on fecal fluid content were recently elucidated.[122] Twelve patients with ileostomies were evaluated to understand the effect of dietary FODMAPs on the nature and volume of ileal effluent and to document perceived changes in ileostomy output. Patients ingested either a high or low FODMAP diet during 4-day periods during this randomized, crossover, single-blind study. Compared to the low FODMAP diet, ileostomy output volume with the high-FODMAP diet was increased by 20% whereas water content and dry weight increased by 20% and 24%, respectively. Participants also perceived effluent consistency as thicker with the low FODMAP diet compared with the high-FODMAP diet. Furthermore, rats fed FODMAPs have been shown to develop more severe colitis after infection with Salmonella species.[123] This is a particularly interesting observation given the mounting evidence to suggest that IBS can occur after an acute gastroenteritis and that one of the most potent predictors of postinfectious IBS is the duration and severity of the index gastroenteritis.[124]

There is a growing body of evidence to support the efficacy of the FODMAP diet in patients with IBS symptoms. Small, early studies reporting promising results with the FODMAP diet in patients with IBS were met with skepticism. Critics were quick to discount the positive results as placebo response or dismiss the diet as impractical.[112,114] Two recent studies provide support for the use of the FODMAP diet in patients with GI symptoms. In a telephone survey study of 72 patients with inflammatory bowel disease (IBD) from Australia, the vast majority of patients were able to reduce FODMAP intake moderately if not completely. Those who adhered to the diet enjoyed impressive improvements (defined as an improvement of at least 5 points on a 21-point balanced scale) in overall abdominal symptoms, pain, bloating, flatulence, and diarrhea at a mean follow-up of 17 months (25th–75th percentiles = 7–26 months). This retrospective study did not report on potential confounders, including disease activity or concurrent medical therapies for IBD. Underscoring some of the practical issues around this diet, when patients were asked about ease of implementing and palatability of the FODMAP diet, they assigned scores of 3 and 2 out of 10, respectively.[125]

A recent randomized, double-blind, quadruple-arm, crossover, placebo-controlled, rechallenge trial in IBS patients and a positive fructose hydrogen breath test result attempted to isolate whether or not the benefits of the FODMAP diet were attributable to exclusion of fructose, fructans or both.[126] All 25 IBS patients included had previously responded to a low FODMAP diet and all 3 subtypes of IBS (diarrhea, constipation, and mixed bowel pattern) were included. After 10 days on a low FODMAP diet, patients were challenged with prepared drinks containing escalating doses of fructose, fructans, fructose/fructan mix, or glucose. Symptoms were assessed daily by 100-mm visual analog scales. Dose-dependent increases in abdominal symptoms, abdominal pain, wind, and bloating were seen with fructose, fructans, and the fructose/fructan mixture arms. Symptom scores were significantly greater for these groups compared with the glucose group. The fructose-fructan mix caused greater symptom severity than did fructose alone. These results suggest that exclusion of both fructose and fructans is likely to be crucial to the benefits of a low FODMAP diet.

The low FODMAP diet differs from most other elimination diets in that no initial attempts are made to identify specific culprit foods. Rather, the FODMAP approach uses a more empiric strategy of initially eliminating or at least significantly reducing all of the most likely culprit foods. In persons who respond to the full elimination phase, specific FODMAP food groups are sequentially reintroduced, allowing determination of the particular foods that the patient cannot tolerate. Given the complexity of the diet, the time necessary to obtain an adequate dietary history, the time needed to explain the intervention, and the need for ongoing dietary counseling, the authors' group believes that the FODMAP diet is best undertaken with the assistance of a trained dietician. For details regarding the practical implementation of the FODMAP diet, readers are directed elsewhere.[112,127] On introducing this diet to a clinical practice, it is natural for providers to initially presume that the complexity of the diet guarantees patient noncompliance. The authors and other investigators have found that IBS patients often desire a more holistic approach to their care. They often are interested in learning about dietary interventions, particularly when symptom onset is related to eating a meal. In support of this statement, a recent survey conducted in more than 1200 IBS patients found that more than 60% of respondents wanted to learn about which foods to avoid.[23] In addition, many IBS patients with meal-related symptoms have tried a variety of dietary restrictions and, often, are already on a highly restricted diet by the time they see a specialist. Unfortunately, haphazard attempts at dietary exclusion are often unsuccessful and potentially dangerous. Such IBS patients have proved that they are highly motivated for dietary interventions and many of them actually express relief when provided with a construct that specifically addresses the foods that they can eat and those that they should avoid.

CONCLUDING COMMENTS

Many of the therapeutic options commonly used for IBS have proved unsatisfactory both to patients and providers, likely due to the inherent complexity and heterogeneity of the disorder. In a subset of patients, diet seems to play a role in the development of symptoms. Many patients are now demanding a more holistic approach to their care. Although dietary interventions may be the low-hanging fruit for such patients, their success is highly dependent on the presence of a motivated patient and caregiver. Despite the fact that gastroenterologists spend more time with their patients than most clinicians,[128] the time required for a complete dietary assessment and overhaul is beyond the capability/resources of even the most dedicated physician. Thus, access to a dietician with expertise and experience with GI disorders, such as IBS, improves the chance of a successful outcome after dietary interventions. Practical considerations aside, dietary intervention as a therapeutic option for IBS is promising. Some of the many questions for future studies include (1) How do individual foods and combinations of foods affect the microbiome, neuroendocrine, and immune function, motility, and sensation of the GI tract? (2) Which subgroups of patients are more or less likely to respond to which type of dietary intervention? (3) What are the most practical ways in which to introduce dietary interventions into clinical practice? (4) Are dietary interventions cost-effective when compared with medical therapies for IBS? (5) Might incremental benefits be derived by combining dietary interventions with medical therapies? Only by answering such questions will we be able to fill in the many blanks that remain in the evolving story of dietary interventions for IBS.

REFERENCES

1. Chey WD, Olden K, Carter E, et al. Utility of the Rome I and Rome II criteria for irritable bowel syndrome in U.S. women. Am J Gastroenterol 2002;97(11): 2803–11.
2. Longstreth GF, Thompson WG, Chey WD, et al. Functional bowel disorders. Gastroenterology 2006;130(5):1480–91.
3. Monsbakken KW, Vandvik PO, Farup PG. Perceived food intolerance in subjects with irritable bowel syndrome—etiology, prevalence and consequences. Eur J Clin Nutr 2005;60(5):667–72.
4. Young E, Stoneham MD, Petruckevitch A, et al. A population study of food intolerance. Lancet 1994;343(8906):1127–30.
5. Locke GR, Zinsmeister AR, Talley NJ, et al. Risk factors for irritable bowel syndrome: role of analgesics and food sensitivities. Am J Gastroenterol 2000; 95(1):157–65.
6. Crespo JF, Rodriguez J. Food allergy in adulthood. Allergy 2003;58(2):98–113.
7. Jarrett M, Visser R, Heitkemper M. Diet triggers symptoms in women with irritable bowel syndrome. The patient's perspective. Gastroenterol Nurs 2001; 24(5):246–52.
8. Bischoff SC, Herrmann A, Manns MP. Prevalence of adverse reactions to food in patients with gastrointestinal disease. Allergy 1996;51(11):811–8.
9. Simrén M, Månsson A, Langkilde AM, et al. Food-related gastrointestinal symptoms in the irritable bowel syndrome. Digestion 2001;63(2):108–15.
10. Dainese R, Galliani EA, De Lazzari F, et al. Discrepancies between reported food intolerance and sensitization test findings in irritable bowel syndrome patients. Am J Gastroenterol 1999;94(7):1892–7.
11. Nanda R, James R, Smith H, et al. Food intolerance and the irritable bowel syndrome. Gut 1989;30(8):1099–104.
12. Jones VA, Shorthouse M, Hunter JO. Food intolerance: a major factor in the pathogenesis of irritable bowel syndrome. Lancet 1982;2(8308):1115–7.
13. Bhat K, Harper A, Gorard DA. Perceived food and drug allergies in functional and organic gastrointestinal disorders. Aliment Pharmacol Ther 2002;16(5): 969–73.
14. Anderson J. The clinical spectrum of food allergy in adults. Clin Exp Allergy 1991;21:304–15.
15. Arslan G, Kahrs GE, Lind R, et al. Patients with subjective food hypersensitivity: the value of analyzing intestinal permeability and inflammation markers in gut lavage fluid. Digestion 2004;70(1):26–35.
16. Iacono G, Cavataio F, Montalto G, et al. Intolerance of cow's milk and chronic constipation in children. N Engl J Med 1998;339(16):1100–4.
17. Stefanini GF, Bazzocchi G, Prati E, et al. Efficacy of oral disodium cromoglycate in patients with irritable bowel syndrome and positive skin prick tests to foods. Lancet 1986;1(8474):207–8.

18. Niec AM, Frankum B, Talley NJ. Are adverse food reactions linked to irritable bowel syndrome? Am J Gastroenterol 1998;93(11):2184–90.
19. Read NW. Food and hypersensitivity in functional dyspepsia. Gut 2002;51(Suppl 1): i50–3.
20. Zar S, Benson MJ, Kumar D. Food-specific serum IgG4 and IgE titers to common food antigens in irritable bowel syndrome. Am J Gastroenterol 2005; 100(7):1550–7.
21. Zar S, Kumar D, Benson MJ. Food hypersensitivity and irritable bowel syndrome. Aliment Pharmacol Ther 2001;15(4):439–49.
22. Saito YA, Locke GR 3rd, Weaver AL, et al. Diet and functional gastrointestinal disorders: a population-based case-control study. Am J Gastroenterol 2005; 100(12):2743–8.
23. Halpert A, Dalton CB, Palsson O, et al. What patients know about irritable bowel syndrome (IBS) and what they would like to know. National survey on patient educational needs in IBS and development and validation of the Patient Educational Needs Questionnaire (PEQ). Am J Gastroenterol 2007;102(9): 1972–82.
24. Camilleri M. Integrated upper gastrointestinal response to food intake. Gastroenterology 2006;131(2):640–58.
25. Stanley S, Wynne K, McGowan B, et al. Hormonal regulation of food intake. Physiol Rev 2005;85(4):1131–58.
26. Dockray GJ. Luminal sensing in the gut: an overview. J Physiol Pharmacol 2003; 54(Suppl 4):9–17.
27. Tack J, Caenepeel P, Corsetti M, et al. Role of tension receptors in dyspeptic patients with hypersensitivity to gastric distention. Gastroenterology 2004; 127(4):1058–66.
28. Vanden Berghe P, Janssen P, Kindt S, et al. Contribution of different triggers to the gastric accommodation reflex in humans. Am J Physiol Gastrointest Liver Physiol 2009;297(5):G902–6.
29. Wiley J, Tatum D, Keinath R, et al. Participation of gastric mechanoreceptors and intestinal chemoreceptors in the gastrocolonic response. Gastroenterology 1988;94(5 Pt 1):1144–9.
30. Sims MA, Hasler WL, Chey WD, et al. Hyperglycemia inhibits mechanoreceptor-mediated gastrocolonic responses and colonic peristaltic reflexes in healthy humans. Gastroenterology 1995;108(2):350–9.
31. Stanghellini V, Borovicka J, Read NW. Feedback regulation and sensation. Frontiers in gastric emptying. Dig Dis Sci 1994;39(Suppl 12):124S–7S.
32. Tanaka T, Katsuma S, Adachi T, et al. Free fatty acids induce cholecystokinin secretion through GPR120. Naunyn Schmiedebergs Arch Pharmacol 2008; 377(4–6):523–7.
33. Karaus M, Niederau C. Effects of CCK-receptor antagonist on colonic motor activity in dogs. Neurogastroenterol Motil 1995;7(2):63–71.
34. Niederau C, Faber S, Karaus M. Cholecystokinin's role in regulation of colonic motility in health and in irritable bowel syndrome. Gastroenterology 1992; 102(6):1889–98.
35. Simren M, Abrahamsson H, Bjornsson ES. An exaggerated sensory component of the gastrocolonic response in patients with irritable bowel syndrome. Gut 2001;48(1):20–7.
36. Simren M, Agerforz P, Bjornsson ES, et al. Nutrient-dependent enhancement of rectal sensitivity in irritable bowel syndrome (IBS). Neurogastroenterol Motil 2007;19(1):20–9.

37. Sabate JM, Gorbatchef C, Flourie B, et al. Cholecystokinin octapeptide increases rectal sensitivity to pain in healthy subjects. Neurogastroenterol Motil 2002;14(6):689–95.
38. Raybould HE. Gut chemosensing: interactions between gut endocrine cells and visceral afferents. Auton Neurosci 2010;153(1–2):41–6.
39. Heizer WD, Southern S, McGovern S. The role of diet in symptoms of irritable bowel syndrome in adults: a narrative review. J Am Diet Assoc 2009;109(7): 1204–14.
40. Rozengurt E, Sternini C. Taste receptor signaling in the mammalian gut. Curr Opin Pharmacol 2007;7(6):557–62.
41. Boesmans W, Owsianik G, Tack J, et al. TRP channels in neurogastroenterology: opportunities for therapeutic intervention. Br J Pharmacol 2011;162:18–37.
42. Skoog SM, Bharucha AE, Camilleri M, et al. Effects of an osmotically active agent on colonic transit. Neurogastroenterol Motil 2006;18(4):300–6.
43. Koutsou GA, Storey DM, Lee A, et al. Dose-related gastrointestinal response to the ingestion of either isomalt, lactitol or maltitol in milk chocolate. Eur J Clin Nutr 1996;50(1):17–21.
44. Schmid HR, Ehrlein HJ. Effects of enteral infusion of hypertonic saline and nutrients on canine jejunal motor patterns. Dig Dis Sci 1993;38(6):1062–72.
45. Marciani L, Cox EF, Hoad CL, et al. Postprandial changes in small bowel water content in healthy subjects and patients with irritable bowel syndrome. Gastroenterology 2010;138(2):469–77, e461.
46. Grabitske HA, Slavin JL. Gastrointestinal effects of low-digestible carbohydrates. Crit Rev Food Sci Nutr 2009;49(4):327–60.
47. Lee KJ, Tack J. Altered intestinal microbiota in irritable bowel syndrome. Neurogastroenterol Motil 2010;22(5):493–8.
48. Cianferoni A, Spergel JM. Food allergy: review, classification and diagnosis. Allergol Int 2009;58(4):457–66.
49. Brandtzaeg P. Food allergy: separating the science from the mythology. Nat Rev Gastroenterol Hepatol 2010;7(9):478.
50. Bock S. Prospective appraisal of complaints of adverse reactions to foods in children during the first 3 years of life. Pediatrics 1987;79:683–8.
51. Sampson HA, Sicherer SH, Birnbaum AH. AGA technical review on the evaluation of food allergy in gastrointestinal disorders. Gastroenterology 2001;120(4): 1026–40.
52. Sampson HA. Update on food allergy. J Allergy Clin Immunol 2004;113(5): 805–19.
53. Bruijnzeel-Koomen C, Ortolani C, Aas K, et al. Adverse reactions to food. Allergy 1995;50(8):623–35.
54. Sicherer SH, Sampson HA. Food allergy. J Allergy Clin Immunol 2010; 125(2 Suppl 2):S116–25.
55. Smith MA, Youngs GR, Finn R. Food intolerance, atopy, and irritable bowel syndrome. Lancet 1985;2(8463):1064.
56. Powell N, Huntley B, Beech T, et al. Increased prevalence of gastrointestinal symptoms in patients with allergic disease. Postgrad Med J 2007;83(977):182–6.
57. Tobin MC, Moparty B, Farhadi A, et al. Atopic irritable bowel syndrome: a novel subgroup of irritable bowel syndrome with allergic manifestations. Ann Allergy Asthma Immunol 2008;100(1):49–53.
58. Roussos A, Koursarakos P, Patsopoulos D, et al. Increased prevalence of irritable bowel syndrome in patients with bronchial asthma. Respir Med 2003; 97(1):75–9.

59. Pires GV, Souza HS, Elia CC, et al. Small bowel of patients with asthma and allergic rhinitis: absence of inflammation despite the presence of major cellular components of allergic inflammation. Allergy Asthma Proc 2004; 25(4):253–9.
60. Kokkonen J, Simila S, Herva R. Gastrointestinal findings in atopic children. Eur J Pediatr 1980;134(3):249–54.
61. Caffarelli C, Cavagni G, Romanini E, et al. Duodenal IgE-positive cells and elimination diet responsiveness in children with atopic dermatitis. Ann Allergy Asthma Immunol 2001;86(6):665–70.
62. Kalimo K, Lammintausta K, Klemi P, et al. Mast cells and IgE in intestinal mucosa in adult atopic dermatitis patients. Br J Dermatol 1988;119(5):579–85.
63. Stefanini GF, Prati E, Albini MC, et al. Oral disodium cromoglycate treatment on irritable bowel syndrome: an open study on 101 subjects with diarrheic type. Am J Gastroenterol 1992;87(1):55–7.
64. Pike MG, Heddle RJ, Boulton P, et al. Increased intestinal permeability in atopic eczema. J Invest Dermatol 1986;86(2):101–4.
65. Jackson PG, Lessof MH, Baker RW, et al. Intestinal permeability in patients with eczema and food allergy. Lancet 1981;1(8233):1285–6.
66. Dunlop SP, Hebden J, Campbell E, et al. Abnormal intestinal permeability in subgroups of diarrhea-predominant irritable bowel syndromes. Am J Gastroenterol 2006;101(6):1288–94.
67. Lillestol K, Helgeland L, Arslan Lied G, et al. Indications of 'atopic bowel' in patients with self-reported food hypersensitivity. Aliment Pharmacol Ther 2010;31(10):1112–22.
68. Ohman L, Simren M. Pathogenesis of IBS: role of inflammation, immunity and neuroimmune interactions. Nat Rev Gastroenterol Hepatol 2010;7(3):163–73.
69. Atkinson W, Sheldon TA, Shaath N, et al. Food elimination based on IgG antibodies in irritable bowel syndrome: a randomised controlled trial. Gut 2004; 53(10):1459–64.
70. Carroccio A, Brusca I, Mansueto P, et al. A cytologic assay for diagnosis of food hypersensitivity in patients with irritable bowel syndrome. Clin Gastroenterol Hepatol 2010;8(3):254–60.
71. Bischoff SC, Mayer J, Wedemeyer J, et al. Colonoscopic allergen provocation (COLAP): a new diagnostic approach for gastrointestinal food allergy. Gut 1997;40(6):745–53.
72. Bentley SJ, Pearson DJ, Rix KJ. Food hypersensitivity in irritable bowel syndrome. Lancet 1983;2(8345):295–7.
73. Petitpierre M, Gumowski P, Girard JP. Irritable bowel syndrome and hypersensitivity to food. Ann Allergy 1985;54(6):538–40.
74. Zwetchkenbaum JF, Burakoff R. Food allergy and the irritable bowel syndrome. Am J Gastroenterol 1988;83(9):901–4.
75. McKee AM, Prior A, Whorwell PJ. Exclusion diets in irritable bowel syndrome: are they worthwhile? J Clin Gastroenterol 1987;9(5):526–8.
76. Ford AC, Talley NJ, Spiegel BM, et al. Effect of fibre, antispasmodics, and peppermint oil in the treatment of irritable bowel syndrome: systematic review and meta-analysis. BMJ 2008;337:a2313.
77. Francis CY, Whorwell PJ. Bran and irritable bowel syndrome: time for reappraisal. Lancet 1994;344(8914):39–40.
78. Bijkerk CJ, de Wit NJ, Muris JW, et al. Soluble or insoluble fibre in irritable bowel syndrome in primary care? Randomised placebo controlled trial. BMJ 2009;339: b3154.

79. King TS, Elia M, Hunter JO. Abnormal colonic fermentation in irritable bowel syndrome. Lancet 1998;352(9135):1187–9.
80. Fasano A, Berti I, Gerarduzzi T, et al. Prevalence of celiac disease in at-risk and not-at-risk groups in the United States: a large multicenter study. Arch Intern Med 2003;163(3):286–92.
81. Green PH, Jabri B. Coeliac disease. Lancet 2003;362(9381):383–91.
82. Ford AC, Chey WD, Talley NJ, et al. Yield of diagnostic tests for celiac disease in individuals with symptoms suggestive of irritable bowel syndrome: systematic review and meta-analysis. Arch Intern Med 2009;169(7):651–8.
83. Saito-Loftus Y, Almazar-Elder A, Larson J, et al. ROME Criteria for Irritable Bowel Syndrome (IBS) should be a quantitative trait and not a qualitative trait. Am J Gastroenterol 2008;103(Suppl 1):S472.
84. Cash B, Lee D, Riddle M, et al. Yield of diagnostic testing in patients with suspected Irritable Bowel Syndrome (IBS): a prospective, U.S. Multi-Center Trial. Am J Gastroenterol 2008;103(Suppl 1):S462.
85. Wahnschaffe U, Schulzke JD, Zeitz M, et al. Predictors of clinical response to gluten-free diet in patients diagnosed with diarrhea-predominant irritable bowel syndrome. Clin Gastroenterol Hepatol 2007;5(7):844–50 [quiz: 769].
86. Verdu EF, Armstrong D, Murray JA. Between celiac disease and irritable bowel syndrome: the "no man's land" of gluten sensitivity. Am J Gastroenterol 2009; 104(6):1587–94.
87. Wahnschaffe U, Ullrich R, Riecken EO, et al. Celiac disease-like abnormalities in a subgroup of patients with irritable bowel syndrome. Gastroenterology 2001; 121(6):1329–38.
88. Loft DE, Nwokolo CU, Ciclitira PJ. The diagnosis of gluten sensitivity and coeliac disease–the two are not mutually inclusive. Eur J Gastroenterol Hepatol 1998; 10(11):911–3.
89. Drossman DA, Camilleri M, Mayer EA, et al. AGA technical review on irritable bowel syndrome. Gastroenterology 2002;123:2108–31. Abstract|PDF (285 K)| View Record in Scopus|Cited By in Scopus (505).
90. Marshall JK, Thabane M, Garg AX, et al. Incidence and epidemiology of irritable bowel syndrome after a large waterborne outbreak of bacterial dysentery. Gastroenterology 2006;131(2):445–50 [quiz: 660].
91. Spiller RC, Jenkins D, Thornley JP, et al. Increased rectal mucosal enteroendocrine cells, T lymphocytes, and increased gut permeability following acute Campylobacter enteritis and in post-dysenteric irritable bowel syndrome. Gut 2000;47(6):804–11.
92. Neal KR, Hebden J, Spiller R. Prevalence of gastrointestinal symptoms six months after bacterial gastroenteritis and risk factors for development of the irritable bowel syndrome: postal survey of patients. BMJ 1997;314(7083):779–82.
93. Pimentel M, Chow EJ, Lin HC. Normalization of lactulose breath testing correlates with symptom improvement in irritable bowel syndrome. A double-blind, randomized, placebo-controlled study. Am J Gastroenterol 2003;98(2):412–9.
94. Gwee KA, Collins SM, Read NW, et al. Increased rectal mucosal expression of interleukin 1beta in recently acquired post-infectious irritable bowel syndrome. Gut 2003;52(4):523–6.
95. Kurppa K, Collin P, Viljamaa M, et al. Diagnosing mild enteropathy celiac disease: a randomized, controlled clinical study. Gastroenterology 2009; 136(3):816–23.
96. Dieterich W, Ehnis T, Bauer M, et al. Identification of tissue transglutaminase as the autoantigen of celiac disease. Nat Med 1997;3(7):797–801.

97. Kaukinen K, Maki M, Partanen J, et al. Celiac disease without villous atrophy: revision of criteria called for. Dig Dis Sci 2001;46(4):879–87.

98. Vande Voort JL, Murray JA, Lahr BD, et al. Lymphocytic duodenosis and the spectrum of celiac disease. Am J Gastroenterol 2009;104(1):142–8.

99. Suchy FJ, Brannon PM, Carpenter TO, et al. National Institutes of Health Consensus Development Conference: lactose intolerance and health. Ann Intern Med 2010;152(12):792–6.

100. Law D, Conklin J, Pimentel M. Lactose intolerance and the role of the lactose breath test. Am J Gastroenterol 2010;105(8).1726–8.

101. Lomer MC, Parkes GC, Sanderson JD. Review article: lactose intolerance in clinical practice–myths and realities. Aliment Pharmacol Ther 2008;27(2): 93–103.

102. Casellas F, Aparici A, Casaus M, et al. Subjective perception of lactose intolerance does not always indicate lactose malabsorption. Clin Gastroenterol Hepatol 2010;8(7):581–6.

103. Brandt LJ, Chey WD, Foxx-Orenstein AE, et al. An evidence-based position statement on the management of irritable bowel syndrome. Am J Gastroenterol 2009;104(Suppl 1):S1–35.

104. Alpers DH. Diet and irritable bowel syndrome. Curr Opin Gastroenterol 2006; 22(2):136–9.

105. Corlew-Roath M, Di Palma JA. Clinical impact of identifying lactose maldigestion or fructose malabsorption in irritable bowel syndrome or other conditions. South Med J 2009;102(10):1010–2.

106. Shaukat A, Levitt MD, Taylor BC, et al. Systematic review: effective management strategies for lactose intolerance. Ann Intern Med 2010;152(12): 797–803.

107. Rumessen JJ, Gudmand-Hoyer E. Functional bowel disease: malabsorption and abdominal distress after ingestion of fructose, sorbitol, and fructose-sorbitol mixtures. Gastroenterology 1988;95(3):694–700.

108. Gibson PR, Newnham E, Barrett JS, et al. Review article: fructose malabsorption and the bigger picture. Aliment Pharmacol Ther 2007;25(4):349–63.

109. Rao SS, Attaluri A, Anderson L, et al. Ability of the normal human small intestine to absorb fructose: evaluation by breath testing. Clin Gastroenterol Hepatol 2007;5(8):959–63.

110. Skoog SM, Bharucha AE, Zinsmeister AR. Comparison of breath testing with fructose and high fructose corn syrups in health and IBS. Neurogastroenterol Motil 2008;20(5):505–11.

111. Choi YK, Kraft N, Zimmerman B, et al. Fructose intolerance in IBS and utility of fructose-restricted diet. J Clin Gastroenterol 2008;42(3):233–8.

112. Shepherd SJ, Gibson PR. Fructose malabsorption and symptoms of irritable bowel syndrome: guidelines for effective dietary management. J Am Diet Assoc 2006;106(10):1631–9.

113. Ledochowski M, Widner B, Bair H, et al. Fructose- and sorbitol-reduced diet improves mood and gastrointestinal disturbances in fructose malabsorbers. Scand J Gastroenterol 2000;35(10):1048–52.

114. Fernandez-Banares F, Rosinach M, Esteve M, et al. Sugar malabsorption in functional abdominal bloating: a pilot study on the long-term effect of dietary treatment. Clin Nutr 2006;25(5):824–31.

115. Austin GL, Dalton CB, Hu Y, et al. A very low-carbohydrate diet improves symptoms and quality of life in diarrhea-predominant irritable bowel syndrome. Clin Gastroenterol Hepatol 2009;7(6):706–708.e1.

116. Goldstein R, Braverman D, Stankiewicz H. Carbohydrate malabsorption and the effect of dietary restriction on symptoms of irritable bowel syndrome and functional bowel complaints. Isr Med Assoc J 2000;2(8):583–7.
117. Fung TT, van Dam RM, Hankinson SE, et al. Low-carbohydrate diets and all-cause and cause-specific mortality: two cohort studies. Ann Intern Med 2010; 153(5):289–98.
118. Gibson PR, Shepherd SJ. Evidence-based dietary management of functional gastrointestinal symptoms: the FODMAP approach. J Gastroenterol Hepatol 2010;25(2):252–8.
119. Ong DK, Mitchell SB, Barrett JS, et al. Manipulation of dietary short chain carbohydrates alters the pattern of gas production and genesis of symptoms in irritable bowel syndrome. J Gastroenterol Hepatol 2010;25(8):1366–73.
120. Argenzio RA, Meuten DJ. Short-chain fatty acids induce reversible injury of porcine colon. Dig Dis Sci 1991;36(10):1459–68.
121. Soret R, Chevalier J, De Coppet P, et al. Short-chain fatty acids regulate the enteric neurons and control gastrointestinal motility in rats. Gastroenterology 2010;138(5):1772–82.
122. Barrett JS, Gearry RB, Muir JG, et al. Dietary poorly absorbed, short-chain carbohydrates increase delivery of water and fermentable substrates to the proximal colon. Aliment Pharmacol Ther 2010;31(8):874–82.
123. Bovee-Oudenhoven IM, ten Bruggencate SJ, Lettink-Wissink ML, et al. Dietary fructo-oligosaccharides and lactulose inhibit intestinal colonisation but stimulate translocation of salmonella in rats. Gut 2003;52(11):1572–8.
124. Thabane M, Simunovic M, Akhtar-Danesh N, et al. Development and validation of a risk score for post-infectious irritable bowel syndrome. Am J Gastroenterol 2009;104(9):2267–74.
125. Gearry R, Irving PM, Barrett JS, et al. Reduction of dietary poorly absorbed short-chain carbohydrates (FODMPAs) improves abdominal symptoms in patients with inflammatory bowel disease—a pilot study. J Crohns Colitis 2009;3:8–14.
126. Shepherd SJ, Parker FC, Muir JG, et al. Dietary triggers of abdominal symptoms in patients with irritable bowel syndrome: randomized placebo-controlled evidence. Clin Gastroenterol Hepatol 2008;6(7):765–71.
127. Catsos P. IBS—free at last!: a revolutionary, new step-by-step method for those who have tried everything. Control IBS symptoms by limiting FODMAPS carbohydrates in your diet. Portland (ME): Pond Cove Press; 2009.
128. Ananthakrishnan AN, McGinley EL, Saeian K. Length of office visits for gastrointestinal disease: impact of physician specialty. Am J Gastroenterol 2010; 105(8):1719–25.

Peripherally Acting Therapies for the Treatment of Irritable Bowel Syndrome

Richard J. Saad, MD

KEYWORDS

- Irritable bowel syndrome • Lubiprostone • Alosetron
- Serotonergic agents

The irritable bowel syndrome (IBS) is a chronic, relapsing, and variably disabling bowel disorder characterized by the presence of abdominal pain or discomfort in association with altered bowel habits. IBS is further subtyped based on the predominant stool pattern into one of IBS with constipation (IBS-C), IBS with diarrhea (IBS-D), or mixed IBS (IBS-M).[1] Given the nature of symptoms related to IBS, gut-acting therapies have been traditionally used and remain among the most common therapies for this chronic condition. Most of these peripheral acting agents, including fiber supplements, laxatives, antidiarrheals, and antispasmodics, are primarily targeted at individual symptoms. The evidence supporting the use of these agents in IBS is largely anecdotal, based on dated studies of marginal methodological quality because high-quality clinical trials are generally lacking. Serotonergic agents and the chloride channel activator lubiprostone have shown efficacy in global as well as various individual symptoms of IBS. Moreover, the clinical evidence supporting the use of these agents is based on data from high-quality clinical trials. The use of serotonergic agents for IBS in the United States is limited to the 5-hydroxytryptamine-3 (5-HT$_3$) antagonist alosetron in the treatment of women with severe IBS-D refractory to traditional therapy.

FIBER SUPPLEMENTS AND LAXATIVES

The use of fiber supplements and laxatives in the treatment of IBS has evolved from the perception of altered gastrointestinal motility as a cause of the abnormal bowel symptoms associated with this heterogeneous condition.[2,3] Specifically, several clinical observations have reported a decrease in bowel motility and a prolonged transit time in patients with IBS-C compared with controls.[4–6] Furthermore, given the proven

Division of Gastroenterology, University of Michigan Health System, 3912 Taubman Center, 1500 East Medical Center Drive, SPC 5362, Ann Arbor, MI 48109, USA
E-mail address: rsaad@umich.edu

Gastroenterol Clin N Am 40 (2011) 163–182
doi:10.1016/j.gtc.2010.12.008
0889-8553/11/$ – see front matter © 2011 Elsevier Inc. All rights reserved.

gastro.theclinics.com

efficacy of fiber supplements and other laxatives in regulating bowel habits and alle-viating constipation, clinicians have traditionally turned to these agents to address the bowel symptoms associated with IBS-C and IBS-M. However, the clinical evidence for this practice is based on limited data because high-quality clinical trials assessing these agents in the treatment of IBS are nearly nonexistent.

Dietary fiber supplements represent a heterogeneous group of complex carbohy-drates that are resistant to hydrolysis during digestion. These nondigested products result in increased stool bulk and water content, effectively decreasing stool consis-tency and increasing stool frequency.[7] Of the various commercially available fiber supplements including psyllium, ispaghula husk, bran (wheat and corn), methylcellu-lose, calcium polycarbophil, and partially hydrolyzed guar gum; psyllium and bran are the best studied in the treatment of IBS. The results of the 6 trials comparing psyl-lium and ispaghula husk (the husk of psyllium seed) with placebo were pooled, yielding a total of 321 patients with IBS, with 161 in the treatment arm.[8] In this pooled analysis, 52% of patients treated with psyllium had persistent IBS symptoms after treatment compared with 64% of those receiving placebo. Although significant heterogeneity existed amongst the studies, the relative risk (RR) of symptoms not improving with psyllium was 0.78 (95% confidence interval [CI] 0.63–0.96) compared with placebo with a number needed to treat (NNT) of 6 (95% CI 3–50). The investigators noted that limiting this analysis to the 5 higher-quality trials resulted in a loss of this significant difference between psyllium and placebo. The pooled analysis of the 5 trials comparing bran with placebo or a low-fiber diet found no difference in treatment outcomes with bran.[8] Guar gum has been assessed (daily dose of 5–10 g) in 2 open trials involving patients with constipation-predominant and diarrhea-predominant IBS, suggesting short-term benefits in gastrointestinal symptoms as well as in quality-of-life (QOL) measures.[9,10] The effects of calcium polycarbophil on IBS have been assessed in 2 clinical trials.[11,12] The first study was a 6-month, placebo-controlled, randomized, double-blind crossover trial in 23 patients with either constipation-predominant IBS or IBS with alternating diarrhea and constipation.[11] Polycarbophil (6 g/d) was preferred over placebo in 71% of patients for treatment of their IBS symptoms. Compared with placebo, polycarbophil was reported to improve ease of bowel movements and relieve symptoms of nausea, pain, and bloating. In the second trial, calcium polycarbophil was given to 26 patients with IBS (14 with IBS-D and 12 with IBS-C).[12] Compared with baseline there was significant improvement in frequency of bowel movement, stool form, and abdominal pain in both IBS subgroups (P<.05). There are no clinical trials assessing the efficacy of methylcellulose in the treatment of IBS.

The clinical trials assessing fiber supplements have been evaluated collectively in several systematic reviews, with varying conclusions. The American College of Gastroenterology (ACG) Task Force recently reported on their findings from an evidence-based systematic review on the effectiveness of fiber supplements in the management of IBS, concluding that "Psyllium hydrophilic mucilliod (ispaghula husk) is moderately effective and can be given a conditional recommendation (Grade 2C) (Table 1). Wheat bran or corn bran is no more effective than placebo in the relief of global symptoms of IBS and cannot be recommended for routine use (Grade 2C). A single study reported improvement with calcium polycarbophil."[13] Using dichotomous outcomes for relief of abdominal pain, improvement in global assessment of IBS symptoms, and improvement in symptom scores, a Cochrane review of 11 studies did not find fiber supplements effective in the treatment of IBS.[14] These investigators cautioned that considerable heterogeneity of patients with IBS existed in the included trials and the effectiveness of fiber supplements have not been completely defined in

Table 1			
Grade recommendations			
Grade of Recommendation	Description of Recommendation	Methodological Quality of Supporting Evidence	Benefit Versus Risk
1A	Strong recommendation based on high-quality evidence	RCTs without important limitations or overwhelming evidence from observational studies	Benefits clearly outweigh risk
1B	Strong recommendation based on moderate-quality evidence	RCTs with important limitations (inconsistent results, methodological flaws, indirect, or imprecise) or exceptionally strong evidence from observational studies	Benefits clearly outweigh risk
1C	Strong recommendation based on low- or very-low-quality evidence	Observational or case studies only	Benefits clearly outweigh risk
2A	Weak recommendation based on high-quality evidence	RCTs without important limitations or overwhelming evidence from observational studies	Benefits closely balanced with risk
2B	Weak recommendation based on moderate-quality evidence	RCTs with important limitations (inconsistent results, methodological flaws, indirect, or imprecise) or exceptionally strong evidence from observational studies	Benefits closely balanced with risk
2C	Strong recommendation based on low- or very-low-quality evidence	Observational or case studies only	Uncertainty in the estimates of benefits and risk

Adapted from Brandt LJ, Chey WD, Foxx-Orenstein AE, et al. An evidence-based position statement on the management of irritable bowel syndrome. Am J Gastroenterol 2009;104(Suppl 1):S10; with permission.

specific IBS subtypes. In an earlier systematic review performed by the ACG Functional Gastrointestinal Disorders Task Force, this panel of experts concluded that bulking agents were not more effective than placebo at relieving the global symptoms of IBS.[15]

The use of laxatives in the treatment of IBS-C has evolved from their known effect on the symptoms of constipation. Only 1 laxative, polyethylene glycol (PEG), has been assessed in the treatment of IBS. This was a sequential study assessing the effects of PEG 3350 on 27 postpubertal adolescents (59% female) with IBS-C (based on Rome II criteria).[16] After 4 weeks of therapy, the group treated with 17 g of PEG 3350 once daily experienced a significant increase in mean bowel movement frequency from 2.07 to 5.04 bowel movements a week ($P<.05$). However, there was no change in mean pain level for the group with the PEG therapy. Regarding laxatives, the ACG Task Force concluded that "PEG laxative was shown to improve stool frequency–but not abdominal pain–in one small sequential study in adolescents with IBS-C."[13]

The fiber supplement psyllium may have some beneficial effects on the symptoms of constipation and alternating bowel habits in patients with IBS-C and IBS-M, respectively. Bran does not seem to offer symptomatic benefit in IBS and the effect of other available fiber supplements remains largely unknown. Potential adverse effects including bloating, abdominal distention, and flatulence may limit use of these agents. Their widespread availability, relative inexpense, and perceived safety make them an attractive treatment options in IBS-C and IBS-M. There are virtually no evidence-based data evaluating traditional laxatives in the treatment of IBS. However, the relative safety, universal availability, and low cost of laxatives make them an attractive therapeutic option for constipation-related complaints in patients with IBS.

ANTIDIARRHEALS

As already noted, there is a general perception that the alterations in bowel habits experienced in IBS are in part a result of altered gastrointestinal motility. Studies around the world have reported accelerated small bowel and colon transit times as well as exaggerated motility patterns in those with IBS-D compared with controls.[4,5,17,18] It is largely a result of these observations that antidiarrheals remain among the more commonly used gut-acting agents used in the treatment of patients with IBS-D.

Of the 2 most commonly used antidiarrheals in the United States, including loperamide and diphenoxylate, only loperamide has been evaluated in randomized controlled trials (RCTs) for the treatment of IBS. A total of 4 studies have been published, all European, none recent, and all containing methodological limitations.[19–22] The first study, from England and published in 1984, was a crossover, placebo-controlled trial involving 28 patients with IBS (75% female).[19] Compared with placebo, 5 weeks of loperamide (dose range of 2–12 mg/d) reduced small bowel ($P>.01$) and whole gut transit time ($P<.01$) and was superior at improving diarrhea ($P<.01$), urgency ($P<.01$), and boborygmi ($P<.05$). There was no improvement in pain with loperamide. Eighteen patients (62%) reported an overall improvement and 9 of them continued therapy for 12 months. The first of 2 Norwegian studies was 1 of 2 double-blind, placebo-controlled trials published in 1987.[20] This study assessed a total of 58 patients with IBS divided into 4 categories: painless diarrhea (n = 16), pain with alternating bowels (n = 21), alternating bowels without pain (n = 12), and constipation with pain (n = 9). Three weeks of loperamide 4 mg once nightly was significantly better than placebo at improving stool frequency and stool consistency in those with painless diarrhea and in those with alternating bowel habits and pain. Loperamide led to significantly fewer days of pain in those with alternating bowel habits and pain. Those with alternating bowel habits and no pain experienced no benefit from loperamide, whereas those with constipation experienced worsening symptoms with loperamide. The other double-blind, placebo-controlled study published in 1987 enrolled 25 Swedish patients with IBS with diarrhea as the predominant symptom.[21] In the 21 patients completing the 13-week treatment period, loperamide (titrated dose ranging from 2 to 8 mg nightly) was superior to placebo at improving stool consistency ($P<.001$), pain ($P<.02$), urgency ($P<.05$), and overall response ($P<.03$). The most recently published study was a double-blind, placebo-controlled trial enrolling 90 Norwegian patients with IBS.[22] Although IBS was not subtyped in this study and 21 patients were not included in the analysis, 5 weeks of loperamide (dose range of 2–6 mg nightly) was superior to placebo at improving stool frequency ($P<.05$), and stool consistency (P<.05). Those receiving loperamide reported an increase in nocturnal abdominal pain compared with placebo (P<.05).

The ACG Task Force recently performed a systematic review of antidiarrheals in the treatment of IBS and concluded that "The antidiarrheal agent loperamide is not more effective than placebo at reducing abdominal pain or global symptoms of IBS, but is an effective agent for treatment of diarrhea, improving stool frequency and stool consistency (Grade 2C). RCTs with other antidiarrheal agents have not been performed. Safety and tolerability data on loperamide are lacking."[13] An earlier systematic review by the ACG Functional Disorders Task Force in 2002 concluded that although none of the trials reported high-quality data, loperamide was an effective treatment of diarrhea, but no more effective than placebo for the treatment of global IBS symptoms or abdominal pain.[23] The investigators further concluded that adverse event data on loperamide were limited and it was safest for use in IBS-D.[23]

ANTISPASMODICS

Abdominal pain or discomfort is a cardinal feature of IBS, a symptom that has been traditionally ascribed to intestinal smooth-muscle spasm. Observation and clinical studies have suggested that an exaggerated motility response of the small bowel and colon to environmental stimuli may be responsible for the symptoms experienced in IBS.[18,24–27] For this reason antispasmodics have been and remain a mainstay of therapy for the symptoms of IBS. Antispasmodics encompass several different drug classes, including antimuscarinics, smooth-muscle relaxants, anticholinergics, and unique agents such as pinaverium, an ammonium derivative with calcium channel blocking action, and trimebutine, a peripheral opiate agonist.[28] Of these various antispasmodics, only 4 specific anticholinergic agents are currently available in the United States: hyoscyamine, dicyclomine, belladonna, and propantheline. Given their mechanism of action, these agents are directed at those subgroups of IBS, with a predominant symptom of abdominal pain and stool patterns that are either mixed or more diarrheal in nature. The anticholinergic properties of these agents restrict their usefulness in clinical practice. Common side effects, including dry mouth, dizziness, blurry vision, confusion (particularly in elderly patients), urinary retention, and constipation, often limit the usefulness of these agents in the treatment of IBS. The propensity of these agents to promote constipation makes them a less attractive option for patients with IBS-C. Further, anticholinergics should be avoided in elderly patients, who are more prone to the development of significant side effects.

Although antispasmodics remain among the most commonly prescribed drugs for IBS, the clinical evidence supporting their use is limited. Of the 4 antispasmodics available in the United States, only dicyclomine has been assessed in placebo-controlled clinical trials involving patients with IBS.[29,30] The first trial was a double-blind, crossover, placebo-controlled trial involving 29 patients divided into a spastic colon group or painless diarrhea group, each receiving 2 weeks of therapy.[29] Although several methodological limitations exist in this study, including the lack of an IBS definition, a crossover study design, inadequate sample size, and short duration of therapy, a dose of dicyclomine 20 mg 3 times was superior to placebo in addressing bowel urgency and relief of pain with urgency. This second trial was a double-blind, placebo-controlled trial showing the superiority of 2 weeks of dicyclomine to placebo in the treatment of 71 patients with IBS with predominant constipation.[30] Despite several methodological limitations associated with this study (only 71 of 97 enrolled patients were analyzed, short treatment period), dicyclomine was superior to placebo with regard to overall improvement of symptoms and decreased abdominal pain.

However, the dose of dicyclomine used in this study (40 mg 4 times daily) led to frequent anticholinergic side effects and is not practically useful in routine clinical practice.

Given the lack of high-quality studies addressing the efficacy of specific antispasmodic agents, attempts to estimate the efficacy of this class of drugs for IBS have been undertaken through systematic review and meta-analysis. The most recent systematic review and meta-analysis of antispasmodics as a class was performed by the ACG IBS Task Force.[13] The Task Force concluded that "Certain antispasmodics (hyoscine, cimetropium, and pinaverium) may provide short-term relief of abdominal pain/discomfort in IBS (Grade 2C). Evidence for long-term efficacy is not available (Grade 2B). Evidence for safety and tolerability are limited (Grade 2C)." The Task Force identified 22 studies suitable for inclusion in their systematic review. Only 1 of these studies involved a drug available in the United States.[30] Three studies evaluated hyoscine, a different preparation than the agent, hyoscyamine, which is available in the United States.[31–33] Drugs not available in the United States that were included in this analysis included otilonium,[34–36] cimetropium,[37,38] pinaverium,[39,40] trimebutine,[41,42] alverine,[43] mebeverine,[44] pirenzipine,[45] prifinium,[46] propinox,[47] and a trimebutine/rociverine combination.[48] Most of these clinical trials are dated, with only 3 of the studies performed in the last 10 years. The Task Force also acknowledged that these clinical trials were collectively fraught with methodological flaws, including diagnostic criteria used, inclusion criteria used, dosing schedule used, duration of therapy studied, study end points used to assess response, and study size (only 3 studies enrolled more than 100 patients). With these limitations in mind, the 22 trials collectively included data from 1778 patients with IBS. The pooled analysis of these studies revealed an RR of symptoms persisting with antispasmodics compared with placebo of 0.68 (95% CI 0.57–0.81) and an NNT of 5 to prevent IBS symptoms from persisting in 1 patient. A pooled analysis was also performed on the 13 studies, including 1379 patients in whom adverse effects were reported. The Task Force acknowledged significant heterogeneity among these patients; however, the RR of a patient experiencing side effects with antispasmodics was 1.62 (95% CI 1.05–2.50), with a number needed to harm with antispasmodics of 18 (95% CI 7–217).

Other systematic reviews have yielded mixed results regarding the efficacy of antispasmodics for IBS. A systematic review has recently been performed on mebeverine in the treatment of IBS.[49] This analysis included the pooled results of 8 randomized clinical trials (6 compared with placebo) involving a total of 555 patients (63% female) of all IBS subtypes. The investigators reported that although well tolerated, the effect of mebeverine on global improvement and the specific symptom of abdominal pain was not statistically significant compared with placebo. A meta-analysis of smooth-muscle relaxants was performed on 23 randomized clinical trials, including the drugs cimetropium, hyoscine, mebeverine, otilium, pinaverium, and trimebutine.[50] Collectively, global improvement and pain relief was reported in 56% and 53%, respectively, by those receiving the smooth-muscle relaxants compared with response rates of 38% and 41%, respectively, in the placebo group (P<.001 in both cases). A smaller systematic review of 16 RCTs evaluating smooth-muscle relaxants reported an NNT of 1.6 to 6.7 to achieve symptom relief in patients with IBS with pain as predominant symptom.[51] In this study, muscle relaxants were found to be efficacious in 13 of the 16 studies, although only 7 studies were considered to be of high quality.

Although the individual studies have primarily involved antispasmodics not available in the United States and have been criticized for their low quality, as a group they have shown efficacy in the treatment of abdominal pain in IBS. These agents are therefore likely to be most effective in those patients with IBS with a predominant symptom of abdominal pain. These agents can worsen constipation and should therefore be used cautiously in patients with IBS with a predominance of constipation.

SEROTONERGIC AGENTS

Serotonin (5-HT) is the neurotransmitter primarily produced and stored in enterochromaffin cells located throughout the intestinal epithelium, with 95% of total body concentration of 5-HT residing in the gastrointestinal tract.[52] Acting through the intrinsic and extrinsic afferent nervous system of the gastrointestinal tract, 5-HT plays an important role in various aspects of gastrointestinal sensory, secretory, absorptive, and motility function.[53] Recent research has identified abnormal serotonergic activity in association with IBS.[54] Several studies describe increased serotonergic activity in association with IBS-D.[55–59] Likewise, a decrease in serotonergic activity has been observed in IBS-C.[57,58] The use of pharmacologic agents targeting serotonin receptors has therefore evolved from these observations of the role of 5-HT in gastrointestinal health and disease. Of the identified serotonin-receptor subtypes, the 5-HT_{1p}, 5-HT_3, 5-HT_4, and 5-HT_7 receptors are the most clinically relevant for gastrointestinal tract functioning.[53] Receptor agonists of 5-HT_1 have been shown to improve gastric accommodation,[60] slow gastric emptying,[61] and stimulate activity of the migratory motor complex.[62] Receptor antagonists of 5-HT_3 have been reported to slow small bowel transit, decrease intestinal secretion, and decrease colonic tone and transit.[53,63–66] Agonists of the 5-HT_4 receptor have shown an ability to accelerate gastric emptying,[67–69] improve gastric accommodation,[70,71] accelerate small bowel transit,[69] accelerate colonic transit,[69] and possibly decrease visceral sensation.[72] No 5-HT_1 or 5-HT_4 receptor agents are approved for the treatment of IBS in the United States or Canada. The 5-HT_4 agonist tegaserod was removed from the market in 2009 for safety issues. The 5-HT_3 antagonist alosetron is available through a restricted-access program for use in women with severe IBS-D who have failed conventional therapies.

Alosetron

Alosetron is the only 5-HT_3 antagonist approved by the US Food and Drug Administration (FDA) for the treatment of IBS-D (**Table 2**). Rigorous, large clinical trials have consistently shown the efficacy of alosetron in the global and individual symptoms of IBS-D in women. A multicenter, placebo-controlled, randomized trial of 647 women with IBS-D or IBS-M reported superiority of alosetron in providing adequate relief of abdominal pain and discomfort compared with placebo for the 3 months of therapy (41% vs 29%).[73] Alosetron also significantly decreased urgency, reduced stool frequency, and increased stool consistency. Constipation occurred in 30% of those taking alosetron compared with 3% in the placebo group. A second multicenter, randomized, placebo-controlled trial of 626 women (71% with IBS-D, 26% with IBS-M) also reported a superiority of alosetron over placebo in providing adequate relief of abdominal pain and discomfort for the 3 months of therapy (43% vs 26%).[74] Alosetron significantly decreased urgency, reduced stool frequency, and increased stool firmness within 1 week of therapy, which persisted throughout the treatment period. Constipation occurred in 25% of those taking alosetron compared with 5% in the placebo group. The pooled effects of alosetron on QOL were also assessed in these 2 clinical trials.[75] Compared with placebo, a significantly higher percentage of those receiving alosetron experienced improvement in 3 QOL domains, including food/diet, social functioning, and role-physical on the validated generic QOL instrument, the SF-36. Another 12-week, randomized, placebo-controlled trial was

Table 2
FDA-approved peripheral acting therapies in the treatment of IBS

Drug	FDA-approved IBS Indication	FDA-approved Dose	Special Prescribing Issues
Alosetron	Treatment of severe IBS-D in women failing conventional therapy	Initial dose of 0.5 mg twice a day for first 4 weeks Can increase to 1 mg twice a day for subsequent 4 weeks	Prescribing provider and patient receiving treatment must participate in a risk management plan Anatomic and biochemical abnormalities of the gastrointestinal tract must be excluded before initiating therapy Treatment must be stopped if no relief of symptoms experienced with 4 weeks of therapy at a dose of 1 mg twice a day
Lubiprostone	Treatment of IBS-C in women aged 18 years or older	8 µg twice a day with food	Women of childbearing potential must have a negative pregnancy test documented before initiating therapy and use contraception while on therapy

performed on 801 women with IBS (98% with IBS-D and 2% with IBS-M) and showed superiority of 1 mg twice a day of alosetron over placebo in adequately controlling urgency (73% vs 57%) and improving the global IBS symptoms (76% vs 44%).[76] Participants in this trial also reported overall treatment satisfaction and satisfaction with 11 specific medication attributes of alosestron.[77]

A 48-week, randomized, placebo-controlled clinical trial has been performed on 714 women with IBS (80% with IBS-D, 20% with more frequent urgency) to assess long-term safety and efficacy of alosetron at a dose of 1 mg twice daily.[78] Those receiving alosetron experienced greater adequate relief of IBS pain in 9 of the 12 months of the study and greater control of urgency in all 12 months compared with placebo. There were no differences in adverse events or serious adverse events between the 2 groups except for constipation occurring more frequently in the alosetron group. A recent randomized, placebo-controlled trial of 705 women with IBS-D has reported efficacy of lower doses of alosetron in providing global improvement in IBS symptoms, adequate relief of IBS pain and discomfort, and improvement in bowel symptoms (0.5 mg and 1 mg total daily dose).[79] Constipation was reported with less frequency in these lower treatment doses (9% on 0.5 mg/d and 16% on 1 mg/d). A dose-ranging, randomized, placebo-controlled trial has recently been performed on 662 men with IBS-D.[80] In this 12-week treatment trial, those receiving 1 mg of alosetron twice daily were more like than those receiving placebo to report adequate relief of pain in discomfort (53% vs 40%). Firmer stool was reported at all doses of alosetron, although there was no significant effect of alosetron on urgency, bowel movement number, or bloating. Constipation was the most common side effect reported, and was dose related, occurring in 15% of those receiving 1 mg twice daily. There was a possible episode of ischemic colitis in a patient receiving alosetron at a dose of 0.5 mg twice daily.

An evidence-based systematic review has been performed by the ACG Task Force on IBS, with the Task Force concluding that "alosetron is more effective than placebo at relieving global IBS in male (Grade 2B) and female (Grade 2A) patients with IBS with diarrhea. Potentially serious side effects including constipation and colonic ischemia occur more commonly in patients treated with alosetron compared with placebo (Grade 2A). The benefits and harms balance for alosetron is most favorable in women with IBS-D who have not responded to conventional therapies (Grade 1B). The quality of evidence for efficacy of $5\text{-}HT_3$ antagonists in IBS is high."[13] The most recent meta-analysis pooled the data from 8 clinical trials of alosetron and 3 clinical trials of the $5\text{-}HT_3$ antagonist cilansetron (which was never marketed).[81] This analysis, which included a total of 7216 patients with IBS, found $5\text{-}HT_3$ antagonists more effective than placebo in treating IBS-D. The RR of IBS symptoms persisting with $5\text{-}HT_3$ antagonists was 0.78 (95% CI 0.71–0.86) compared with placebo.

Alosetron was initially approved for the treatment of women with IBS-D in February 2000 and subsequently withdrawn from the US marketplace in November 2000 because of the infrequent occurrence of significant side effects, including severe complications of constipation and ischemic colitis. During this postmarketing period, 80 cases of ischemic colitis and 100 cases of serious complications of constipation had been reported. These postmarketing surveillance data were later reviewed by an expert panel, which reported a postadjudication rate of 1.1 cases of ischemic colitis per 1000 patient-years of alosetron use and 0.66 cases of serious complications of constipation with 1000 patient-years of alosetron use.[82] A small number of hospitalizations, surgical interventions, and deaths were identified in affected patients taking alosetron. The panel also reported an increased rate of ischemic colitis in the alosetron treatment group compared with the placebo group in a pooled analysis of the available clinical trials (0.15% vs 0.0%, $P = .03$). In the clinical trial dataset, there was no difference in the occurrence of serious side effects between the alosetron and placebo groups, and all cases of ischemic colitis were reversible without long-term sequelae.

Largely as a consequence of phone calls and letters from patients, alosetron was reapproved by the FDA in June 2002 for the treatment of women with severe IBS-D failing to respond to conventional therapies. It is available for this specific indication through a risk management plan that includes specific dosing instructions, an educational program for prescribing physicians and patients to improve awareness and management of constipation and ischemic colitis, and a standardized patient monitoring program while on therapy. Alosetron is initially prescribed at a dose of 0.5 mg once or twice daily. After 4 weeks of therapy, this dose can be increased to a maximum of 1 mg twice daily if well tolerated and a higher dose is needed for symptom management. If adequate relief of IBS-D symptoms has not occurred after 4 weeks of therapy at a dose of 1 mg twice daily, alosetron should be discontinued. The complication risk of alosetron under this risk management plan has been carefully monitored since reapproval. Safety data from November 2002 to June 2008 including 203,939 prescriptions for 29,072 patients were recently reported.[83] Compared with the postmarketing period before the withdrawal of alosetron, this analysis found a reduction in the absolute numbers of cases of ischemic colitis and complications of constipation, but no significant differences in the incidence rates for either complication (0.95 and 0.36 cases per 1000 patient-years, respectively). All cases were of short duration, with improvement after prompt withdrawal of alosetron under this risk management plan. There were no episodes of mesenteric ischemia, bowel perforation, surgical intervention, need for transfusion, toxic megacolon, or death.

Tegaserod

Tegaserod was the only 5-HT$_4$ receptor agonist available in North America for the treatment of women with IBS-C until it was voluntarily withdrawn from the market in 2009. Tegaserod is a selective 5-HT$_4$ receptor partial agonist approved in 2002 for the treatment of women with IBS-C. The efficacy and tolerability of tegaserod in the treatment of women with IBS-C was initially reported in 3 multicenter, double-blind, placebo-controlled trials involving more than 3000 patients from the Western hemisphere.[84–86] These pivotal clinical trials consistently reported the superiority of tegaserod over placebo at improving global IBS symptoms and individual symptoms of abdominal pain, stool frequency, stool consistency, straining, and bloating. The results led to the FDA's approval of tegaserod in April 2002 for short-term use in women suffering from IBS-C. The precise reason for the effect of tegaserod on the global symptoms of IBS has remained incompletely defined. In preclinical trials tegaserod has had promotility effects in the small and large intestine[87–90] and modulation of visceral sensation.[72,91–93] There was evidence to suggest tegaserod was also effective in the treatment of women with IBS-M.[94]

The safety and tolerability of tegaserod was reported in multiple large 12-week clinical trials[84,85,95,96] as well as a 12-month safety trial.[97] The most commonly reported side effects included diarrhea, headache, and abdominal pain. Tegaserod was designated as a pregnancy category B drug by the FDA. Of the 31 pregnancies occurring during the clinical trials, there was a nonsignificant increased miscarriage rate of 17% (4/23) in women receiving tegaserod versus 12% (1/8) in the placebo group (not significant). No pregnancy-related complications were reported in the clinical trials. Although there were no reports of ischemic colitis in the clinical trials, 26 cases of possible colonic ischemia were reported during postmarketing surveillance, with an estimated incidence of 7 to 8 cases of colonic ischemia per 100,000 patient-years of tegaserod use.[98] This finding led to the addition of a precaution on tegaserod labeling regarding the risk of colonic ischemia.

On March 30, 2007 the sales and marketing of tegaserod were suspended after a review of the clinical trials database uncovered unexpected increased incidence of cardiovascular and cerebrovascular events in the tegaserod treatment group compared with those taking placebo.[99] A pooled analysis had been performed on clinical trials involving tegaserod. This analysis revealed a total of 13 cardiovascular ischemic events (3 myocardial infarctions, 1 sudden cardiac death, 6 cases of unstable angina, and 3 cerebrovascular accidents) in 11,614 patients treated with tegaserod compared with 1 event in the 7031 patients receiving placebo. Although the event rates were low (0.1% in the tegaserod group compared with 0.01% in the placebo group), the difference was found to be statistically significant ($P = .02$). Furthermore, it was reported that all patients experiencing a cardiovascular ischemic event were either at risk or had a history of cardiovascular disease before study enrollment. The significance and explanation for this discrepancy remain unknown. There has been speculation that tegaserod may induce platelet aggregation through actions on 5-HT$_4$ receptors found on platelets.[100] Several studies have used various patient databases to assess for increased cardiovascular ischemic events in those prescribed tegaserod. A case-control study involving more than 18,000 patients from the Intermountain Healthcare database in Utah identified 12 cardiovascular events in 2603 patients receiving tegaserod versus 54 cardiovascular events in 15,618 matched controls.[101] This finding yielded an incidence rate of 0.46% in tegaserod users versus an incidence rate of 0.35% in controls (odds ratio = 1.27, 95% CI 0.68–2.38, $P = .46$). Investigators concluded that no association between tegaserod use and cardiovascular events was identified in their study. An observational cohort study was also performed on more than 100,000 patients using the Ingenix Research Database Mart, a US health insurance claims database.[102] In this study researchers found no increase in cardiovascular ischemic events in those taking tegaserod versus matched controls over a period of 6 months (cardiovascular RR = 1.14 [95% CI 0.83–1.56], stroke RR = 1.09 [95% CI 0.49–2.02]). Despite the results of these retrospective database studies, no clear conclusions have been reached regarding the cardiovascular safety profile of tegaserod. Tegaserod remained available in the United States for a short time through a restrictive compassionate program. Tegaserod was completely removed from the market in 2009 and is no longer available in the United States or Canada. There are no plans by the manufacturer to reintroduce tegaserod to the market.

LUBIPROSTONE

Lubiprostone is the only chloride channel activator with FDA approval for the management of IBS-C (see **Table 2**). Lubiprostone is an oral bicyclic fatty acid derivative of prostaglandin E_1. It is a potent and highly selective activator of the type-2 chloride channel (ClC-2) located on the apical side of human intestinal epithelial cells.[103] ClC-2 is a voltage-gated transmembrane chloride channel that regulates chloride ion transport across the cellular membrane.[104] ClC-2 is found in cells throughout the body and throughout the gastrointestinal tract.[105] Primary functions of ClC-2 channels include maintenance of the membrane potential of the cell, regulation of pH and cell volume, and regulation of chloride ion channel transport and fluid secretion. Through dose-dependent ClC-2 activation, lubiprostone promotes a net flow of chloride ions across the apical membrane of epithelial cells. This process leads to passive paracellular movement of sodium ions and water and a resultant net increase in fluid secretion into the lumen of the intestine.[103] These physiologic effects are felt to underlie the clinical benefits of lubiprostone.

Initial studies investigating the effects of lubiprostone in healthy adults reported an acceleration of small bowel transit and colonic transit and an increase in frequency of bowel movement.[106,107] Three RCTs involving a total of 688 adults reported the efficacy of lubiprostone in the treatment of chronic idiopathic constipation.[108–110] In these trials, lubiprostone was consistently found to be superior to placebo at increasing the number of weekly spontaneous bowel movements. Lubiprostone was also effective in improving stool consistency, straining, constipation severity, bloating, and treatment effectiveness. The most commonly reported side effects included nausea, headache, and diarrhea. A pooled analysis of 91 patients meeting diagnostic criteria for IBS-C from the 2 phase III constipation trials revealed significant improvements in constipation symptoms as well as abdominal symptoms with lubiprostone compared with placebo.[111] This observation led to further evaluation of lubiprostone in the treatment of IBS-C.

The efficacy and tolerability of lubiprostone have been assessed in several high-quality RCTs. A phase II, dose-ranging, double-blind, placebo-controlled trial was performed in 194 adults meeting Rome II criteria for IBS (92% female, 83% White).[112] In this trial, participants were randomized to 1 of 4 12-week treatment arms: placebo, lubiprostone 8 μg twice daily, lubiprostone 16 μg twice daily, or lubiprostone 24 μg twice daily. All 3 doses of lubiprostone were superior to placebo with regard to frequency of spontaneous bowel movement ($P \leq .0499$), constipation severity ($P \leq .0056$), stool consistency ($P < .0001$), and straining ($P \leq .0094$) in each of the

3 months of treatment. Those randomized to lubiprostone also experienced significantly less abdominal discomfort/pain than those receiving placebo at months 1 and 2 (P = .0431 and P = .0336, respectively). Bloating was significantly improved with lubiprostone versus placebo at months 1 and 2 (P = .0298 and P = .0398, respectively). Adverse events were greatest in those taking 16 μg twice daily or 24 μg twice daily. The 8-μg dose taken twice daily had the best efficacy and safety profile, and was therefore the dose selected for further study in subsequent phase III clinical trials.

Two phase III 12-week, multicenter, double-blind, randomized, placebo-controlled trials further evaluated lubiprostone in a total of 1167 patients (92% female) meeting the Rome II criteria for IBS-C.[113] In these trials, participants were randomized in 2:1 fashion to receive lubiprostone 8 μg twice a day (n = 780) or placebo (n = 387). The studies used a rigorous and previously untested primary end point. For this end point, participants used a 7-point balanced Likert scale to answer the following question: "How would you rate your relief of IBS symptoms (abdominal pain/discomfort, bowel habits, and other IBS symptoms) over the past week compared with how you felt before you entered the study?" Those reporting at least moderate relief in 4 of 4 weeks or significant relief in 2 of 4 weeks were considered monthly responders. An overall responder had to be a monthly responder in 2 of the 3 months of the clinical trial. This rigorous end point was designed to minimize the placebo effect. In these 2 phase III trials, those on lubiprostone were nearly twice as likely to be responders as those on placebo (18% vs 10%, P = .001). Lubiprostone was also superior to placebo in improving individual IBS symptoms, including abdominal discomfort/pain, stool consistency, straining, constipation severity, and QOL. The most common treatment-related side effects were nausea (8%), diarrhea (6%), and abdominal pain (5%). There was no difference in serious side effects between those taking lubiprostone and placebo (1% in both groups). The results of these 2 large well-designed clinical trials led to the FDA's approval in April 2008 for the use of lubiprostone in the treatment of women aged 18 years and older suffering from IBS-C.

Since the FDA's approval of lubiprostone in the treatment of IBS-C, several additional studies reported in abstract form have further characterized the effects of lubiprostone on IBS-C symptoms. A 36-week open-labeled extension trial using lubiprostone 8 μg twice daily was performed in 476 participants from the 2 initial phase III clinical trials.[114] Using the same primary end point as in the initial phase III trials, those receiving lubiprostone during the initial 12-week phase III trial experienced an increase in response from 15% to 37% and those initially receiving placebo experienced an increase in response from 8% to 31% at the conclusion of the 36-week extension period. Diarrhea (4.8%) and nausea (3.5%) were the most commonly reported side effects in this extension trial. No treatment-related serious side effects were reported during the 48 weeks of therapy. A withdrawal trial was also performed on selected participants from 1 of the pivotal phase III clinical trials.[115] Those receiving lubiprostone for the initial 12 weeks were randomly assigned to continue on lubiprostone 8 μg twice daily for an additional 4 weeks or given placebo. The response rate at 16 weeks was 38% in those continued on lubiprostone and 40% in those switched to placebo. This curious finding might be explained by residual benefits of lubiprostone extending beyond its discontinuation or regression to the mean in the placebo group. A retrospective analysis of data from the 2 phase III trials was performed to determine which individual IBS symptoms were most responsible for the global improvement in IBS.[116] The findings of this study suggested that the beneficial effects of lubiprostone on multiple IBS symptoms were responsible for its efficacy for global IBS-C symptoms. The effects of lubiprostone on QOL measures were assessed through a retrospective analysis of data from the initial 2 phase III clinical trials.[117] This analysis revealed significant improvement in the QOL domains of health worry (*P* = .025) and body image (*P* = .015), with a trend for improvement in overall IBS-QOL score and domains of social reaction, food avoidance, and dysphoria in those receiving lubiprostone compared with those receiving placebo.

The efficacy of lubiprostone in the treatment of IBS-C was critically evaluated by the ACG IBS Task Force.[13] An evidence-based systematic review was performed, with the Task Force concluding that "Lubiprostone in a dose of 8µg twice daily is more effective than placebo in relieving global IBS symptoms in women with IBC-S (Grade 1B rating)." Lubiprostone is contraindicated in patients with mechanical bowel obstruction and should be avoided in patients with preexisting diarrhea. In addition to the side effects of nausea, diarrhea, and headache, there have been postmarketing reports of dyspnea. This side effect has been specifically described as "chest tightness" or "difficulty taking a breath" occurring within an hour of taking the first dose. The dyspnea typically resolves over several hours but sometimes reoccurs with subsequent dosing. Similar symptoms were reported in the clinical trials. This adverse event occurred more frequently in those with chronic constipation receiving 24 µg twice daily than those with IBS-C receiving 8 µg twice daily (>2.5% vs 0.4%, respectively). Although not considered a serious event, the potential for dyspnea has been added in safety labeling under "warnings and precautions." Lubiprostone carries a pregnancy category C rating because of fetal demise in guinea pig studies. The manufacturer recommends documentation of a negative pregnancy test before initiation of therapy and use of contraception while taking lubiprostone in women capable of childbearing. The ACG Task Force also concluded a need for further studies in men with IBS-C before a recommendation for use in this population.

SUMMARY

A variety of peripheral acting agents, including fiber supplements, laxatives, antidiarrheals, antispasmodics, the serotonergic antagonist alosetron, and the chloride channel activator lubiprostone, are used in the treatment of IBS. Fiber supplements, laxatives, antidiarrheals, and antispasmodics are most effective on specific individual symptoms associated with this syndrome. The evidence supporting the use of these agents in IBS is largely anecdotal, although they are generally safe and well tolerated. On the other hand, alosetron and lubiprostone have shown efficacy in the global as well as individual symptoms of IBS in high-quality clinical trials. Alosetron has a restricted FDA indication for treatment of women with severe IBS-D refractory to traditional therapy. For safety purposes, alosetron can be prescribed only through a specific risk management program. Lubiprostone is approved only for the treatment of women aged 18 years or older suffering from IBS-C. Because of safety related to the fetus, lubiprostone cannot be taken during pregnancy.

REFERENCES

1. Longstreth GF, Thompson WG, Chey WD, et al. Functional bowel disorders. Gastroenterology 2006;130(5):1480–91.
2. Sadik R, Bjornsson E, Simren M. The relationship between symptoms, body mass index, gastrointestinal transit and stool frequency in patients with irritable bowel syndrome. Eur J Gastroenterol Hepatol 2010;22(1):102–8.
3. Camilleri M. Motor function in irritable bowel syndrome. Can J Gastroenterol 1999;13(Suppl A):8A–11A.

4. Manabe N, Wong BS, Camilleri M, et al. Lower functional gastrointestinal disorders: evidence of abnormal colonic transit in a 287 patient cohort. Neurogastroenterol Motil 2010;22(3):293, e82.
5. Deiteren A, Camilleri M, Burton D, et al. Effect of meal ingestion on ileocolonic and colonic transit in health and irritable bowel syndrome. Dig Dis Sci 2010; 55(2):384–91.
6. Cann PA, Read NW, Brown C, et al. Irritable bowel syndrome: relationship of disorders in the transit of a single solid meal to symptom patterns. Gut 1983; 24(5):405–11.
7. Stevens J, VanSoest PJ, Robertson JB, et al. Comparison of the effects of psyllium and wheat bran on gastrointestinal transit time and stool characteristics. J Am Diet Assoc 1988;88(3):323–6.
8. Ford AC, Talley NJ, Spiegel BM, et al. Effect of fibre, antispasmodics, and peppermint oil in the treatment of irritable bowel syndrome: systematic review and meta-analysis. BMJ 2008;337:a2313.
9. Parisi GC, Zilli M, Miani MP, et al. High-fiber diet supplementation in patients with irritable bowel syndrome (IBS): a multicenter, randomized, open trial comparison between wheat bran diet and partially hydrolyzed guar gum (PHGG). Dig Dis Sci 2002;47(8):1697–704.
10. Parisi G, Bottona E, Carrara M, et al. Treatment effects of partially hydrolyzed guar gum on symptoms and quality of life of patients with irritable bowel syndrome. A multicenter randomized open trial. Dig Dis Sci 2005;50(6):1107–12.
11. Toskes PP, Connery KL, Ritchey TW. Calcium polycarbophil compared with placebo in irritable bowel syndrome. Aliment Pharmacol Ther 1993;7(1):87–92.
12. Chiba T, Kudara N, Sato M, et al. Colonic transit, bowel movements, stool form, and abdominal pain in irritable bowel syndrome by treatments with calcium polycarbophil. Hepatogastroenterology 2005;52(65):1416–20.
13. Brandt LJ, Chey WD, Foxx-Orenstein AE, et al. An evidence-based position statement on the management of irritable bowel syndrome. Am J Gastroenterol 2009;104(Suppl 1):S1–35.
14. Quartero AO, Meineche-Schmidt V, Muris J, et al. Bulking agents, antispasmodic and antidepressant medication for the treatment of irritable bowel syndrome. Cochrane Database Syst Rev 2005;2:CD003460.
15. American College of Gastroenterology Functional Gastrointestinal Disorders Task Force. Evidence-based position statement on the management of irritable bowel syndrome in North America. Am J Gastroenterol 2002;97(11 Suppl):S1–5.
16. Khoshoo V, Armstead C, Landry L. Effect of a laxative with and without tegaserod in adolescents with constipation predominant irritable bowel syndrome. Aliment Pharmacol Ther 2006;23(1):191–6.
17. Lee OY. Asian motility studies in irritable bowel syndrome. J Neurogastroenterol Motil 2010;16(2):120–30.
18. Chey WY, Jin HO, Lee MH, et al. Colonic motility abnormality in patients with irritable bowel syndrome exhibiting abdominal pain and diarrhea. Am J Gastroenterol 2001;96(5):1499–506.
19. Cann PA, Read NW, Holdsworth CD, et al. Role of loperamide and placebo in management of irritable bowel syndrome (IBS). Dig Dis Sci 1984;29(3):239–47.
20. Hovdenak N. Loperamide treatment of the irritable bowel syndrome. Scand J Gastroenterol Suppl 1987;130:81–4.
21. Lavo B, Stenstam M, Nielsen AL. Loperamide in treatment of irritable bowel syndrome–a double-blind placebo controlled study. Scand J Gastroenterol Suppl 1987;130:77–80.

22. Efskind PS, Bernklev T, Vatn MH. A double-blind placebo-controlled trial with loperamide in irritable bowel syndrome. Scand J Gastroenterol 1996;31(5): 463–8.
23. Brandt LJ, Bjorkman D, Fennerty MB, et al. Systematic review on the management of irritable bowel syndrome in North America. Am J Gastroenterol 2002; 97(11 Suppl):S7–26.
24. Drossman DA, Camilleri M, Mayer EA, et al. AGA technical review on irritable bowel syndrome. Gastroenterology 2002;123(6):2108–31.
25. Kellow JE, Phillips SF. Altered small bowel motility in irritable bowel syndrome is correlated with symptoms. Gastroenterology 1987;92(6):1885–93.
26. Clemens CH, Samsom M, Roelofs JM, et al. Association between pain episodes and high amplitude propagated pressure waves in patients with irritable bowel syndrome. Am J Gastroenterol 2003;98(8):1838–43.
27. Fukudo S, Kanazawa M, Kano M, et al. Exaggerated motility of the descending colon with repetitive distention of the sigmoid colon in patients with irritable bowel syndrome. J Gastroenterol 2002;37(Suppl 14):145–50.
28. Talley NJ. Pharmacologic therapy for the irritable bowel syndrome. Am J Gastroenterol 2003;98(4):750–8.
29. Irritable colon syndrome treated with an antispasmodic drug. Practitioner 1976; 217(1298):276–80.
30. Page JG, Dirnberger GM. Treatment of the irritable bowel syndrome with Bentyl (dicyclomine hydrochloride). J Clin Gastroenterol 1981;3(2):153–6.
31. Ritchie JA, Truelove SC. Treatment of irritable bowel syndrome with lorazepam, hyoscine butylbromide, and ispaghula husk. Br Med J 1979;1(6160): 376–8.
32. Nigam P, Kapoor KK, Rastog CK, et al. Different therapeutic regimens in irritable bowel syndrome. J Assoc Physicians India 1984;32(12):1041–4.
33. Schafer E, Ewe K. [The treatment of irritable colon. Efficacy and tolerance of buscopan plus, buscopan, paracetamol and placebo in ambulatory patients with irritable colon]. Fortschr Med 1990;108(25):488–92 [in German].
34. Glende M, Morselli-Labate AM, Battaglia G, et al. Extended analysis of a double-blind, placebo-controlled, 15-week study with otilonium bromide in irritable bowel syndrome. Eur J Gastroenterol Hepatol 2002;14(12):1331–8.
35. Baldi F, Corinaldesi R, Ferrarini F. Clinical and functional evaluation of octilonium bromide in irritable bowel syndrome. A double blind controlled trial. Clin Trials J 1983;20:77–88.
36. Castiglione F, Daniele B, Mazzacca G. Therapeutic strategy for the irritable bowel syndrome. Ital J Gastroenterol 1991;23(8 Suppl 1):53–5.
37. Centonze V, Imbimbo BP, Campanozzi F, et al. Oral cimetropium bromide, a new antimuscarinic drug, for long-term treatment of irritable bowel syndrome. Am J Gastroenterol 1988;83(11):1262–6.
38. Passaretti S, Guslandi M, Imbimbo BP, et al. Effects of cimetropium bromide on gastrointestinal transit time in patients with irritable bowel syndrome. Aliment Pharmacol Ther 1989;3(3):267–76.
39. Levy C, Charbonnier A, Cachin M. [Pinaverium bromide and functional colonic disease (double-blind study)]. Sem Hop Ther 1977;53(7–8):372–4 [in French].
40. Delmont J. [The value of adding an antispasmodic musculotropic agent in the treatment of painful constipation in functional colopathies with bran. Double-blind study]. Med Chir Dig 1981;10(4):365–70 [in French].
41. Moshal MG, Herron M. A clinical trial of trimebutine (Mebutin) in spastic colon. J Int Med Res 1979;7(3):231–4.

42. Fielding JF. Double blind trial of trimebutine in the irritable bowel syndrome. Ir Med J 1980;73(10):377–9.
43. Mitchell SA, Mee AS, Smith GD, et al. Alverine citrate fails to relieve the symptoms of irritable bowel syndrome: results of a double-blind, randomized, placebo-controlled trial. Aliment Pharmacol Ther 2002;16(6):1187–95.
44. Kruis W, Weinzierl M, Schussler P, et al. Comparison of the therapeutic effect of wheat bran, mebeverine and placebo in patients with the irritable bowel syndrome. Digestion 1986;34(3):196–201.
45. Gilvarry J, Kenny A, Fielding JF. The non-effect of pirenzepine in dietary resistant irritable bowel syndrome. Ir J Med Sci 1989;158(10):262.
46. Piai G, Mazzacca G. Prifinium bromide in the treatment of the irritable colon syndrome. Gastroenterology 1979;77(3):500–2.
47. Di Girolamo G, de los Santos AR, Marti ML, et al. Propinox in intestinal colic: multicenter randomized prospective double-blind study of three doses of propinox vs. placebo in acute intestinal colic pain. Int J Clin Pharmacol Res 2000; 20(1–2):31–40.
48. Ghidini O, Zenari L, Guilarte N, et al. Effects of short-term treatment with coenzyme A or sulodexide on plasma lipids in patients with hypertriglyceridemia (type IV) or mixed hyperlipemia (type IIb). Int J Clin Pharmacol Ther Toxicol 1986;24(7):390–6.
49. Darvish-Damavandi M, Nikfar S, Abdollahi M. A systematic review of efficacy and tolerability of mebeverine in irritable bowel syndrome. World J Gastroenterol 2010;16(5):547–53.
50. Poynard T, Regimbeau C, Benhamou Y. Meta-analysis of smooth muscle relaxants in the treatment of irritable bowel syndrome. Aliment Pharmacol Ther 2001; 15(3):355–61.
51. Jailwala J, Imperiale TF, Kroenke K. Pharmacologic treatment of the irritable bowel syndrome: a systematic review of randomized, controlled trials. Ann Intern Med 2000;133(2):136–47.
52. Keszthelyi D, Troost FJ, Masclee AA. Understanding the role of tryptophan and serotonin metabolism in gastrointestinal function. Neurogastroenterol Motil 2009;21(12):1239–49.
53. Gershon MD, Tack J. The serotonin signaling system: from basic understanding to drug development for functional GI disorders. Gastroenterology 2007;132(1): 397–414.
54. Coates MD, Mahoney CR, Linden DR, et al. Molecular defects in mucosal serotonin content and decreased serotonin reuptake transporter in ulcerative colitis and irritable bowel syndrome. Gastroenterology 2004;126(7):1657–64.
55. Bearcroft CP, Perrett D, Farthing MJ. Postprandial plasma 5-hydroxytryptamine in diarrhoea predominant irritable bowel syndrome: a pilot study. Gut 1998; 42(1):42–6.
56. Houghton LA, Atkinson W, Whitaker RP, et al. Increased platelet depleted plasma 5-hydroxytryptamine concentration following meal ingestion in symptomatic female subjects with diarrhoea predominant irritable bowel syndrome. Gut 2003;52(5):663–70.
57. Dunlop SP, Coleman NS, Blackshaw E, et al. Abnormalities of 5-hydroxytryptamine metabolism in irritable bowel syndrome. Clin Gastroenterol Hepatol 2005; 3(4):349–57.
58. Atkinson W, Lockhart S, Whorwell PJ, et al. Altered 5-hydroxytryptamine signaling in patients with constipation- and diarrhea-predominant irritable bowel syndrome. Gastroenterology 2006;130(1):34–43.

59. Zuo XL, Li YQ, Yang XZ, et al. Plasma and gastric mucosal 5-hydroxytryptamine concentrations following cold water intake in patients with diarrhea-predominant irritable bowel syndrome. J Gastroenterol Hepatol 2007;22(12): 2330–7.

60. Coulie B, Tack J, Sifrim D, et al. Role of nitric oxide in fasting gastric fundus tone and in 5-HT1 receptor-mediated relaxation of gastric fundus. Am J Physiol 1999; 276(2 Pt 1):G373–7.

61. Coulie B, Tack J, Maes B, et al. Sumatriptan, a selective 5-HT1 receptor agonist, induces a lag phase for gastric emptying of liquids in humans. Am J Physiol 1997;272(4 Pt 1):G902–8.

62. Tack J, Coulie B, Wilmer A, et al. Actions of the 5-hydroxytryptamine 1 receptor agonist sumatriptan on interdigestive gastrointestinal motility in man. Gut 1998; 42(1):36–41.

63. Talley NJ, Phillips SF, Haddad A, et al. GR 38032F (ondansetron), a selective 5HT3 receptor antagonist, slows colonic transit in healthy man. Dig Dis Sci 1990;35(4):477–80.

64. Zighelboim J, Talley NJ, Phillips SF, et al. Visceral perception in irritable bowel syndrome. Rectal and gastric responses to distension and serotonin type 3 antagonism. Dig Dis Sci 1995;40(4):819–27.

65. Delvaux M, Louvel D, Mamet JP, et al. Effect of alosetron on responses to colonic distension in patients with irritable bowel syndrome. Aliment Pharmacol Ther 1998;12(9):849–55.

66. Houghton LA, Foster JM, Whorwell PJ. Alosetron, a 5-HT3 receptor antagonist, delays colonic transit in patients with irritable bowel syndrome and healthy volunteers. Aliment Pharmacol Ther 2000;14(6):775–82.

67. Baeyens R, Reyntjens A, Verlinden M. Cisapride accelerates gastric emptying and mouth-to-caecum transit of a barium meal. Eur J Clin Pharmacol 1984; 27(3):315–8.

68. Staniforth DH, Pennick M. Human pharmacology of renzapride: a new gastrokinetic benzamide without dopamine antagonist properties. Eur J Clin Pharmacol 1990;38(2):161–4.

69. Degen L, Petrig C, Studer D, et al. Effect of tegaserod on gut transit in male and female subjects. Neurogastroenterol Motil 2005;17(6):821–6.

70. Tack J, Broeckaert D, Coulie B, et al. The influence of cisapride on gastric tone and the perception of gastric distension. Aliment Pharmacol Ther 1998;12(8): 761–6.

71. Tack J, Vos R, Janssens J, et al. Influence of tegaserod on proximal gastric tone and on the perception of gastric distension. Aliment Pharmacol Ther 2003; 18(10):1031–7.

72. Coffin B, Farmachidi JP, Rueegg P, et al. Tegaserod, a 5-HT4 receptor partial agonist, decreases sensitivity to rectal distension in healthy subjects. Aliment Pharmacol Ther 2003;17(4):577–85.

73. Camilleri M, Northcutt AR, Kong S, et al. Efficacy and safety of alosetron in women with irritable bowel syndrome: a randomised, placebo-controlled trial. Lancet 2000;355(9209):1035–40.

74. Camilleri M, Chey WY, Mayer EA, et al. A randomized controlled clinical trial of the serotonin type 3 receptor antagonist alosetron in women with diarrhea-predominant irritable bowel syndrome. Arch Intern Med 2001;161(14):1733–40.

75. Watson ME, Lacey L, Kong S, et al. Alosetron improves quality of life in women with diarrhea-predominant irritable bowel syndrome. Am J Gastroenterol 2001; 96(2):455–9.

76. Lembo T, Wright RA, Bagby B, et al. Alosetron controls bowel urgency and provides global symptom improvement in women with diarrhea-predominant irritable bowel syndrome. Am J Gastroenterol 2001;96(9):2662–70.
77. Olden K, DeGarmo RG, Jhingran P, et al. Patient satisfaction with alosetron for the treatment of women with diarrhea-predominant irritable bowel syndrome. Am J Gastroenterol 2002;97(12):3139–46.
78. Chey WD, Chey WY, Heath AT, et al. Long-term safety and efficacy of alosetron in women with severe diarrhea-predominant irritable bowel syndrome. Am J Gastroenterol 2004;99(11):2195–203.
79. Krause R, Ameen V, Gordon SH, et al. A randomized, double-blind, placebo-controlled study to assess efficacy and safety of 0.5 mg and 1 mg alosetron in women with severe diarrhea-predominant IBS. Am J Gastroenterol 2007; 102(8):1709–19.
80. Chang L, Ameen VZ, Dukes GE, et al. A dose-ranging, phase II study of the efficacy and safety of alosetron in men with diarrhea-predominant IBS. Am J Gastroenterol 2005;100(1):115–23.
81. Ford AC, Brandt LJ, Young C, et al. Efficacy of 5-HT3 antagonists and 5-HT4 agonists in irritable bowel syndrome: systematic review and meta-analysis. Am J Gastroenterol 2009;104(7):1831–43 [quiz: 1844].
82. Chang L, Chey WD, Harris L, et al. Incidence of ischemic colitis and serious complications of constipation among patients using alosetron: systematic review of clinical trials and post-marketing surveillance data. Am J Gastroenterol 2006;101(5):1069–79.
83. Chang L, Tong K, Ameen V. Ischemic colitis and complications of constipation associated with the use of alosetron under a risk management plan: clinical characteristics, outcomes, and incidences. Am J Gastroenterol 2010;105(4): 866–75.
84. Muller-Lissner SA, Fumagalli I, Bardhan KD, et al. Tegaserod, a 5-HT(4) receptor partial agonist, relieves symptoms in irritable bowel syndrome patients with abdominal pain, bloating and constipation. Aliment Pharmacol Ther 2001; 15(10):1655–66.
85. Novick J, Miner P, Krause R, et al. A randomized, double-blind, placebo-controlled trial of tegaserod in female patients suffering from irritable bowel syndrome with constipation. Aliment Pharmacol Ther 2002;16(11):1877–88.
86. Lefkowitz M, Shi Y, Heggland J, et al. Tegaserod rapidly improves abdominal pain, bloating and bowel function in patients with C-IBS [abstract]. Gut 2000; 47(Suppl 3):A217.
87. Grider JR, Foxx-Orenstein AE, Jin JG. 5-Hydroxytryptamine4 receptor agonists initiate the peristaltic reflex in human, rat, and guinea pig intestine. Gastroenterology 1998;115(2):370–80.
88. Nguyen A, Camilleri M, Kost LJ, et al. SDZ HTF 919 stimulates canine colonic motility and transit in vivo. J Pharmacol Exp Ther 1997;280(3):1270–6.
89. Degen L, Matzinger D, Merz M, et al. Tegaserod, a 5-HT4 receptor partial agonist, accelerates gastric emptying and gastrointestinal transit in healthy male subjects. Aliment Pharmacol Ther 2001;15(11):1745–51.
90. Prather CM, Camilleri M, Zinsmeister AR, et al. Tegaserod accelerates orocecal transit in patients with constipation-predominant irritable bowel syndrome. Gastroenterology 2000;118(3):463–8.
91. Jiao HM, Xie PY. Tegaserod inhibits noxious rectal distention induced responses and limbic system c-Fos expression in rats with visceral hypersensitivity. World J Gastroenterol 2004;10(19):2836–41.

92. Schikowski A, Thewissen M, Mathis C, et al. Serotonin type-4 receptors modulate the sensitivity of intramural mechanoreceptive afferents of the cat rectum. Neurogastroenterol Motil 2002;14(3):221–7.

93. Sabate JM, Bouhassira D, Poupardin C, et al. Sensory signalling effects of tegaserod in patients with irritable bowel syndrome with constipation. Neurogastroenterol Motil 2008;20(2):134–41.

94. Chey WD, Pare P, Viegas A, et al. Tegaserod for female patients suffering from IBS with mixed bowel habits or constipation: a randomized controlled trial. Am J Gastroenterol 2008;103(5):1217–25.

95. Kellow J, Lee OY, Chang FY, et al. An Asia-Pacific, double blind, placebo controlled, randomised study to evaluate the efficacy, safety, and tolerability of tegaserod in patients with irritable bowel syndrome. Gut 2003;52(5): 671–6.

96. Nyhlin H, Bang C, Elsborg L, et al. A double-blind, placebo-controlled, randomized study to evaluate the efficacy, safety and tolerability of tegaserod in patients with irritable bowel syndrome. Scand J Gastroenterol 2004;39(2): 119–26.

97. Tougas G, Snape WJ Jr, Otten MH, et al. Long-term safety of tegaserod in patients with constipation-predominant irritable bowel syndrome. Aliment Pharmacol Ther 2002;16(10):1701–8.

98. Schoenfeld P. Review article: the safety profile of tegaserod. Aliment Pharmacol Ther 2004;20(Suppl 7):25–30.

99. Thompson CA. Novartis suspends tegaserod sales at FDA's request. Am J Health Syst Pharm 2007;64(10):1020.

100. Serebruany VL, Mouelhi ME, Pfannkuche HJ, et al. Investigations on 5-HT4 receptor expression and effects of tegaserod on human platelet aggregation in vitro. Am J Ther 2010;17(6):543–52.

101. Anderson JL, May HT, Bair TL, et al. Lack of association of tegaserod with adverse cardiovascular outcomes in a matched case-control study. J Cardiovasc Pharmacol Ther 2009;14(3):170–5.

102. Loughlin J, Quinn S, Rivero E, et al. Tegaserod and the risk of cardiovascular ischemic events: an observational cohort study. J Cardiovasc Pharmacol Ther 2010;15(2):151–7.

103. Cuppoletti J, Malinowska DH, Tewari KP, et al. SPI-0211 activates T84 cell chloride transport and recombinant human ClC-2 chloride currents. Am J Physiol Cell Physiol 2004;287(5):C1173–83.

104. Suzuki M, Morita T, Iwamoto T. Diversity of Cl(-) channels. Cell Mol Life Sci 2006; 63(1):12–24.

105. Lipecka J, Bali M, Thomas A, et al. Distribution of ClC-2 chloride channel in rat and human epithelial tissues. Am J Physiol Cell Physiol 2002;282(4):C805–16.

106. Ueno R. Multiple, escalating, oral-dose study to assess the safety, tolerance and pharmacodynamic profile of lubiprostone in normal healthy volunteers [abstract]. Neurogastroenterol Motil 2005;17(4):626.

107. Camilleri M, Bharucha AE, Ueno R, et al. Effect of a selective chloride channel activator, lubiprostone, on gastrointestinal transit, gastric sensory, and motor functions in healthy volunteers. Am J Physiol Gastrointest Liver Physiol 2006; 290(5):G942–7.

108. Johanson JF, Ueno R. Lubiprostone, a locally acting chloride channel activator, in adult patients with chronic constipation: a double-blind, placebo-controlled, dose-ranging study to evaluate efficacy and safety. Aliment Pharmacol Ther 2007;25(11):1351–61.

109. Johanson JF, Morton D, Geenen J, et al. Multicenter, 4-week, double-blind, randomized, placebo-controlled trial of lubiprostone, a locally-acting type-2 chloride channel activator, in patients with chronic constipation. Am J Gastroenterol 2008;103(1):170–7.
110. Barish CF, Drossman D, Johanson JF, et al. Efficacy and safety of lubiprostone in patients with chronic constipation. Dig Dis Sci 2010;55(4):1090–7.
111. Johanson J, Wahle A, Ueno R. Efficacy and safety of lubiprostone in a subgroup of constipation patients diagnosed with irritable bowel syndrome with constipation (IBS-C) [abstract]. Am J Gastroenterol 2006;101:s491.
112. Johanson JF, Drossman DA, Panas R, et al. Clinical trial: phase 2 study of lubiprostone for irritable bowel syndrome with constipation. Aliment Pharmacol Ther 2008;27(8):685–96.
113. Drossman DA, Chey WD, Johanson JF, et al. Clinical trial: lubiprostone in patients with constipation-associated irritable bowel syndrome–results of two randomized, placebo-controlled studies. Aliment Pharmacol Ther 2009;29(3): 329–41.
114. Chey WD, Drossman D, Scott C, et al. Lubiprostone is effective and well tolerated through 48 weeks of treatment in adults with irritable bowel syndrome and constipation [abstract]. Gastroenterology 2008;134(4 Suppl 1):A215.
115. Chey WD, Saad RJ, Panas R, et al. Discontinuation of lubiprostone treatment for irritable bowel syndrome with constipation is not associated with symptom increase or recurrence: results from a randomized withdrawal study [abstract]. Gastroenterology 2008;134(4 Suppl 1):A401.
116. Chey WD, Drossman D, Scott C, et al. What symptoms drive global symptom improvement with lubiprostone in patients with irritable bowel syndrome and constipation: data from two multicenter, randomized, placebo-controlled trials [abstract]. Gastroenterology 2008;134(4 Suppl 1):A28.
117. Drossman D, Chey WD, Scott C, et al. Health-related quality of life in adults with irritable bowel syndrome with constipation: results of a combined analysis of two phase 3 studies with lubiprostone [abstract]. Gastroenterology 2008; 134(4 Suppl 1):A469.

Centrally Acting Therapies for Irritable Bowel Syndrome

Madhusudan Grover, MD[a], Douglas A. Drossman, MD[b],*

KEYWORDS

- Irritable bowel syndrome • Treatment • Psychotropic agents
- Antidepressants • Behavioral treatments

A more recent expansion in our understanding of irritable bowel syndrome (IBS) is leading to important therapeutic gains. The traditional concept of abnormal motility has been insufficient to explain the symptoms and pathogenesis of IBS and other functional GI disorders (FGIDs). We now recognize that visceral hypersensitivity (enhanced perception of peripheral signals), infection/inflammation, and psychological factors that alter brain-gut axis function are all operative in understanding these disorders.[1] Modalities like brain imaging and brain-gut neurotransmitter research demonstrate a dysregulated brain-gut axis at peripheral, spinal, or supraspinal levels, all of which together contribute toward IBS and other FGID symptoms.[2,3] For example, neurotransmitters like serotonin (5 HT), norepinephrine (NE), corticotrophin-releasing factor (CRF), and opioids, among others, modify both motility and sensation in the gut. This has made centrally acting treatments (psychotropic agents and behavioral treatments) a particularly attractive treatment strategy because of their modulation of 5-HT and NE pathways causing overarching effects on the brain-gut axis in addition to their use for managing associated psychological disturbances that are commonly associated with these disorders.[4]

The use of psychotropic agents for FGIDs has grown significantly in the past 2 decades.[5] Nowadays, at least every 1 in 8 patients with IBS is offered an antidepressant.[6] A recent pharmacy database study from the United Kingdom has shown that patients prescribed ongoing therapy for presumed IBS are 2 to 4 times more likely to be prescribed central nervous system (CNS)-acting drugs than

The authors have no disclosures.
a Division of Gastroenterology and Hepatology, Mayo Clinic, 200 First Street Southwest, Rochester, MN 55905, USA
b Division of Gastroenterology and Heptology, UNC Center for Functional GI and Motility Disorders, 4150 Bioinformatics, CB 7080, University of North Carolina, Chapel Hill, NC 27599-7080, USA
* Corresponding author.
E-mail address: drossman@med.unc.edu

Gastroenterol Clin N Am 40 (2011) 183–206
doi:10.1016/j.gtc.2010.12.003
0889-8553/11/$ – see front matter © 2011 Elsevier Inc. All rights reserved.

controls.[7] These included antidepressants, anxiolytics, antipsychotics, and hypno-sedatives. In a study from Sweden, after anti-acids, antidepressants were the most commonly used drug category reported by IBS patients.[8] In a recent survey of around 2000 IBS patients, about 31% reported antidepressant use.[9] However, it still remains a challenging strategy because of insufficient understanding and the complex nature of these disorders, lack of well-designed drug studies, and variability among the treatment efficacy end points.[10]

This article describes the rationale, mechanisms, efficacy, side-effects, practical aspects involving use of psychotropics, and behavioral treatments in IBS and other FGIDs with focus on some of the more recent work in this field.

BIOPSYCHOSOCIAL CONSTRUCT OF IRRITABLE BOWEL SYNDROME AND ROLE OF PSYCHOLOGICAL FACTORS

In the biomedical model of medicine, IBS is often considered at the "functional" end of the "functional-organic" spectrum where a disorder is characterized by absence of detectable structural abnormalities using traditional diagnostic techniques, such as endoscopy or imaging. In the past 2 decades, there has been a surge in the research in the area of motility, brain imaging, and neurotransmitters, which has helped define the "brain-gut axis." As a result, pathophysiological understanding of IBS has increased, leading to organification of a "functional" disorder.[11–13] In fact, IBS can be best conceptualized with a biopsychosocial construct where an influence of central nervous system at spinal and supraspinal levels results in sensory and motor dysfunction of the GI tract. The trigger can be peripheral (eg, GI infection, abdominal surgery) or central (eg, history of abuse) but psychosocial factors often play an important role in perpetuation and clinical manifestation of this disorder through centrally mediated pathways. The influence of these factors becomes increasingly significant with increasing severity of these disorders.

Psychosocial factors can play a vital role at any and all stages in the natural history of IBS, being responsible for predisposition, precipitation, and perpetuation of symptoms and illness behavior. In one series, up to three-fourths of patients with FGID seeking care at a tertiary care referral center meet diagnostic criteria for a psychiatric disorder, most commonly anxiety and depression,[14] although in general the prevalence is much lower for patients seen in primary care or even general gastroenterology practice.[15] A history of major stressful life events, such as sexual abuse, separation, and personal losses are common in IBS, particularly for patients with more severe symptoms who perpetuate the severity via maladaptive illness behavior (catastrophizing).[16,17] Abuse, life stress, and poor or maladaptive coping can directly influence symptom severity, health-related quality of life (HRQOL), and response to treatment.[18] Feelings of distress in response to the GI condition can have adverse effects on psychological state or health status independent of presence of a preexisting psychiatric diagnosis. Furthermore, a negative workup, incomplete understanding, and an unsatisfactory explanation from the physician lead to constant worry, fear, and anxiety and often perpetuates the symptom severity.[19] Postinfectious (PI)-IBS provides an ideal example of psychological factors on IBS disease process.[20] Psychosocial distress at the time of infection has been shown to be an independent predictor of later development of PI-IBS. Stress has been proposed to act by overarching effects on inflammation and the brain-gut axis in PI-IBS.

In addition, a subgroup of patients with IBS, particularly with more severe and refractory symptoms, report many non-GI symptoms, and some have hypothesized the existence of broader neurophysiological processes (eg, so called "somatization") in up to 15% to 45% of patients with IBS.[21] In effect, these patients have central dysregulation of pain regulatory pathways[22] and often have comorbid problems such as fibromyalgia, chronic fatigue, or chronic generalized pain. This understanding has important implications on using centrally acting treatments, alone or in combination, to target this broader polysymptomatic process with FGIDs and even predicting response to these agents. These individuals may set lower thresholds for symptom reporting and often turn out to be "nonresponders" to a variety of different, especially peripherally based, pharmacologic interventions.[23]

RATIONALE FOR THE USE OF PSYCHOTROPIC AGENTS AND BEHAVIORAL THERAPIES

Most widely used psychotropic agents in IBS and other FGIDs are antidepressants, especially tricyclic antidepressants (TCAs). The rationale for the use of these agents in IBS is highlighted in **Box 1**. In spite of significant heterogeneity in study designs and treatment end points, several reviews and meta-analyses have shown both pain reduction and global improvement as potential benefits of antidepressants in IBS and other FGIDs.[24,25] A recent American College of Gastroenterology–funded meta-analysis showed significantly decreased relative risk of persistent IBS symptoms with antidepressant treatment.[24] Others have estimated an overall improvement in IBS with an odds ratio of 2.6 to 4.2.[26] On average, 3 to 4 patients needed to be treated with an antidepressant to improve 1 patient's symptom.[24,26] Up to 80% of patients with IBS appear to have moderate to greater physician-rated benefits in an open-label clinical practice, and adherence to antidepressants is higher than for other treatments.[6,27] The peripheral effects of these agents on the gut may be of secondary importance considering that most patients treated with antidepressants have failed treatment with conventional gut-acting agents. In addition, studies on therapeutic effects of antidepressants on visceral hypersensitivity are mixed.[28,29] Also, treatment satisfaction with TCAs[30] or selective serotonin reuptake inhibitors (SSRIs)[31,32] has not been consistently correlated with reduction in the pain ratings. Overall, the benefit with these agents, especially SSRIs seems to correlate more with improvement in global measures of well-being rather than improvements in pain ratings. This improvement in global distress is still therapeutic, as morbidity associated with FGIDs is linked to

---

Box 1
Potential benefits for use of psychopharmacological agents in FGIDs

Central effects:

1. Alters central pain perception: analgesia or antihyperalgesia.

2. Therapeutic effects on mood: to manage general anxiety, hypervigilance, symptom-related anxiety, agoraphobia, and increased stress responsiveness.

3. Treatment of associated psychiatric disorders: depression, posttraumatic stress disorder, somatization.

4. Treatment of associated sleep disturbances.

Peripheral effects:

1. Peripheral analgesic effects: alters visceral afferent signaling.

2. Effect in GI physiology (motility and secretion) via effects on cholinergic, noradrenergic, and serotonergic pathways.

3. Smooth muscle effects on viscera, eg, gastric fundic relaxation.

global distress in the form of social impairment, work absenteeism, and other functional limitations.

The concept of neuroplasticity with loss of cortical neurons in psychiatric trauma, and neurogenesis (ie, regrowth of neurons) with clinical treatment, also provides rationalization for the use of central treatments. Functional MRI studies have shown reduced neuron density in cortical brain regions involved in emotional and pain regulation in patients with pain disorder[33] and with IBS.[34] Notably, recent data suggest that antidepressant (and possibly psychological) treatments may restore lost neurons. Levels of brain-derived neurotrophic factor, a precursor of neurogenesis, increase with antidepressant treatment and correlate with longer periods of treatment and with the degree of recovery from depression.[35] Furthermore, the longer patients are treated with antidepressants, the lower is the frequency of relapse or recurrence of the depression.[36] These findings provide insight into neuronal growth regulation in key areas of the central pain matrix and provide new and important opportunities for research and patient care using antidepressants for treatment of IBS.[37]

PSYCHOTROPIC AGENTS

Four major classes of psychotropic agents of interest and investigation in IBS are tricyclic antidepressants (TCAs), selective serotonin reuptake inhibitors (SSRIs), serotonin-norepinephrine reuptake inhibitors (SNRIs), and atypical antipsychotics. Among these, TCAs and SSRIs have been most widely studied. However, other agents, especially SNRIs, are gaining popularity for treatment for other chronic pain conditions such as fibromyalgia and are likely to be further explored in IBS and other FGIDs.

Tricyclic Antidepressants

The tricyclic antidepressants (TCAs) are the most rigorously studied class of psychotropic agents used in IBS. The results of some of the recent randomized controlled trials (RCTs) are summarized in **Table 1**. The reason for marginal intention-to-treat effects in our large study was because one-fourth of the patients dropped out from the treatment arm, primarily because of side effects. However, a per protocol post hoc analysis showed a 20% effect size margin.[30] Clouse and colleagues[27] reported managing 138 patients with IBS with antidepressants in whom TCAs were used 130 times, newer agents 39 times, and anxiolytics 47 times. Improvement occurred in 89% and complete remission in 61% of patients. For the most part, despite methodological problems in designing good studies with antidepressants, there is evidence of treatment benefit with TCAs, providing patients are able to stay on medication.

TCAs reduce pain sensitivity in chronic neuropathic animal models, more effectively than SSRIs.[44] In animal studies, they reduce the frequency of nerve impulses evoked by noxious distension in the colon.[44,45] The analgesic properties are also likely contributed by alpha-adrenergic, sodium channel blockade, and N-methyl D-aspartate (NMDA) antagonistlike action.[46] Their effect on visceral perception has been mixed.[47] A recent study showed that TCAs do not have significant effects on gastric motor function or satiation post nutrient challenge in healthy individuals.[48] In another recent proof on concept study, amitriptyline appeared to decrease stress-induced rectal hypersensitivity in patients with IBS, thus providing mechanistic insights of potential disease-modifying actions of TCAs.[49]

The lack of substantive data on peripheral analgesic properties of TCAs in humans suggests that the more pronounced effects are on central pain modulation. In functional MRI studies, the mid cingulate cortex (MCC) is activated during painful rectal

Table 1
Recent studies on use of TCAs in IBS

Citation	Drug	Sample	Study Design	Outcome
Drossman et al,[30] 2003	Desipramine	Women; moderate to severe IBS (n = 431)	12 weeks Multicenter, comparator-controlled RCT	Per-protocol analysis: desipramine superior to placebo; intention-to-treat analysis: not significant. With dosages up to 150 mg, there is no relationship between total dose or plasma level and the clinical response.[38]
Otaka et al,[39] 2005	Amitriptyline	Refractory Functional Dyspepsia (n = 14)	4 weeks Double-blind RCT	Amitriptyline showed 66.7% efficacy in famotidine-failed group and 75.0% efficacy in the mosapride-failed group.
Morgan et al,[40] 2005	Amitriptyline	Women with severe IBS (n = 19)	4 weeks RCT	During stress, amitriptyline reduced pain-related cerebral activations in the perigenual ACC and the left posterior parietal cortex.
Vahedi et al,[41] 2008	Amitriptyline	IBS-D (n = 50)	8 weeks Double-blind RCT	Lower incidence of loose stool and feeling of incomplete defecation. Increased report of "loss of all symptoms" compared with placebo (68% vs 28%)
Bahar et al,[42] 2008	Amitriptyline	Adolescent IBS (n = 33)	13 weeks Double-blind RCT	Improved overall quality of life. Reduction in IBS diarrhea. Improved abdominal pain.
Abdul-Baki et al,[43] 2009	Imipramine	IBS (n = 107)	12 weeks RCT	Higher global symptom relief. Improvements in SF-36 scales.

Abbreviations: ACC, anterior cingulate cortex; IBS, irritable bowel syndrome; RCT, randomized controlled trial; TCA, tricyclic antidepressant.

distensions in patients with IBS. This activation is associated with poor clinical status in severe IBS and there is reduced activation with clinical improvement.[50] Those with IBS and abuse report more pain, greater MCC activation, and reduced activity of anterior cingulate cortex (ACC), which is implicated in pain inhibition and arousal.[51] Furthermore, amitriptyline reduced brain activation during pain in the perigenual (limbic) ACC and parietal association cortex during stress.[40]

Side effects depend on the class of TCAs but for the most part include sedation, anticholinergic (constipation, tachycardia, urinary retention, and xerostomia), and CNS side effects (insomnia, agitation, nightmares). TCAs can slow both small bowel and colonic transit.[52] However, the side-effect profiles vary because of differences in the postsynaptic receptor affinities. In general, secondary amine TCAs (eg, desipramine, nortriptyline) are better tolerated than tertiary amine TCAs (eg, amitriptyline, imipramine) because of their lower antihistaminic and anticholinergic properties.[5]

Selective Serotonin Reuptake Inhibitors

The main action of selective serotonin reuptake inhibitors (SSRIs) is to selectively inhibit the re-uptake of 5HT and block the 5HT transporter protein at the level of presynaptic nerve endings, increasing synaptic concentration of 5HT. These agents have effects on animal somatic pain models, although weaker than the TCAs.[44] Activation of opioid descending spinal pathways is another proposed mechanism of action. Data on visceral pain perception with SSRIs is mixed and central nociceptive effects of SSRIs have not been studied. **Table 2** summarizes some of the recent RCTs on use of SSRIs in FGIDs.

SSRIs can be used to augment the overall benefit of TCAs through their effect on anxiety, or in sufficient dosages in treating psychiatric comorbidities. Although they are reported to show analgesic effect in neuropathic pain, back pain, and migraines, the studies do not show an independent effect of SSRIs on GI pain.[58]

In summary, SSRIs may help in treating FGIDs because (1) they improve global well-being and some GI-specific symptoms (independent of the effects on depression); (2) they have anxiolytic properties and can target social phobia, agoraphobia, and symptom-related anxiety; (3) they may augment the analgesic effects of other agents (TCAs); and (4) they treat psychiatric comorbidities. In contrast to the dose ranging needed with TCAs, SSRIs do not require much dose readjustment because of selective receptor affinity for 5HT. Thus, diarrhea may be a side effect, and SSRIs may benefit patients with constipation. Within the SSRI class, paroxetine has more muscarinic effect and may be useful for those with predominant diarrhea. Fluoxetine has a longer half-life and fewer withdrawal effects and may be selected if poor compliance is an issue. Side effects include agitation, hostility, and suicidality.

Serotonin-Norepinephrine Reuptake Inhibitors

The serotonin-norepinephrine reuptake inhibitors (SNRIs), including venlafaxine, duloxetine, and desvenlafaxine, may potentially be as effective as the TCAs, owing to their dual blockade of reuptake of NE and 5HT receptors. Currently these agents are gaining increased use for other somatic painful conditions such as fibromyalgia.

Duloxetine

This is the only SNRI agent that has been studied for the treatment of IBS. In a 12-week open-label study of 15 nondepressed patients with IBS, duloxetine (60 mg daily dosage) appeared to be effective for pain, severity of illness, quality of life, loose stool, work and family disability, and anxiety. Seven patients withdrew from the study reporting adverse effects, most notably constipation.[59] It lacks activity at muscarinic, histamine, and adrenergic sites, thus avoids side effects seen with TCAs. Most common side effects are nausea, dry mouth, and constipation. It can also rarely cause nonspecific elevation of liver enzymes.

Venlafaxine

This agent inhibits both 5HT and NE reuptake and can increases stimulated pain threshold.[60] However, higher dosages are needed to achieve pain benefit. It is also a mild inhibitor of dopamine reuptake. It can improve postprandial accommodation of the proximal stomach and may be used for treating functional dyspepsia.[61] However, a recent multicenter RCT did not identify any benefit in functional dyspepsia.[62] It has also been shown to decrease the sensitivity of colon to rectal distension.[63] Nausea is a side effect to consider. Venlafaxine can be started at 37.5 mg or 75 mg and titrated up to achieve maximum effect.

Desvenlafaxine

Desvenlafaxine is related to venlafaxine in molecular structure and has recently been released for treatment of depression. Its benefit for painful GI conditions has not yet been studied.

Milnacipran

Milnacipran also belongs to the SNRI class and is currently used in the treatment of fibromyalgia. This agent can also potentially be used in pain-related chronic GI conditions such as IBS.

Atypical Antipsychotics

Atypical antipsychotics have gained wide acceptance for treatment of bipolar disorder and schizophrenia because of their efficacy and low toxicity. They can also be beneficial in lower dosages for patients with FGIDs because of their analgesic properties (alone or in synergism with antidepressants[64]) and their sedative and anxiolytic effects. They can enhance a more normal sleep architecture.[65] Recently, we have used a low-dose atypical antipsychotic agent (eg, quetiapine 25–100 mg) with dopaminergic actions for augmenting treatment in our patients with FGIDs. Preliminary data from our clinic show that about 50% of patients with severe IBS and functional abdominal pain syndrome, who previously failed antidepressants and who are prescribed quetiapine with an antidepressant, stay on it, and most of those who do stay on it achieve some benefit.[66] Olanzapine, another drug of this class, has shown promise for treating nausea and vomiting in patients with cancer.[67]

BEHAVIORAL THERAPIES

The forms of behavioral therapies studied in IBS include cognitive behavior therapy (CBT), relaxation training, psychodynamic interpersonal therapy (PIT), hypnotherapy, mindfulness meditation, and multicomponent psychotherapies. The rationale for their use is summarized in **Box 2**.

Cognitive Behavior Therapy

Cognitive behavior therapy (CBT) is based on social learning theory, which recognizes that behavior is shaped as a result of its social consequences. It focuses on ways to increase or decrease thoughts and behaviors. With treatment of the IBS, it typically consists of 3 components: cognitive change where patients learn to recognize the relationship between their beliefs and symptoms, addressing thoughts, behaviors, and responses that result from their experiences, and changing behavior by teaching

Table 2
Recent studies on the use of SSRIs in IBS

Citation	Drug	Sample	Study Design	Outcome
Creed et al,[31] 2003	Paroxetine	Severe IBS (n = 257)	3 months Multicenter Parallel RCT	Improved physical component of SF-36 (QOL) scale. Decreased health care costs at 1-year follow-up. Decreased severity and number of days in pain.
Kuiken et al,[28] 2003	Fluoxetine	IBS (n = 40)	6 weeks Double-blind placebo-controlled RCT	Improved abdominal pain score (53% vs 26%) showing trends toward significance. Patients on fluoxetine were more likely to continue with the drug (84% vs 37%). Significant reduction in abdominal pain in patients with gut hypersensitivity.
Tabas et al,[32] 2004	Paroxetine	IBS (n = 110)	12 weeks Double-blind placebo-controlled RCT	Improved overall well-being. Increased desire to continue medication. Less IBS-related anxiety. Decreased food avoidance. Benefit seen in nondepressed.
Vahedi et al,[53] 2005	Fluoxetine	IBS-C (n = 44)	12 weeks Double-blind RCT	Decreased abdominal discomfort and bloating. Increased frequency of bowel movements and decreased stool consistency. Insignificant reduction in the mean number of symptoms per patient.

Tack et al,[54] 2006	Citalopram	IBS patients (n = 23)	6 weeks Double-blind placebo-controlled RCT	Improved abdominal pain and bloating. Less impact of symptoms on daily life and improved overall well-being. Effects independent of psychologic and colonic sensory-motor function.
Talley et al,[55] 2008	Imipramine and Citalopram	IBS patients (n = 51)	12 week Multicenter double-blind parallel-group RCT	Imipramine improved bowel symptom severity rating for interference and distress. Imipramine improved depression and SF-36 (mental component) score. Neither imipramine nor citalopram significantly improved Rome III global IBS end point (adequate relief).
Masand et al,[56] 2009	Paroxetine (controlled release)	IBS patients (n = 72)	12 week Double-blind RCT	No significant differences in composite pain scores (primary outcomes). Higher proportion of responders in treatment group per clinical global improvement scale (secondary outcome).
Ladabaum et al,[57] 2010	Citalopram	Nondepressed IBS patients (n = 54)	4 weeks Double-blind RCT	Not superior to placebo in achieving global relief, specific symptom, or QOL improvement.

Abbreviations: IBS, irritable bowel syndrome; QOL, quality of life; RCT, randomized controlled trial; SSRI, selective serotonin reuptake inhibitor.

> **Box 2**
> **Targets for behavioral treatments in FGIDs**
>
> 1. To establish a rational model of illness: reframe maladaptive beliefs
> 2. To reduce overresponsiveness to stress, eg, stress and autonomic reactivity
> 3. To reduce or modify maladaptive psychological responses: catastrophizing, symptom-specific anxiety, shame/guilt
> 4. To reduce or modify maladaptive behaviors, eg, agoraphobia, seeking diagnostic studies

relaxation and stress-management strategies. The specific content of the therapy is based on a biopsychosocial assessment of the patient's background and current difficulties. For example, if a history of sexual abuse interferes with adaptation to the disorder, factors related to the abuse will be discussed. Several studies have looked at CBT for IBS (**Table 3**), but with significant heterogeneity. Various ways to implement CBT (group, individual, therapist based, Internet based) have been assessed. In 2 recent separate analyses, early response (4 weeks) and maladaptive coping have been shown to be predictive of sustained response.[78,79] It has been shown that CBT has a direct effect on global IBS symptom improvement, independent of its effects on distress, and symptom improvements are not moderated by variables reflecting the mental well-being of patients with IBS.[80] Symptom benefit with CBT may be mediated through changes in neural activity of cortical-limbic regions that subserve hypervigilance and emotion regulation.[81]

Relaxation Training

Relaxation techniques are to train patients to counteract physiologic sequelae of stress or anxiety. Five recent studies have assessed efficacy of relaxation therapy in IBS (**Table 4**). Although there has been significant heterogeneity in the study designs, relaxation alone or in combination with CBT and other therapies can be beneficial for IBS symptoms.

Psychodynamic Interpersonal Therapy

Psychodynamic interpersonal therapy (PIT) focuses on the impact of GI symptoms on a person's feelings and relationships. Unlike CBT, the emphasis is on addressing the person's feelings and inner mood states as they relate to flare-ups of symptoms rather than modifying thoughts or cognitions. Bowel disorders have an impact on relationships and family life in a way that can become counterproductive and even damaging for the person with bowel problems and his or her family. PIT looks at the whole marital/relationship system or family system where appropriate, and it can help address and manage issues related to previous sexual/physical abuse. Problems or difficulties with emotions or relationships are brought alive in the sessions, and possible solutions tried and tested out with the therapist, before transference to real-life situations. At the end of the therapy, the patient is provided with a detailed personal letter outlining the key points of therapy, plans for the future, and ways to cope with bowel symptoms should they recur.[87] The key to success is the development of a trusting and supportive relationship with the treating therapist. Interpersonal psychotherapy has been used with success in the treatment of refractory IBS by Guthrie and colleagues,[88] where improvement in symptoms and lesser disability and health care use were reported.[89] Creed and colleagues,[31] when comparing usual medical treatment to paroxetine to PIT, found that paroxetine and PIT significantly reduced pain scores and improved HRQOL compared with usual medical treatment. However, only the psychotherapy group had a reduction in health care cost in the 1-year follow-up period. A recent study by Hyphantis and colleagues[90] has suggested that improvement in interpersonal problems is associated with improved psychosocial distress and improved health status following psychotherapy in patients with IBS.

Hypnotherapy

The essence of hypnotherapy is to create a relaxing, calming environment that allows the patient to refocus away from uncomfortable symptoms and toward a more pleasant perception of his or her current state. It capitalizes on the use of heightened suggestibility, where the patient becomes receptive to viewing his or her symptoms in a more refocused and positive way. Hypnotherapy has been shown to be effective for the treatment of IBS[91] and a recent review concluded that hypnosis has a favorable impact on refractory IBS symptoms.[92] One approach directs the patient away from experiencing uncomfortable sensations such as pain toward more positive interpretations of the sensations such as a gentle "flowing" of their bowels. Its long-term efficacy in IBS[93] and functional dyspepsia[94] has been shown. Thus, hypnotherapy is becoming increasingly recognized as a viable treatment modality for IBS.[93,95] The mechanism is unclear, although there is some evidence that it reduces gut contractility and normalizes pain thresholds after balloon rectal distension,[96] although this has not been confirmed by others.[97] Some have demonstrated changes similar to that after CBT[98] with reduction in anxiety and somatization scores[97] without physiologic changes in the gut. The median response rate to hypnosis treatment is 87%, bowel symptoms can generally be expected to improve by about half, psychological symptoms and life functioning improve after treatment, and therapeutic gains are likely long lasting.[92]

Mindfulness Meditation

As compared with relaxation, which is a passive state of mind, mindfulness meditation is an active, yet relaxed state of consciousness. A recent, open, 10-week pilot study showed significant reduction in symptoms, which were sustained at follow-up.[99] Another recent study has demonstrated feasibility to undertake a rigorous RCT of mindfulness training for people with IBS, using a standardized protocol adapted for those experiencing IBS.[100] More investigations are expected exploring mindfulness meditation in IBS in the future.

Multicomponent Psychotherapies

Three studies have compared multicomponent psychological therapy to control therapy or physicians' "usual management."[101-103] IBS symptoms persisted in 55 (51.9%) of 106 of those assigned to multicomponent psychological therapy compared with 80 (76.2%) of 105 of those allocated to control therapy or physicians' "usual management." These results suggest a potential role for multicomponent psychotherapy in the treatment of IBS.

PRACTICAL STRATEGIES ON WHEN AND HOW TO USE CENTRALLY ACTING TREATMENTS

Fig. 1 conceptualizes a stepwise algorithm for treatment of IBS across the severity of symptoms. For most patients with mild to moderate symptoms, there are environmental- and gut-related factors (eg, dietary, infection, bowel injury, hormonal factors) that "turn up" afferent excitation system. For milder symptoms, lifestyle and dietary changes may be sufficient. For more moderate symptoms, medications that act on

Table 3
Recent studies on the use of CBT in IBS

Citation	Therapy	Sample	Study Design	Outcome
Greene et al,[68] 1994	CBT	IBS patients (n = 20)	8 weeks RCT	Significant symptom reduction (80% vs 10% of the monitoring group). Results sustained at 3-month follow-up.
Payne and Blanchard,[69] 1995	CBT	IBS patients (n = 34)	8 weeks Triple arm RCT	Significantly greater reductions in individual GI symptoms and composite GI symptom index change compared with wait list or support group. Results maintained at 3-month follow-up.
Vollmer et al,[70] 1998	CBT	IBS patients (n = 32)	8 weeks Triple-arm RCT	Significantly greater GI composite symptom score reduction as compared with monitoring. No differences in group and individual cognitive treatment groups.
Drossman et al,[30] 2003	CBT	Women; moderate to severe IBS (n = 431)	12 weeks Multicenter RCT	On intention-to-treat analysis, CBT significantly more effective than education alone. Number needed to treat was 3.
Tkachuk et al,[71] 2003	CBT (group therapy)	Refractory IBS (n = 28)	9 weeks	Significant improvement with CBT than weekly telephone contact on posttreatment global measures and daily diary pain scores at 3-month follow-up. Significant improvement in psychological distress and health-related quality of life.
Kennedy et al,[72] 2006	CBT (nurse delivered)	Moderate or severe IBS (resistant to the antispasmodic mebeverine) (n = 149)	6 weeks RCT	Benefit on symptom severity compared with mebeverine alone (persisting at 3 and 6 months after therapy but not later). Persistent (12-month) significant benefit on the work and social adjustment scale.

Blanchard et al,[73] 2007	CBT (group based)	At least moderately severe IBS (n = 202)	8 weeks RCT with active control	Both group CBT and psychoeducational support (active control) were superior to intensive symptom monitoring in long and short term but none was superior to another.
Sanders et al,[74] 2007	CBT (self-administered)	IBS (n = 28)	10 weeks Crossover RCT	Self-help CBT group significantly decreased composite GI symptom scores in comparison with the wait list, but not in QOL scales.
Lackner et al,[75] 2008	CBT (10-session, therapist-administered vs 4-session, patient-administered)	Moderate or severe IBS (n = 71)	10 weeks RCT	At week 12, both CBT versions were significantly superior to wait list in the percentage of participants reporting adequate relief and improvement of symptoms. CBT-treated patients reported significantly improved QOL and IBS symptom severity but not psychological distress relative to wait list.
Hunt et al,[76] 2009	Internet-based brief CBT	IBS (n = 54)		Treatment completers experienced statistically and clinically significant declines in IBS symptoms and improvements in QOL.
Moss-Morris et al,[77] 2010	CBT-based self-management program	IBS (n = 64)	8 weeks RCT	At 2-, 3-, and 6-month follow-up, significantly more reported symptom relief in the self-management group compared with usual treatment; 83% showed significant change in IBS severity scales compared with 49% in the control group at 8 months.

Abbreviations: CBT, cognitive behavior therapy; IBS, irritable bowel syndrome; QOL, quality of life; RCT, randomized controlled trial.

Table 4
Recent studies on the use of relaxation training or therapy in IBS

Citation	Therapy	Sample	Study Design	Outcome
Blanchard et al,[82] 1993	Progressive muscle relaxation	IBS patients (n = 16)	8 weeks RCT	Significant (≥50%) reduction in baselines symptom score compared with symptom monitoring.
Keefer et al,[83] 2001	Relaxation response meditation	IBS patients (n = 16)	6 weeks Controlled treatment study	Significant (≥50%) improvement in IBS composite primary reduction scores compared with symptom monitoring. Improved flatulence, belching, bloating, and diarrhea. Effects persisted at 3-month follow-up.
Boyce et al,[84] 2003	CBT and relaxation therapy	IBS patients (n = 105)	8 weeks Triple-arm RCT	Cognitive behavior and relaxation therapy not to be superior to standard care alone.
Van der Veek et al,[85] 2007	Relaxation training	IBS patients (n = 98)	3 months RCT	IBS symptom severity significantly reduced in relaxation training group compared with standard medical care at 3, 6, and 12 months, Improved QOL. Reduced frequency of doctor visits.
Lahmann et al,[86] 2010	Functional relaxation	IBS patients (n = 80)	5 weeks RCT	Impairment in impairment-severity score (IS). Effects remained stable at 3-month follow-up.

Abbreviations: CBT, cognitive behavior therapy; IBS, irritable bowel syndrome; QOL, quality of life; RCT, randomized controlled trial.

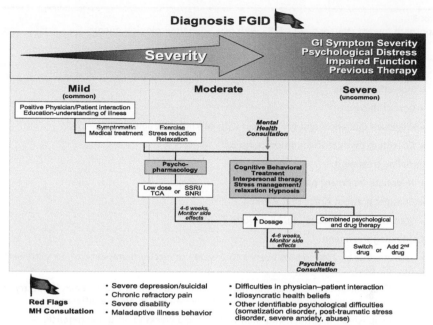

Fig. 1. Treatment algorithm for patients with FGIDs. "Red flags" are indications for considering early referral to a mental health professional. There is a range of intensity of psychological approaches to treatment and intensity of treatment is matched with the severity of FGID. (*From* Grover M, Drossman DA. Psychopharmacologic and behavioral treatments for functional gastrointestinal disorders. Gastrointest Endosc Clin N Am 2009;19(1):151–70, vii–viii; with permission.)

the gut (eg, anticholinergics, peripheral 5HT agents) can be considered. On the opposite end are the 20% of patients who suffer from severe IBS characterized by increased levels of pain, poorer HRQOL, higher levels of health care use, more psychosocial difficulties, and a higher frequency of psychiatric comorbidities. Because these patients are usually refractory to first- and second-line therapies,[18] they require behavioral (eg, CBT, PIT, hypnosis, stress-management/relaxation) or psychotropic agents or a combination of these two. **Fig. 1** also lists some of the red flags that warrant referral to and comanagement with a mental health person, such as a psychotherapist. Notably, many of these treatments can be used in addition to gut-acting agents.

Box 3 summarizes a general approach for prescribing psychotropic agents in IBS. An effective physician-patient relationship is crucial in the management of IBS with psychotropic agents. A positive physician-patient interaction has been related to reduced use of ambulatory health services by patients with IBS.[104] The choice of the agent depends on specific symptoms targeted, side-effect profile, and past experience with antidepressants. The therapeutic benefit may take 4 to 6 weeks to achieve; however, side effects may be reported within 1 to 2 weeks.[105] Starting at a low dose and a closer follow-up, especially in the first week, may increase compliance. It is important to "set the stage" by summarizing the long-term treatment plan and expectations before starting these agents. Global outcomes such as daily function, coping, QOL, and emotional well-being should be emphasized rather than specific GI symptoms. It is important to explain the use of these agents in the context of GI health

---

Box 3
Approach toward management of IBS with psychopharmacological agents

1. Choice of the agent:
   - Specific symptom treated
   - Side-effect profile
   - Cost of the drug
   - Previous experiences and preferences with psychotropic agents
   - Coexisting psychiatric conditions targeted

2. Initiating treatment:
   - Negotiate treatment plan
   - Consider previous drugs that worked
   - Start with a low dosage (eg, 25 mg/d of TCA)

3. Continuing treatment:
   - Escalate dose by 25% to 50% every 1 to 2 weeks to receive therapeutic effect with least possible dose.
   - Watch for side effects. Counsel that most of them disappear in 1 to 2 weeks. If not, try to continue same or lower dose from same class before switching to a different class.
   - Follow-up within first week and then within 2 to 3 weeks to ensure adherence.
   - Gauge treatment benefit with improvement in coping, daily function, QOL, and emotional state.
   - If a poor initial response:

     Re-address patient concerns

     Switch to a different class

     Combination therapies (eg, SSRI+TCA, pharmacologic and psychological treatment)

     If needed, psychiatry consultation for pharmacotherapy.
   - Increase dosages up to full psychiatric dosages if patient can tolerate before discontinuing.
   - If there is no benefit in 6 to 8 weeks on higher dosages, alternate strategies (eg, adding psychological treatment or referral) should be sought.
   - Depending on the response and side effects, another agent with different mechanism of action can be added to augment treatment efficacy and minimize side effects.

4. Stopping treatment: Continue treatment at minimum effective dosages for 6 to 12 months. Long-term therapy may be warranted for some patients. Gradual taper to prevent withdrawal symptoms.

From Grover M, Drossman DA. Psychopharmacologic and behavioral treatments for functional gastrointestinal disorders. Gastrointest Endosc Clin N Am 2009;19(1):151–70, vii–viii; with permission.

---

and share your willingness to continue to work on the patients as they undergo these treatments. Some of the issues with prescribing these agents are a suboptimal dose or failure to escalate dose if the response is poor, there is nonadherence, or if there is a delayed response.[5] Depending on the response and side effects, another agent with different mechanism of action can be added to augment treatment efficacy and minimize side effects. **Table 5** summarizes the class effect of various

Table 5
Class effects of psychotropic agents

	TCAs	SSRIs	SNRIs
Agents	Amitriptyline Imipramine Doxepin Desipramine Nortriptyline	Fluoxetine Sertraline Paroxetine Citalopram Escitalopram	Duloxetine Venlafaxine
Dose range	10–50 mg 10–200 mg (Desipramine)	10–40 mg 25–100 mg (Sertraline)	30–90 mg (Duloxetine) 75–225 (Venlafaxine)
Potential benefits			
Peripheral pain modulation	++	?	++
Central anti-nociception	+++	+	+++
Anxiolysis			
Motility			
Visceral pain	+	+++	+
Sleep	++	+	?
Psychiatric comorbidities	+++ ++ ++ (high doses)	? — +++	? ? +++
Adverse effects	Sedation Constipation Dry mouth/eyes Weight gain Hypotension Sexual dysfunction	Insomnia Diarrhea Night sweats Weight loss Agitation Sexual dysfunction	Nausea Agitation Dizziness Fatigue Liver dysfunction

Time to action	Few days–2 weeks
	  (low doses)
	2–6 weeks
	  (high doses)
		4–6 weeks	4–6 weeks

Efficacy	Good	Moderate	Not well studied
Dose adjustments	Required	Usually Not	Required

Abbreviations: SNRI, serotonin-norepinephrine reuptake inhibitor; SSRI, selective serotonic reuptake inhibitor; TCA, Tricyclic antidepressant; +, weak effect; ++, moderate effect, +++, strong effect.

From Grover M, Drossman DA. Psychopharmacologic and behavioral treatments for functional gastrointestinal disorders. Gastrointest Endosc Clin N Am 2009;19(1):151–70, vii–viii; with permission.

psychotropic agents. Patients with high degrees of somatization tolerate medication side effects poorly, and the overall effectiveness of the medication regimen is impaired. Some investigators have suggested starting with even a lower dose (10 mg of TCA) and escalating slowly in these individuals.[5] Patients with a good response can be successfully maintained on antidepressant medications for months to years and tapering the dosage before withdrawing minimizes the likelihood of withdrawal syndromes.

Failure to maintain treatment occurs in nearly a quarter of outpatients given antidepressants for FGIDs.[106] Somatization features[21] and presence of depression[30] or anxiety most significantly interfered with treatment by predicting side effects, poor treatment response, and premature antidepressant discontinuation. Patients less likely to have a good outcome with antidepressant therapy are those with constipation-predominant IBS, patients with objective indicators of gastrointestinal motility delay, patients with medical comorbidities exacerbated by antidepressant medications, and patients with somatization disorder.[5,30] Management algorithms should include specific strategies targeted at patients with these risk factors and poor treatment adherence.[107]

SUMMARY

As we expand our understanding of etiopathogenesis and clinical manifestations of IBS, the use of centrally acting psychopharmacological and behavioral treatments is expected to grow. Psychosocial factors play a key role in the natural history of IBS, especially at the moderate to severe end of the spectrum. Although better designed treatment trials are needed and in spite of significant heterogeneity among available studies, the evidence favors the use of both psychopharmacological and behavioral therapies. To enhance the therapeutic effect and improve adherence to treatment, an effective physician-patient relationship is essential and guidelines for this can be found elsewhere.[108] Future work in the management of IBS will lead to the evaluation of multicomponent treatments (eg, the common combination of psychotherapy and pharmacotherapy) and physician treatment behaviors.

REFERENCES

1. Drossman DA, Camilleri M, Mayer EA, et al. AGA technical review on irritable bowel syndrome. Gastroenterology 2002;123(6):2108–31.
2. Mayer EA, Naliboff BD, Craig AD. Neuroimaging of the brain-gut axis: from basic understanding to treatment of functional GI disorders. Gastroenterology 2006;131(6):1925–42.
3. Spiller R. Recent advances in understanding the role of serotonin in gastrointestinal motility in functional bowel disorders: alterations in 5-HT signalling and metabolism in human disease. Neurogastroenterol Motil 2007;19(Suppl 2): 25–31.
4. Mayer EA, Tillisch K, Bradesi S. Review article: modulation of the brain-gut axis as a therapeutic approach in gastrointestinal disease. Aliment Pharmacol Ther 2006;24(6):919–33.
5. Clouse RE, Lustman PJ. Use of psychopharmacological agents for functional gastrointestinal disorders. Gut 2005;54(9):1332–41.
6. Whitehead WE, Levy RL, von KM, et al. The usual medical care for irritable bowel syndrome. Aliment Pharmacol Ther 2004;20(11/12):1305–15.
7. Canavan JB, Bennett K, Feely J, et al. Significant psychological morbidity occurs in irritable bowel syndrome: a case-control study using a pharmacy reimbursement database. Aliment Pharmacol Ther 2009;29(4):440–9.
8. Faresjo A, Grodzinsky E, Johansson S, et al. Self-reported use of pharmaceuticals among patients with irritable bowel syndrome in primary care. J Manag Care Pharm 2008;14(9):870–7.
9. Drossman DA, Morris CB, Schneck S, et al. International survey of patients with IBS: symptom features and their severity, health status, treatments, and risk taking to achieve clinical benefit. J Clin Gastroenterol 2009;43(6):541–50.
10. Camilleri M, Mangel AW, Fehnel SE, et al. Primary endpoints for irritable bowel syndrome trials: a review of performance of endpoints. Clin Gastroenterol Hepatol 2007;5(5):534–40.

11. Drossman DA. Presidential address: gastrointestinal illness and the biopsychosocial model. Psychosom Med 1998;60(3):258–67.
12. Drossman DA. The "organification" of functional GI disorders: implications for research. Gastroenterology 2003;124(1):6–7.
13. Grover M, Herfarth H, Drossman DA. The functional-organic dichotomy: postinfectious irritable bowel syndrome and inflammatory bowel disease-irritable bowel syndrome. Clin Gastroenterol Hepatol 2009;7(1):48–53.
14. Lydiard RB. Irritable bowel syndrome, anxiety, and depression: what are the links? J Clin Psychiatry 2001;62(Suppl 8):38–45.
15. Drossman DA. The functional gastrointestinal disorders and the Rome III process. Gastroenterology 2006;130(5):1377–90.
16. Drossman DA, Li Z, Leserman J, et al. Health status by gastrointestinal diagnosis and abuse history. Gastroenterology 1996;110(4):999–1007.
17. Drossman DA, Talley NJ, Olden KW, et al. Sexual and physical abuse and gastrointestinal illness: review and recommendations. Ann Intern Med 1995;123(10):782–94.
18. Drossman DA, Whitehead WE, Toner BB, et al. What determines severity among patients with painful functional bowel disorders? Am J Gastroenterol 2000;95(4):974–80.
19. Posserud I, Agerforz P, Ekman R, et al. Altered visceral perceptual and neuroendocrine response in patients with irritable bowel syndrome during mental stress. Gut 2004;53(8):1102–8.
20. Drossman DA. Mind over matter in the postinfective irritable bowel. Gut 1999;44(3):306–7.
21. North CS, Downs D, Clouse RE, et al. The presentation of irritable bowel syndrome in the context of somatization disorder. Clin Gastroenterol Hepatol 2004;2(9):787–95.
22. Drossman DA. Brain imaging and its implications for studying centrally targeted treatments in IBS: a primer for gastroenterologists. Gut 2005;54(5):569–73.
23. North CS, Hong BA, Alpers DH. Relationship of functional gastrointestinal disorders and psychiatric disorders: implications for treatment. World J Gastroenterol 2007;13(14):2020–7.
24. Ford AC, Talley NJ, Schoenfeld PS, et al. Efficacy of antidepressants and psychological therapies in irritable bowel syndrome: systematic review and meta-analysis. Gut 2009;58(3):367–78.
25. Jailwala J, Imperiale TF, Kroenke K. Pharmacologic treatment of the irritable bowel syndrome: a systematic review of randomized, controlled trials. Ann Intern Med 2000;133(2):136–47.
26. Lesbros-Pantoflickova D, Michetti P, Fried M, et al. Meta-analysis: the treatment of irritable bowel syndrome. Aliment Pharmacol Ther 2004;20(11–12):1253–69.
27. Clouse RE, Lustman PJ, Geisman RA, et al. Antidepressant therapy in 138 patients with irritable bowel syndrome: a five-year clinical experience. Aliment Pharmacol Ther 1994;8(4):409–16.
28. Kuiken SD, Tytgat GN, Boeckxstaens GE. The selective serotonin reuptake inhibitor fluoxetine does not change rectal sensitivity and symptoms in patients with irritable bowel syndrome: a double blind, randomized, placebo-controlled study. Clin Gastroenterol Hepatol 2003;1(3):219–28.
29. Siproudhis L, Dinasquet M, Sebille V, et al. Differential effects of two types of antidepressants, amitriptyline and fluoxetine, on anorectal motility and visceral perception. Aliment Pharmacol Ther 2004;20(6):689–95.

30. Drossman DA, Toner BB, Whitehead WE, et al. Cognitive-behavioral therapy versus education and desipramine versus placebo for moderate to severe functional bowel disorders. Gastroenterology 2003;125(1):19–31.

31. Creed F, Fernandes L, Guthrie E, et al. The cost-effectiveness of psychotherapy and paroxetine for severe irritable bowel syndrome. Gastroenterology 2003; 124(2):303–17.

32. Tabas G, Beaves M, Wang J, et al. Paroxetine to treat irritable bowel syndrome not responding to high-fiber diet: a double-blind, placebo-controlled trial. Am J Gastroenterol 2004;99(5):914–20.

33. Valet M, Gundel H, Sprenger T, et al. Patients with pain disorder show gray-matter loss in pain-processing structures: a voxel-based morphometric study. Psychosom Med 2009;71(1):49–56.

34. Blankstein U, Chen J, Diamant NE, et al. Altered brain structure in irritable bowel syndrome: potential contributions of pre-existing and disease-driven factors. Gastroenterology 2010;138(5):1783–9.

35. Brunoni AR, Lopes M, Fregni F. A systematic review and meta-analysis of clinical studies on major depression and BDNF levels: implications for the role of neuroplasticity in depression. Int J Neuropsychopharmacol 2008;11(8):1169–80.

36. Geddes JR, Carney SM, Davies C, et al. Relapse prevention with antidepressant drug treatment in depressive disorders: a systematic review. Lancet 2003; 361(9358):653–61.

37. Drossman DA. Beyond tricyclics: new ideas for treating patients with painful and refractory functional gastrointestinal symptoms. Am J Gastroenterol 2009; 104(12):2897–902.

38. Halpert A, Dalton CB, Diamant NE, et al. Clinical response to tricyclic antidepressants in functional bowel disorders is not related to dosage. Am J Gastroenterol 2005;100(3):664–71.

39. Otaka M, Jin M, Odashima M, et al. New strategy of therapy for functional dyspepsia using famotidine, mosapride and amitriptyline. Aliment Pharmacol Ther 2005;21(Suppl 2):42–6.

40. Morgan V, Pickens D, Gautam S, et al. Amitriptyline reduces rectal pain related activation of the anterior cingulate cortex in patients with irritable bowel syndrome. Gut 2005;54(5):601–7.

41. Vahedi H, Merat S, Momtahen S, et al. Clinical trial: the effect of amitriptyline in patients with diarrhoea-predominant irritable bowel syndrome. Aliment Pharmacol Ther 2008;27(8):678–84.

42. Bahar RJ, Collins BS, Steinmetz B, et al. Double-blind placebo-controlled trial of amitriptyline for the treatment of irritable bowel syndrome in adolescents. J Pediatr 2008;152(5):685–9.

43. Abdul-Baki H, El Hajj II, Elzahabi L, et al. A randomized controlled trial of imipramine in patients with irritable bowel syndrome. World J Gastroenterol 2009; 15(29):3636–42.

44. Bomholt SF, Mikkelsen JD, Blackburn-Munro G. Antinociceptive effects of the antidepressants amitriptyline, duloxetine, mirtazapine and citalopram in animal models of acute, persistent and neuropathic pain. Neuropharmacology 2005; 48(2):252–63.

45. Su X, Gebhart GF. Effects of tricyclic antidepressants on mechanosensitive pelvic nerve afferent fibers innervating the rat colon. Pain 1998;76(1–2):105–14.

46. Willert RP, Woolf CJ, Hobson AR, et al. The development and maintenance of human visceral pain hypersensitivity is dependent on the N-methyl-D-aspartate receptor. Gastroenterology 2004;126(3):683–92.

47. Gorelick AB, Koshy SS, Hooper FG, et al. Differential effects of amitriptyline on perception of somatic and visceral stimulation in healthy humans. Am J Physiol 1998;275(3 Pt 1):G460–6.

48. Choung RS, Cremonini F, Thapa P, et al. The effect of short-term, low-dose tricyclic and tetracyclic antidepressant treatment on satiation, postnutrient load gastrointestinal symptoms and gastric emptying: a double-blind, randomized, placebo-controlled trial. Neurogastroenterol Motil 2008;20(3):220–7.

49. Thoua NM, Murray CD, Winchester WJ, et al. Amitriptyline modifies the visceral hypersensitivity response to acute stress in the irritable bowel syndrome. Aliment Pharmacol Ther 2009;29(5):552–60.

50. Drossman DA, Ringel Y, Vogt BA, et al. Alterations of brain activity associated with resolution of emotional distress and pain in a case of severe irritable bowel syndrome. Gastroenterology 2003;124(3):754–61.

51. Ringel Y, Drossman DA, Leserman JL, et al. Effect of abuse history on pain reports and brain responses to aversive visceral stimulation: an FMRI study. Gastroenterology 2008;134(2):396–404.

52. Gorard DA, Libby GW, Farthing MJ. Influence of antidepressants on whole gut and orocaecal transit times in health and irritable bowel syndrome. Aliment Pharmacol Ther 1994;8(2):159–66.

53. Vahedi H, Merat S, Rashidioon A, et al. The effect of fluoxetine in patients with pain and constipation-predominant irritable bowel syndrome: a double-blind randomized-controlled study. Aliment Pharmacol Ther 2005;22(5):381–5.

54. Tack J, Broekaert D, Fischler B, et al. A controlled crossover study of the selective serotonin reuptake inhibitor citalopram in irritable bowel syndrome. Gut 2006;55(8):1095–103.

55. Talley NJ, Kellow JE, Boyce P, et al. Antidepressant therapy (imipramine and citalopram) for irritable bowel syndrome: a double-blind, randomized, placebo-controlled trial. Dig Dis Sci 2008;53(1):108–15.

56. Masand PS, Pae CU, Krulewicz S, et al. A double-blind, randomized, placebo-controlled trial of paroxetine controlled-release in irritable bowel syndrome. Psychosomatics 2009;50(1):78–86.

57. Ladabaum U, Sharabidze A, Levin TR, et al. Citalopram provides little or no benefit in nondepressed patients with irritable bowel syndrome. Clin Gastroenterol Hepatol 2010;8(1):42–8.

58. Creed F. How do SSRIs help patients with irritable bowel syndrome? Gut 2006; 55(8):1065–7.

59. Brennan BP, Fogarty KV, Roberts JL, et al. Duloxetine in the treatment of irritable bowel syndrome: an open-label pilot study. Hum Psychopharmacol 2009;24(5): 423–8.

60. Bradley RH, Barkin RL, Jerome J, et al. Efficacy of venlafaxine for the long term treatment of chronic pain with associated major depressive disorder. Am J Ther 2003;10(5):318–23.

61. Chial HJ, Camilleri M, Burton D, et al. Selective effects of serotonergic psychoactive agents on gastrointestinal functions in health. Am J Physiol Gastrointest Liver Physiol 2003;284(1):G130–7.

62. van Kerkhoven LA, Laheij RJ, Aparicio N, et al. Effect of the antidepressant venlafaxine in functional dyspepsia: a randomized, double-blind, placebo-controlled trial. Clin Gastroenterol Hepatol 2008;6(7):746–52 [quiz: 718].

63. Chial HJ, Camilleri M, Ferber I, et al. Effects of venlafaxine, buspirone, and placebo on colonic sensorimotor functions in healthy humans. Clin Gastroenterol Hepatol 2003;1(3):211–8.

64. Fishbain DA, Cutler RB, Lewis J, et al. Do the second-generation "atypical neuroleptics" have analgesic properties? A structured evidence-based review. Pain Med 2004;5(4):359–65.

65. Hamner MB, Deitsch SE, Brodrick PS, et al. Quetiapine treatment in patients with posttraumatic stress disorder: an open trial of adjunctive therapy. J Clin Psychopharmacol 2003;23(1):15–20.

66. Grover M, Dorn SD, Weinland SR, et al. Atypical antipsychotic quetiapine in the management of severe refractory functional gastrointestinal disorders. Dig Dis Sci 2009;54(6):1284–91.

67. Passik SD, Lundberg J, Kirsh KL, et al. A pilot exploration of the antiemetic activity of olanzapine for the relief of nausea in patients with advanced cancer and pain. J Pain Symptom Manage 2002;23(6):526–32.

68. Greene B, Blanchard EB. Cognitive therapy for irritable bowel syndrome. J Consult Clin Psychol 1994;62(3):576–82.

69. Payne A, Blanchard EB. A controlled comparison of cognitive therapy and self-help support groups in the treatment of irritable bowel syndrome. J Consult Clin Psychol 1995;63(5):779–86.

70. Vollmer A, Blanchard EB. Controlled comparison of individual versus group cognitive therapy for irritable bowel syndrome [abstract]. Behav Ther 1998;29:19–23.

71. Tkachuk GA, Graff LA, Martin GL. Randomized controlled trial of cognitive-behavioral group therapy for irritable bowel syndrome in a medical setting [abstract]. J Clin Psychol Med Settings 2003;10:57–69.

72. Kennedy TM, Chalder T, McCrone P, et al. Cognitive behavioural therapy in addition to antispasmodic therapy for irritable bowel syndrome in primary care: randomised controlled trial. Health Technol Assess 2006;10(19):1–67, ii–iv, ix–x.

73. Blanchard EB, Lackner JM, Sanders K, et al. A controlled evaluation of group cognitive therapy in the treatment of irritable bowel syndrome. Behav Res Ther 2007;45(4):633–48.

74. Sanders KA, Blanchard EB, Sykes MA. Preliminary study of a self-administered treatment for irritable bowel syndrome: comparison to a wait list control group. Appl Psychophysiol Biofeedback 2007;32(2):111–9.

75. Lackner JM, Jaccard J, Krasner SS, et al. Self-administered cognitive behavior therapy for moderate to severe irritable bowel syndrome: clinical efficacy, tolerability, feasibility. Clin Gastroenterol Hepatol 2008;6(8):899–906.

76. Hunt MG, Moshier S, Milonova M. Brief cognitive-behavioral Internet therapy for irritable bowel syndrome. Behav Res Ther 2009;47(9):797–802.

77. Moss-Morris R, McAlpine L, Didsbury LP, et al. A randomized controlled trial of a cognitive behavioural therapy-based self-management intervention for irritable bowel syndrome in primary care. Psychol Med 2010;40(1):85–94.

78. Lackner JM, Gudleski GD, Keefer L, et al. Rapid response to cognitive behavior therapy predicts treatment outcome in patients with irritable bowel syndrome. Clin Gastroenterol Hepatol 2010;8(5):426–32.

79. Reme SE, Kennedy T, Jones R, et al. Predictors of treatment outcome after cognitive behavior therapy and antispasmodic treatment for patients with irritable bowel syndrome in primary care. J Psychosom Res 2010;68(4):385–8.

80. Lackner JM, Jaccard J, Krasner SS, et al. How does cognitive behavior therapy for irritable bowel syndrome work? A mediational analysis of a randomized clinical trial. Gastroenterology 2007;133(2):433–44.

81. Lackner JM, Lou CM, Mertz HR, et al. Cognitive therapy for irritable bowel syndrome is associated with reduced limbic activity, GI symptoms, and anxiety. Behav Res Ther 2006;44(5):621–38.

82. Blanchard EB, Greene B, Scharff L, et al. Relaxation training as a treatment for irritable bowel syndrome. Biofeedback Self Regul 1993;18(3):125–32.
83. Keefer L, Blanchard EB. The effects of relaxation response meditation on the symptoms of irritable bowel syndrome: results of a controlled treatment study. Behav Res Ther 2001;39(7):801–11.
84. Boyce PM, Talley NJ, Balaam B, et al. A randomized controlled trial of cognitive behavior therapy, relaxation training, and routine clinical care for the irritable bowel syndrome. Am J Gastroenterol 2003;98(10):2209–18.
85. van der Veek PP, van Rood YR, Masclee AA. Clinical trial: short- and long-term benefit of relaxation training for irritable bowel syndrome. Aliment Pharmacol Ther 2007;26(6):943–52.
86. Lahmann C, Rohricht F, Sauer N, et al. Functional relaxation as complementary therapy in irritable bowel syndrome: a randomized, controlled clinical trial. J Altern Complement Med 2010;16(1):47–52.
87. Howlett S, Guthrie E. Use of farewell letters in the context of brief psychodynamic-interpersonal therapy with irritable bowel syndrome patients [abstract]. Br J Psychother 2001;18(1):52–67.
88. Guthrie E, Creed F, Dawson D, et al. A controlled trial of psychological treatment for the irritable bowel syndrome. Gastroenterology 1991;100(2):450–7.
89. Hamilton J, Guthrie E, Creed F, et al. A randomized controlled trial of psychotherapy in patients with chronic functional dyspepsia. Gastroenterology 2000; 119(3):661–9.
90. Hyphantis T, Guthrie E, Tomenson B, et al. Psychodynamic interpersonal therapy and Improvement in interpersonal difficulties in people with severe irritable bowel syndrome. Pain 2009;145(1–2):196–203.
91. Whorwell PJ, Prior A, Faragher EB. Controlled trial of hypnotherapy in the treatment of severe refractory irritable-bowel syndrome. Lancet 1984;2(8414): 1232–4.
92. Whitehead WE. Hypnosis for irritable bowel syndrome: the empirical evidence of therapeutic effects. Int J Clin Exp Hypn 2006;54(1):7–20.
93. Gonsalkorale WM, Miller V, Afzal A, et al. Long term benefits of hypnotherapy for irritable bowel syndrome. Gut 2003;52(11):1623–9.
94. Calvert EL, Houghton LA, Cooper P, et al. Long-term improvement in functional dyspepsia using hypnotherapy. Gastroenterology 2002;123(6):1778–85.
95. Gonsalkorale WM, Houghton LA, Whorwell PJ. Hypnotherapy in irritable bowel syndrome: a large-scale audit of a clinical service with examination of factors influencing responsiveness. Am J Gastroenterol 2002;97(4):954–61.
96. Lea R, Houghton LA, Calvert EL, et al. Gut-focused hypnotherapy normalizes disordered rectal sensitivity in patients with irritable bowel syndrome. Aliment Pharmacol Ther 2003;17(5):635–42.
97. Palsson OS, Turner MJ, Johnson DA, et al. Hypnosis treatment for severe irritable bowel syndrome: investigation of mechanism and effects on symptoms. Dig Dis Sci 2002;47(11):2605–14.
98. Gonsalkorale WM, Toner BB, Whorwell PJ. Cognitive change in patients undergoing hypnotherapy for irritable bowel syndrome. J Psychosom Res 2004;56(3):271–8.
99. Ljotsson B, Andreewitch S, Hedman E, et al. Exposure and mindfulness based therapy for irritable bowel syndrome—an open pilot study. J Behav Ther Exp Psychiatry 2010;41(3):185–90.
100. Gaylord SA, Whitehead WE, Coble RS, et al. Mindfulness for irritable bowel syndrome: protocol development for a controlled clinical trial. BMC Complement Altern Med 2009;9:24.

101. Blanchard EB, Schwarz SP, Suls JM, et al. Two controlled evaluations of multi-component psychological treatment of irritable bowel syndrome. Behav Res Ther 1992;30(2):175–89.

102. Heitkemper MM, Jarrett ME, Levy RL, et al. Self-management for women with irritable bowel syndrome. Clin Gastroenterol Hepatol 2004;2(7):585–96.

103. Schwarz SP, Blanchard EB, Neff DF. Behavioral treatment of irritable bowel syndrome: a 1-year follow-up study. Biofeedback Self Regul 1986;11(3):189–98.

104. Owens DM, Nelson DK, Talley NJ. The irritable bowel syndrome: long-term prognosis and the physician-patient interaction. Ann Intern Med 1995;122(2): 107–12.

105. Wald A. Psychotropic agents in irritable bowel syndrome. J Clin Gastroenterol 2002;35(Suppl 1):S53–7.

106. Prakash C, Clouse RE. Long-term outcome from tricyclic antidepressant treatment of functional chest pain. Dig Dis Sci 1999;44(12):2373–9.

107. Sayuk GS, Elwing JE, Lustman PJ, et al. Predictors of premature antidepressant discontinuation in functional gastrointestinal disorders. Psychosom Med 2007; 69(2):173–81.

108. Chang L, Drossman DA. Optimizing patient care: the psychosocial interview in the irritable bowel syndrome. Clin Perspect Gastroenterol 2002;5(6):336–41.

Therapies Aimed at the Gut Microbiota and Inflammation: Antibiotics, Prebiotics, Probiotics, Synbiotics, Anti-inflammatory Therapies

Eamonn M.M. Quigley, MD, FRCP, FRCPI

KEYWORDS

• Gut microbiota • Antibiotics • Prebiotics • Synbiotics
• Anti-inflammatories

Several recent observations have raised the possibility that disturbances in the gut microbiota and/or a low-grade inflammatory state may contribute to symptomatology and even, perhaps, the etiology of irritable bowel syndrome (IBS), if not in all sufferers, possibly in some subpopulations. Consequent on these hypotheses and also as a result of blind trial and error by the patient and the physician, several quite unexpected therapeutic categories have found their way into the armamentarium of those who care for IBS sufferers. Before these new (to IBS) agents (eg, probiotics, prebiotics, antibiotics, and anti-inflammatory agents) are discussed, one should first consider the context in which such therapeutic strategies are being considered. The logical place to begin is the microbiota.

THE NORMAL MICROBIOTA: AN ESSENTIAL FACTOR IN HEALTH

The human gastrointestinal (GI) microflora (now more usually referred to as the microbiota) is a complex ecosystem of approximately 300 to 500 bacterial species comprising nearly 2 million genes (the microbiome). Indeed, the number of bacteria within the gut is about 10 times that of all of the cells in the human body. At birth, the entire intestinal tract is sterile; bacteria enter the gut with the first feed.[1] Following infancy, the composition of the intestinal microbiota remains relatively constant

Department of Medicine, Alimentary Pharmabiotic Centre, Cork University Hospital, University College Cork, Clinical Sciences Building, Cork, Ireland
E-mail address: e.quigley@ucc.ie

Gastroenterol Clin N Am 40 (2011) 207–222
doi:10.1016/j.gtc.2010.12.009
0889-8553/11/$ – see front matter © 2011 Elsevier Inc. All rights reserved.

gastro.theclinics.com

thereafter. When disturbed, the microbiota has a remarkable capacity to restore itself and to return to exactly the same state as it was in before.[2]

Because of the normal motility of the intestine (peristalsis) and the antimicrobial effects of gastric acid, the stomach and proximal small intestine contain relatively small numbers of bacteria in healthy subjects; jejunal cultures may not detect any bacteria in as many as 33% of subjects. The microbiology of the terminal ileum represents a transition zone between the jejunum containing predominantly facultative anaerobes and the dense population of anaerobes found in the colon. Bacterial colony counts may be as high as 10^9 colony-forming units (CFU)/mL in the terminal ileum immediately proximal to the ileocecal valve, with a predominance of Gram-negative organisms and anaerobes. On crossing into the colon, the bacterial concentration and variety of the enteric microbiota change dramatically. Concentrations as high as 10^{12} CFU/mL may be found, comprised mainly of anaerobes such as *Bacteroides, Porphyromonas, Bifidobacterium, Lactobacillus,* and *Clostridium*, with anaerobic bacteria outnumbering aerobic bacteria by a factor of 100 to 1000 to 1.[3] The predominance of anaerobes in the colon reflects the fact that oxygen concentrations in the colon are very low; the microbiota has simply adapted to survive in this hostile environment.

It must be emphasized, however, that the true size and diversity of the human microbiota are largely unknown. The application of modern technologies—genomics, metagenomics, and metabolomics—to the study of the colonic microbiota has the potential to expose the true diversity and metabolic profile of the microbiota and the real extent of changes in disease.[4] Techniques based on 16S rDNA sequences have revealed that the diversity of the human microbiota is much greater than previously thought and that most bacterial sequences correspond to unculturable sequences and novel bacteria.[5] At any given level of the gut, the composition of the microbiota also demonstrates variation along its diameter, with certain bacteria tending to be adherent to the mucosal surface while others predominate in the lumen; studies that rely on the analysis of the fecal microbiota alone may miss the impact of an important population of organisms, those closely adherent to the mucosa.[5] In people, the composition of the microbiota is also influenced by age, diet, socioeconomic conditions and, above all, the use of antibiotics. Studies purporting to identify variations in the microbiota in disease states must, accordingly, be interpreted with great care and some degree of skepticism.

The normal enteric bacterial microbiota influences various intestinal functions and plays a key role in nutrition, maintaining the integrity of the epithelial barrier, and the development of mucosal immunity.[6] The relationship between the host's immune system and nonpathogenic constituents of the microbiota is important in protecting the host from colonization by pathogenic species. In this regard, intestinal bacteria produce various substances, ranging from relatively nonspecific fatty acids and peroxides to highly specific bacteriocins, which can inhibit or kill other, potentially pathogenic, bacteria.[7]

THE GUT MICROBIOTA IN DISEASE

The key role of the microbiota in health is only beginning to be understood and it has only been in very recent years that the true extent of the consequences of disturbances in the microbiota, or in the interaction between the microbiota and the host, to health has been recognized.[6,8] Some of these are relatively obvious; for example, when many components of the normal microbiota are eliminated or suppressed by a course of broad-spectrum antibiotics, the stage is set for other organisms that may be pathogenic to step in and cause disease. The classical example of this is antibiotic-associated diarrhea and its deadliest manifestation, *Clostridium difficile* colitis.[9] Similar perturbations in the microbiota are thought to be involved in a devastating form of intestinal inflammation that may occur in newborn and, especially, premature, infants: necrotizing enterocolitis.[10] In other situations, bacteria may simply be where they should not be; if intestinal motility is impaired and/or gastric acid secretion abolished, an environment conducive to the proliferation—in the small intestine—of organisms that are normally confined to the colon results. Small intestinal bacterial overgrowth (SIBO) can significantly disturb both the digestion and absorption of food and the products of digestion.[11] Alternatively, when the immunologic interaction between the microbiota is disturbed, the host may, for example, begin to recognize the constituents of the normal microbiota, not as friend, but as foe and may mount an inappropriate inflammatory response that ultimately may lead to conditions such as inflammatory bowel disease.[12] Injury to the intestinal epithelium, regardless of cause, renders the gut wall leaky and permits luminal bacteria (in whole or in part) to gain access to the submucosal compartments or even to the systemic circulation with the associated potential to cause catastrophic sepsis. This mechanism is thought to account for many of the infections that occur in the critically ill patient in the intensive care unit, for example. Most recently, qualitative changes in the microbiota have been invoked in the pathogenesis of a global epidemic: obesity.[13–15]

PROBIOTICS

Probiotics, derived from the Greek and meaning "for life," are defined as live organisms that, when ingested in adequate amounts, exert a health benefit to the host. There are several commercially available supplements containing viable microorganisms with probiotic properties. The most commonly used probiotics are lactic acid bacteria and nonpathogenic yeasts. Although probiotics have been proposed for use in inflammatory, infectious, neoplastic, and allergic disorders, the ideal probiotic strain, for use in any of these indications, has yet to be identified. The interpretation of available data on probiotics is further confounded by variability in strain selection, dose, delivery vehicle, and evaluation of viability and efficacy.[16]

Probiotics were first described by Metchnikoff in 1908 based on his observations on the longevity of individuals who lived in a certain part of Bulgaria and which he attributed to their ingestion, on a regular basis, of a fermented milk product. Over the years since then, many products have appeared on health food store and supermarket shelves throughout the world that include the term probiotic in their label. Very few fulfill the definition provided:

They may not contain live organisms or have not been adequately tested to ensure that the organisms will survive in the conditions (eg, room temperature) or for the length of time (days, weeks, or months) that is claimed.

They may not confer health benefit, because either, they have never been tested on people or because what tests have been preformed have been inadequate or even negative.

Other issues of quality control continue to complicate the probiotic area. Does the product actually contain the organism and the dose of that organism that the label claims that it contains? Unfortunately, when researchers have analyzed some store products, they have found, not only that organisms claimed to be alive were actually dead, but that the product contained organisms (including pathogens) that it was not supposed to contain.

Some probiotic companies have gone to considerable efforts to ensure that their products do contain the very organisms and in the precise dose that are claimed. These products can guarantee the survival of live organisms over the time and in the conditions specified on the label. Whether these same products can provide the health benefits that they claim can only be deduced from a critical assessment of the medical literature. Fortunately, more and higher quality clinical trials are being performed and can guide the consumer on the optimal product for a given condition. This latter point is critically important; no two probiotics are the same! Even within the same species, different strains may have vastly different and even contrasting effects. Although probiotics have been proposed for use in inflammatory, infectious, neoplastic, and allergic disorders, the ideal probiotic strain for many of these indications has yet to be defined, although progress continues in this area. While probiotic cocktails also have been advocated to maximize effect, it should be noted that some probiotic combinations have been shown to prove antagonistic, rather than synergistic, in certain situations.

Right now the consumer finds it impossible to assess the validity of the many claims made for probiotics. This dilemma stems, in large part, from the manner in which they are regulated. Despite the fact that probiotics are advocated for the management of disease, they are regulated, in most jurisdictions, in a manner that is more akin to a food than a pharmaceutical. This situation may change very soon, as agencies in both the United States and in Europe are currently re-evaluating the status of these products. Deliberations by the European Food Safety Authority on health claims for probiotics pursuant to European Union Regulation 1924/2006[17] will undoubtedly set a much higher standard for all health claims relating to nutritional products, including probiotics.

One of the areas of most active research pertains to the mechanism of action of probiotics.[7] The interaction between a probiotic strain or cocktail of strains/species must be examined in the context of those interactions that normally take place between the microbiota and the host, as well as between individual components of the microbiota. How does the host differentiate between friend and foe? What interactions between the constituents of the microbiota favor the growth of some bacteria but not others? The complexities of microbiota–host and microbe–microbe interactions continue to be unraveled. With regard to the former, the important roles of pattern recognition receptors [PRRs, such as Toll-like receptors [TLRs], signaling pathways, immune responses, and the secretion of antimicrobial peptides such as defensins and chemokines by the epithelium all appear to play important roles.[3,18] Administered probiotics appear to be able, if only transiently and for the duration of their administration, to influence the composition and function of the intestinal microbiota.[19–21] It appears plausible to suggest that effects that are primarily metabolic in nature should occur primarily in that site of greatest microbial metabolic activity, the colon, whereas probiotic effects that are mediated through immune engagement should take place in those areas where immune tissue is most dense, the distal small intestine. Using novel reporter systems, the locations of niche environments for administered probiotics are beginning to be defined in animal models.[22] While many of the factors, such as secretion of antimicrobial peptides, quorum sensing, possession of certain metabolic pathways, competition for resources, bacterial motility, and adherence properties, to name but a few,[19,23] which have been identified as relevant to competition within the microbiota, are undoubtedly directly relevant to the survival and proliferation of an administered probiotic, very little direct research has been preformed on these issues in people.

If the probiotic survives its hazardous journey through the intestine and manages to establish a niche within the microbiota, how does it exert its health-benefiting effects?

For answers, one again must rely largely on animal work, with some limited data from people. Possible modes of action revealed in such studies include competitive metabolic interactions with pathogens, production of chemical products (bacteriocins) that directly inhibit other bacteria or viruses, inhibition of bacterial movement across the gut wall (translocation), enhancement of mucosal barrier function, and signaling with the epithelium and immune system to modulate the inflammatory/immune response.[7,16,24,25] Probiotics also may produce other chemicals, including neurotransmitters that are normally found in the bowel, which can modify other gut functions, such as motility[26,27] or sensation.[28] The whole area of the production of biologically active products by probiotic organisms promises to be one of the most exciting areas of research in this field and may yet prove relevant to their efficacy in IBS. It is evident that various probiotics have different potency in relation to any one of these actions; some are avid producers of antibacterial peptides and may become active participants in the fight against certain infections,[29,30] while others are potent anti-inflammatory agents.[4] Still other probiotics have been shown to enhance epithelial barrier function through direct effects on mucin expression, proteins of the cytoskeleton, and intercellular tight junctions[31] and indirect effects emanating from interactions between the bacterium, the mucosa and the mucosa-associated lymphoid tissue.[3] The potent anti-inflammatory effects of some probiotics have clearly emphasized how the therapeutic potential of these agents may extend beyond their ability to displace other organisms and has led to their evaluation in inflammatory bowel disease.[32] In an experimental animal (interleukin [IL]-10 knockout) model of colitis, for example, one group of researchers found that both a *Lactobacillus* and a *Bifidobacterium* produced a marked and parallel reduction in inflammation in the colon and cecum and in the production of the proinflammatory cytokines interferon (IFN)-γ, tumor necrosis factor (TNF)-α, and IL-12, while levels of the anti-inflammatory cytokine transforming growth factor (TGF)-β were maintained.[33] Similar effects have been demonstrated for the probiotic cocktail VSL#3 in experimental models of colitis; these anti-inflammatory effects could, indeed, be transmitted by bacterial DNA alone.[34] What is very exciting is the observation, again in an animal model, of the ability of orally administered probiotics to exert anti-inflammatory effects at sites well distant from the gut such as in an inflamed joint.[35] While the focus of this article is on the gut and on digestive disorders, the latter experiments illustrate the ability of strategies that manipulate the microbiota to alter immune function at distal sites and provide an experimental basis for clinical observations on the efficacy of probiotic therapy in allergic disorders, for example. For many probiotics, their mechanism of action in a given disease state, or in health, is likely to be multifactorial.

PROBIOTICS IN IBS

While experimental observations suggest potential benefits for probiotics in various GI, pancreatic, and liver disorders, solid clinical data are confined to three main areas: infection, inflammatory bowel disease,[36–38] and IBS.[39,40] The latter will be discussed here.

Reflecting, perhaps, the paucity of truly disease-modifying therapies that are available to relieve the disorder, irritable bowel sufferers commonly have recourse to the use of complimentary and alternative medical remedies and practices.[41] Foremost among such approaches have been various dietary manipulations, including exclusion diets, and various dietary supplements. In Europe, in particular, where several such products are advertised widely for their general immune-boosting and health-enhancing properties, probiotics have been widely used as dietary supplements by

IBS patients. Recently, based on data from the experimental laboratory, as well as some evidence from clinical trials, the concept of probiotic use in IBS has begun to wind its way into the realm of conventional medicine. While probiotics have been used on an empiric basis for some time in the management of IBS, several recent developments provide a more logical basis for their use in this context.[42] These include the clear recognition that IBS may be induced by bacterial gastroenteritis (postinfectious IBS) and that qualitative and quantitative changes in the microbiota, as well as immune dysfunction, may be prevalent in IBS, in general.

Up to the year 2000, a small number of studies evaluated the response of IBS to probiotic preparations, and, while results between studies were difficult to compare because of differences in study design, probiotic dose and strain, there was some, but by no means consistent, evidence of symptom improvement.

Further studies, since then, have assessed the response to a number of well-characterized organisms and have produced discernible trends. Thus, several organisms, such as *Lactobacillus GG, L plantarum, L acidophilus, L casei*, the probiotic cocktail VSL#3, and *Bifidobacterium animalis*, have been shown to alleviate individual IBS symptoms, such as bloating, flatulence, and constipation. Only a few products, however, have been shown to affect pain and global symptoms in IBS.[43–47] Among these, *B infantis* 35,624 has attracted particular attention.[47] In the first study with this organism, superiority was shown over both a *Lactobacillus* and placebo for each of the cardinal symptoms of the IBS (abdominal pain/discomfort, distension/bloating, and difficult defecation), as well as for a composite score.[48] A larger, 4-week duration, dose-ranging study of the same *Bifidobacterium* in over 360 community-based subjects with IBS confirmed efficacy for this organism in a dose of 10^8. Again, all of the primary symptoms of IBS were significantly improved, and a global assessment of IBS symptoms at the end of therapy revealed a greater than 20% therapeutic gain for the effective dose of the probiotic over placebo (**Fig. 1**).[49]

Further large, long-term, randomized controlled trials of this *Bifidobacterium* and other strains are warranted in IBS, and detailed explorations of its mechanism(s) of action are indicated.

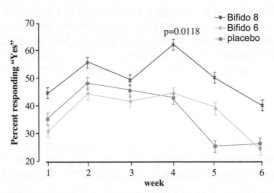

Fig. 1. Subjects global assessment of relief of irritable bowel syndrome (IBS) symptoms in response to *Bifidobacterium infantis* 35,624 in doses of 10^6 or 10^8 or placebo during a 6-week study (4 weeks treatment and 2 weeks wash-out). Note significant increase in percentage of positive responders to the question "Do you feel better now compared with before treatment?" among those randomized to *B infantis* 35,624 in a dose of 10^8 in comparison to the other 2 groups. (*Data from* Whorwell PJ, Altringer L, Morel J, et al. Efficacy of an encapsulated probiotic *Bifidobacterium infantis* 35,624 in women with irritable bowel syndrome. Am J Gastroenterol 2006;101:326–33.)

Several factors, including a reduction in gas production,[50–52] changes in bile salt conjugation, an antibacterial or antiviral effect (in the case of postinfectious IBS), the promotion of motility,[53] effects on mucus secretion, or even an antiinflammatory effect[48] could be relevant to the benefits of specific probiotic strains in IBS.

SAFETY

Many different species and strains and preparations of probiotics have been used for decades and by millions of healthy and diseased individuals, yet definitive data on safety are scanty. In a review In 2006, Boyle and colleagues concluded that although probiotics have an excellent overall safety record, they should be used with caution in certain patient groups, particularly neonates born prematurely or with immune deficiency.[54] They reviewed case reports of instances of abscesses and endocarditis in relation to probiotic use; in many instances the probiotic cultured from the infected tissue was most likely an innocent contaminant rather than the real pathogen. Fears that live probiotic organisms might translocate across the gut and lead to systemic sepsis have also been allayed by the absence of such reports from studies among patients with inflammatory bowel disease and other situations where the intestinal barrier may be compromised. Two notes of caution must be mentioned. The first relates to reports of septicemia occurring among infants with short bowel syndrome,[55,56] and the second to instances of increased mortality among patients with severe acute pancreatitis who had been administered a probiotic cocktail through a nasoenteric tube. These deaths were associated, not with sepsis, but with intestinal ischemla whose etiology remains unclear.[57]

PREBIOTICS AND SYNBIOTICS

Prebiotics are defined as nondigestible, but fermentable, foods that beneficially affect the host by selectively stimulating the growth and activity of one species or a limited number of species of bacteria in the colon. Compared with probiotics, which introduce exogenous bacteria into the human colon, prebiotics stimulate the preferential growth of a limited number of health-promoting species already residing in the colon and, especially, but not exclusively, lactobacilli and bifidobacteria. The oligosaccharides in human breast milk are considered the prototypic prebiotic as they facilitate the preferential growth of bifidobacteria and lactobacilli, in the colon, among exclusively breast-fed neonates; this phenomenon may well account for some of the immunologic and other benefits that accrue to breast-fed infants.[58]

The only prebiotics for which sufficient data have been generated to allow an evaluation of their possible classification as functional food ingredients are the inulin-type fructans, which are linked by β (2–1) bonds that limit their digestion by upper intestinal enzymes, and fructo-oligosaccharides. Both are present in significant amounts in many edible fruits and vegetables, including wheat, onion, chicory, garlic, leeks, artichokes, and bananas. Because of their chemical structure, prebiotics are not absorbed in the small intestine but are fermented, in the colon, by endogenous bacteria to energy and metabolic substrates, with lactic and short-chain carboxylic acids as end products of the fermentation.

Most of the evidence regarding the potential health benefits of prebiotics is derived from experimental animal studies and human trials in small numbers of subjects; there are insufficient, prospective, adequately powered studies in GI disease to permit definitive conclusions to be drawn; some recent studies suggest that prebiotics that have been designed to produce quite selective changes in the composition of the microbiota[59] may have benefits in IBS.[60] It must also be remembered that substances, such as fiber, fiber supplements and lactulose, for example, which have been widely employed in the treatment of constipation, exert prebiotic effects.[61]

Synbiotics, defined as a combination of a probiotic and a prebiotic, aim to increase the survival and activity of proven probiotics in vivo, as well as stimulating indigenous bifidobacteria and lactobacilli. Again, data for efficacy in human disease are scanty, although there have been some small trials in IBS that suggest some promise.[62–65]

ANTIBIOTICS

Although antibiotics have been identified in population studies as a risk factor for the development of IBS, the suggestion that some IBS subjects might harbor SIBO led to clinical trials of these agents in this disorder.[66–70] In a subsequent study that did not document bacterial overgrowth, Pimentel and colleagues treated IBS patients with the poorly absorbed antibiotic rifaximin.[71] Some IBS patients demonstrated a prolonged response (up to 10 weeks) to a short course of this antibiotic. As pointed out in an accompanying editorial, there were, however, several limitations to this study that reduced its impact.[72] In a recently reported multicenter phase 2 study, 388 diarrhea-associated IBS subjects were randomized to either rifaximin in a dose of 550 mg twice a day or placebo for 14 days, followed by another 14 days on placebo alone and then 2 weeks follow-up. During treatment, at 4 weeks and at 12 weeks, those randomized to rifaximin had a modest 8% to 13% therapeutic gain for adequate relief of global IBS symptoms and a rather disappointing 4% to 8% gain for relief of bloating.[73,74] These encouraging results have been reproduced and even bettered in two large multicenter trials which have been recently published.[75] These trials, showed a 9% therapeutic gain for adequate relief of IBS symptoms and a 9.9% therapeutic gain for adequate relief of bloating for rifaximin in a dose of 550 mg three times daily over placebo among a total of 1260 patients with nonconstipated IBS.[75]

The eradication of SIBO, as initially proposed, may not be the sole explanation for these responses, which could also be explained on the basis of a suppression of fermenting bacteria in the colon,[76,77] or indeed, by a multitude of other consequences of altering the colonic microbiota. These results notwithstanding, one must remain reluctant, pending long-term studies, to recommend a prolonged course of antibiotic therapy to any population regardless of the safety profile of a given antibiotic. It also needs to be remembered that relapse rates following discontinuation of rifaximin therapy are high among patients with SIBO (not necessarily associated with IBS),[78] and while such recurrences can be treated successfully by further courses of antibiotic,[79] the advisability of repeated courses of antibiotics in any condition must questioned.

Nevertheless, the consistency of this effect of this antibiotic on IBS symptomatology, albeit modest, is compelling and demands that one address how it is mediating these benefits. Who are the responders, and why do they respond? What is the mechanism of action, and where is this action exerted? The answers to these questions must provide valuable insights into IBS, in general.

ANTI-INFLAMMATORY AGENTS

The other new concept that may, ultimately, lead to new therapeutic approaches to IBS is the suggestion that a low-grade inflammatory, or immune-activated, state may exist in IBS. For many who work in this area, the assumption is that these immunologic phenomena represent the host's normal or abnormal response to a luminal stimulus, such as the microbiota. The story here begins with a clinical observation.

Clinicians who have dealt with IBS for several years will have seen patients, formerly in perfect health, who, following exposure to gastroenteritis, have gone on to develop frank

IBS; the concept of postinfectious IBS (PI-IBS) has now been described in considerable detail in several large series.[80,81] Various clinical and demographic factors have been shown to increase the risk for the development of IBS following bacterial gastroenteritis: female gender, past history of anxiety or depression, more severe clinical course of gastroenteritis, and a persistent inflammatory response in the colonic mucosa. Most recently, some genetic factors that seem to predispose to postinfectious IBS have been identified.[82] Interestingly, the genes implicated codes for interleukins and epithelial barrier factors considered relevant to the pathogenesis of IBS, in general.[83]

The other area that has revealed a convergence of factors that seem to be relevant to the pathogenesis of both IBS and IBD is that of the host immune response. Clearly central to the development and course of IBD, mucosal and systemic immune responses are now generating considerable interest in IBS. With some consistency, elevated levels of the proinflammatory cytokines IL-6 and IL-8 have been demonstrated in the peripheral circulation in IBS.[84–86] Others have examined various components of the mucosal immune response and have variably demonstrated activation of mast cell[87–91] and lymphocyte populations,[92–95] as well as increased epithelial barrier permeability,[96,97] altered expression of cytokine-related genes,[98,99] upregulation of TLRs,[100] and increased levels of β-defensin 2.[101] Involvement of TLRs and β-defensin 2, coupled with reports of variations in the composition of the microbiota,[102,103] provides support for engagement of the microbiota with the host immune system in IBS.

Evidence for or against anti-inflammatory agents in the therapy of IBS remains scanty, and appropriately powered randomized controlled trials employing meaningful clinical endpoints have not been performed. In one study, Dunlop and colleagues[104] assessed the impact of prednisolone administered in a dose of 30 mg daily for 3 weeks to 29 patients with postinfectious IBS. Although lamina propria T-lymphocyte counts in the colon decreased significantly, no changes in enterochromaffin cell numbers were noted, and most importantly, there was no symptom response. More recently, Corinaldesi and colleagues[105] performed a randomized, double-blind, placebo-controlled trial to assess the impact of 8 weeks of therapy with oral mesalazine administered in a dose of 2.4 g daily to unselected IBS patients. Mesalazine therapy resulted in a significant decrease in mucosal immune cells and, especially, mast cells, and was accompanied by an improvement in general wellbeing. However, there was no significant treatment-related improvement in abdominal pain, bloating, or bowel habit.

Klooker and colleagues[106] addressed the potential contribution of mast cells and their products in a randomized, placebo-controlled trial of ketotifen, the mast cell stabilizer and histamine H_1 receptor antagonist, in IBS. Prior studies had suggested potential benefits in IBS and related conditions following the administration of disodium cromoglycate.[107–109] In contrast to prior studies,[87–91] Klooker and colleagues[106] failed to demonstrate either increased numbers of mast cells or tryptase release at baseline among IBS subjects. Furthermore, while ketotifen had exerted positive influences on both visceral hypersensitivity and symptoms, these effects were unrelated to effects on the release of either tryptase or histamine. The mechanism of this symptomatic response remains unclear.

SUMMARY

Two, perhaps related, areas of human biology have begun to impact on IBS: the microbiome and mucosal immunology. Both deserve more investigation. Over the next few years studies of the complex ecology, the gut microbiota, and its interaction to the human host via the mucosal immune system will not only unlock the secrets of several important human diseases, but will lead, through successful mining and modulation of the microbiota, to new therapeutic approaches.[110] Before approaches to modify the microbiota or the host immune response by any agent can be advocated for widespread use in IBS, more clinical studies are needed to address, not merely efficacy, but also safety[111] and mechanism of action.[112] The latter may lead to some valuable clues to the etiology of this challenging disorder.

REFERENCES

1. Palmer C, Bik EM, DiGiulio DB, et al. Development of the human infant intestinal microbiota. PLoS Biol 2007;5:1556–73.
2. Guarner F, Malagelada JR. Gut flora in health and disease. Lancet 2003;361:512–9.
3. Neish AS. Microbes in gastrointestinal health and disease. Gastroenterology 2009;136:65–80.
4. Hattori M, Taylor TD. The human intestinal microbiome: a new frontier of human biology. DNA Res 2009;16:1–12.
5. Eckburg PB, Bik EM, Bernstein CN, et al. Diversity of the human intestinal microbial flora. Science 2005;308:1635–8.
6. Shanahan F. The host–microbe interface within the gut. Best Pract Res Clin Gastroenterol 2002;16:915–31.
7. O'Hara AM, Shanahan F. Gut microbiota: mining for therapeutic potential. Clin Gastroenterol Hepatol 2007;5:274–84.
8. Isolauri E, Salminen S, Ouwehand AC. Microbial–gut interactions in health and disease. Probiotics. Best Pract Res Clin Gastroenterol 2004;18:299–313.
9. Kelly CP, LaMont JT. Clostridium difficile—more difficult than ever. N Engl J Med 2008;359:1932–40.
10. Neu J, Mshvildadze M, Mai V. A roadmap for understanding and preventing necrotizing enterocolitis. Curr Gastroenterol Rep 2008;10:450–7.
11. Quigley EMM, Abu-Shanab A. The diagnosis of small intestinal bacterial overgrowth: the challenges persist! Expert Rev Gastroenterol Hepatol 2009;3:77–87.
12. Sartor RB, Muehlbauer M. Microbial host interactions in IBD: implications for pathogenesis and therapy. Curr Gastroenterol Rep 2007;9:497–507.
13. Tilg H, Moschen AR, Kaser A. Obesity and the microbiota. Gastroenterology 2009;136:1476–83.
14. Turnbaugh PJ, Ley RE, Mahowald MA, et al. An obesity-associated gut microbiome with increased capacity for energy harvest. Nature 2006;444:1027–31.
15. Zhang H, DiBaise JK, Zuccolo A, et al. Human gut microbiota in obesity and after gastric bypass. Proc Natl Acad Sci U S A 2009;106:2365–70.
16. Shanahan F. Probiotics: a perspective on problems and pitfalls. Scand J Gastroenterol Suppl 2003;237:34–6.
17. Available at: http://eur-lex.europa.eu/LexUriServ/LexUriServ.do?uri=CELEX:32006R1924R(01):EN: NOT. Accessed November 8, 2010.
18. Kotarsky K, Sitnik KM, Stenstad H, et al. A novel role for constitutively expressed epithelial-derived chemokines as antibacterial peptides in the intestinal mucosa. Nat Immunol 2010;3:40–8.
19. O'Toole PW, Cooney JC. Probiotic bacteria influence the composition and function of the intestinal microbiota. Interdiscip Perspsect Infect Dis 2008;2008:175285.
20. Bonetti A, Morelli L, Campominos E. Assessment of the persistence in the human intestinal tract of two probiotic Lactobacilli *Lactobacillus salivarius* I 1794 and *Lactobacillus paracasei* I 1688. Microb Ecol Health Dis 2002;4:229–33.

21. Engelbrektson AL, Korzenik JR, Sanders ME, et al. Analysis of treatment effects on the microbial ecology of the human intestine. FEMS Microbiol Ecol 2006;57: 239–50.

22. Cronin M, Sleator RD, Hill C, et al. Development of a luciferase-based reporter system to monitor *Bifidobacterium breve* UCC2003 persistence in mice. BMC Microbiol 2008;8:161.

23. Hibbing ME, Fuqua C, Parsek MR, et al. Bacterial competition: surviving in the microbial jungle. Nat Rev Microbiol 2010;8:15–25.

24. Preidis GA, Versalovic J. Targeting the human microbiome with antibiotics, probiotics, and prebiotics: gastroenterology enters the metagenomics era. Gastroenterology 2009;136:2015–31.

25. Zeng J, Li YQ, Zuo XL, et al. Clinical trial: effect of active lactic acid bacteria on mucosal barrier function in patients with diarrhoea-predominant irritable bowel syndrome. Aliment Pharmacol Ther 2008;28:994–1002.

26. Quigley EMM. Bacteria: a new player in gastrointestinal motility disorders—infections, bacterial overgrowth, and probiotics. Gastroenterol Clin North Am 2007;36: 735–48.

27. Bueno L, de Ponti F, Fried M, et al. Serotonergic and nonserotonergic targets in the pharmacotherapy of visceral hypersensitivity. Neurogastroenterol Motil 2007;19(Suppl 1):89–119.

28. Rousseaux C, Thuru X, Gelot A, et al. Lactobacillus acidophilus modulates intestinal pain and induces opioid and cannabinoid receptors. Nat Med 2007; 13:35–7.

29. Corr SC, Li Y, Riedel CU, et al. Bacteriocin production as a mechanism for the anti-infective activity of *Lactobacillus salivarius* UCC118. Proc Natl Acad Sci U S A 2007;104:7617–21.

30. Cotter PD, O'Connor PM, Draper LA, et al. Posttranslational conversion of L-serines to D-alanines is vital for optimal production and activity of the lantibiotic lactlcin 3147. Proc Natl Acad Sci U S A 2005;102:18584–9.

31. Ait-Belgnaoui A, Han W, Lamine F, et al. *Lactobacillus farciminis* treatment suppresses stress-induced visceral hypersensitivity: a possible action through interaction with epithelial cells cytoskeleton contraction. Gut 2006; 55:1090–4.

32. Dunne C, Murphy L, Flynn S, et al. Probiotics: from myth to reality. Demonstration of functionality in animal models of disease and in human clinical trials. Antonie Van Leeuwenhoek 1999;76:279–92.

33. McCarthy J, O'Mahony L, O'Callaghan L, et al. Double-blind, placebo-controlled trial of two probiotic strains in interleukin 10 knockout mice and mechanistic link with cytokine balance. Gut 2003;52:975–80.

34. Rachmilewitz D, Katakura K, Karmeli F, et al. Toll-like receptor 9 signaling mediates the anti-inflammatory effects of probiotics in murine experimental colitis. Gastroenterology 2004;126:520–8.

35. Sheil B, McCarthy J, O'Mahony L, et al. Is the mucosal route of administration essential for probiotic function? Subcutaneous administration is associated with attenuation of murine colitis and arthritis. Gut 2004;53:694–700.

36. Ewaschuk JB, Tejpar QZ, Soo I, et al. The role of antibiotic and probiotic therapies in current and future management of inflammatory bowel disease. Curr Gastroenterol Rep 2006;8:486–98.

37. Gionchetti P, Rizzello F, Helwig U, et al. Prophylaxis of pouchitis onset with probiotic therapy: a double-blind, placebo-controlled trial. Gastroenterology 2003; 124:1202–9.

38. Mimura T, Rizzello F, Helwig U, et al. Once daily high-dose probiotic therapy (VSL#3) for maintaining remission in recurrent or refractory pouchitis. Gut 2004;53:108–14.

39. NASPGHAN Nutrition Report Committee, Michail S, Sylvester F, et al. Clinical efficacy of probiotics: review of the evidence with focus on children. J Pediatr Gastroenterol Nutr 2006;43:550–7.

40. Floch MH, Walker WA, Guandalini S, et al. Recommendations for probiotic use—2008. J Clin Gastroenterol 2008;42(Suppl 2):S104–8.

41. Hussein Z, Quigley EM. Complementary and alternative medicine in irritable bowel syndrome. Aliment Pharmacol Ther 2006;15:465–71.

42. Quigley EMM, Flourie B. Probiotics in irritable bowel syndrome: a rationale for their use and an assessment of the evidence to date. Neurogastroenterol Motil 2007;19:166–72.

43. Nikfar S, Rahimi R, Rahimi F, et al. Efficacy of probiotics in irritable bowel syndrome: a meta-analysis of randomized, controlled trials. Dis Colon Rectum 2008;51:1775–80.

44. McFarland LV, Dublin S. Meta-analysis of probiotics for the treatment of irritable bowel syndrome. World J Gastroenterol 2008;14:2650–61.

45. Hoveyda N, Heneghan C, Mahtani KR, et al. A systematic review and meta-analysis: probiotics in the treatment of irritable bowel syndrome. BMC Gastroenterol 2009;9:15.

46. Moayyedi P, Ford AC, Talley NJ, et al. The efficacy of probiotics in the therapy of irritable bowel syndrome: a systematic review. Gut 2010;59(3):325–32.

47. Brenner DM, Moeller MJ, Chey WD, et al. The utility of probiotics in the treatment of irritable bowel syndrome: a systematic review. Am J Gastroenterol 2009; 104(4):1033–49 [quiz: 1050].

48. O'Mahony L, McCarthy J, Kelly P, et al. A randomized, placebo-controlled, double-blind comparison of the probiotic bacteria *Lactobacillus* and *Bifidobacterium* in irritable bowel syndrome (IBS): symptom responses and relationship to cytokine profiles. Gastroenterology 2005;128:541–51.

49. Whorwell PJ, Altringer L, Morel J, et al. Efficacy of an encapsulated probiotic *Bifidobacterium infantis* 35624 in women with irritable bowel syndrome. Am J Gastroenterol 2006;101:326–33.

50. Biarti B, Matterelli P. The family bifidobacteria. In: Dworkin M, Fallow S, Rosenberg E, et al, editors. The prokaryotes. New York: Springer; 2001. p. 1–70.

51. Sen S, Mulan MM, Parker TJ, et al. Effect of *Lactobacillus plantarum* 299V on colonic fermentation and symptoms of irritable bowel syndrome. Dig Dis Sci 2002;47:2615–20.

52. Barrett JS, Canale KE, Gearry RB, et al. Probiotic effects on intestinal fermentation patterns in patients with irritable bowel syndrome. World J Gastroenterol 2008;14:5020–4.

53. Agrawal A, Houghton LA, Morris J, et al. Clinical trial: the effects of a fermented milk product containing *Bifidobacterium lactis* DN-173-010 on abdominal distension and gastrointestinal transit in irritable bowel syndrome with constipation. Aliment Pharmacol Ther 2008. [Epub ahead of print].

54. Boyle RJ, Robins-Browne RM, Tang MLK. Probiotic use in clinical practice: what are the risks? Am J Clin Nutr 2006;83:1256–64.

55. Kunz AN, Noel JM, Fairchok MP. Two cases of *Lactobacillus* bacteremia during probiotic treatment of short gut syndrome. J Pediatr Gastroenterol Nutr 2004;38:457–8.

56. DeGroote MA, Frank DN, Dowell E, et al. *Lactobacillus rhamnosus* GG bacteremia associated with probiotic use in a child with short gut syndrome. Pediatr Infect Dis J 2005;24:278–80.
57. Besselink MG, van Santvoort HC, Buskens E, et al. Probiotic prophylaxis in predicted severe acute pancreatitis: a randomised, double-blind, placebo-controlled trial. Lancet 2008;371:651–9.
58. Depeint F, Tzprtzis G, Vulevic J, et al. Prebiotic evaluation of a novel galacto-oligosaccheride mixture produced by the enzymatic activity of *Bifidobacterium bifidum* NCIMB 44171, In healthy humans: a randomized, double-blind, crossover, placebo-controlled intervention study. Am J Clin Nutr 2008;87:785–91.
59. Vos AP, M'Rabert L, Stahl B, et al. Immunomodulatory effects and potential working mechanisms of orally applied nondigestible carbohydrates. Crit Rev Immunol 2007;27:97–140.
60. Silk DBA, Davis A, Vulevic J, et al. Clinical trial: the effects of a trans-galactooligosaccheride on faecal microbiota and symptoms in irritable bowel syndrome. Aliment Pharmacol Ther 2009;29:508–18.
61. Bouhnik Y, Neut C, Raskine L, et al. Prospective, randomized, parallel-group trial to evaluate the effects of lactulose and polyethylene glycol-4000 on colonic flora in chronic idiopathic constipation. Aliment Pharmacol Ther 2004;19: 889–99.
62. Andriulli A, Neri M, Loguercio C, et al. Clinical trial on the efficacy of a new symbiotic formulation, Flortec, in patients with irritable bowel syndrome: a multicenter, randomized study. J Clin Gastroenterol 2008;42:S218–23.
63. Colecchia A, Vestito A, La Rocca A, et al. Effect of a symbiotic preparation on the clinical manifestations of irritable bowel syndrome, constipation-variant. Results of an open, uncontrolled multicenter study. Minerva Gastroenterol Dietol 2006;52:349–58.
64. Tsuchiya J, Barreto R, Okura R, et al. Single-blind follow-up study on the effectiveness of a symbiotic preparation in irritable bowel syndrome. Chin J Dig Dis 2004;5:169–74.
65. Dughera L, Elia C, Navino M, et al. Effects of symbiotic preparations on constipated irritable bowel syndrome symptoms. Acta Biomed 2007;78:111–6.
66. Pimentel M, Chow EJ, Lin HC. Eradication of small bowel bacterial overgrowth reduces symptoms of irritable bowel syndrome. Am J Gastroenterol 2000;95: 3503–6.
67. Pimentel M, Chow E, Lin H. Normalization of lactulose breath testing correlates with symptom improvement in irritable bowel syndrome: a double-blind, randomized, placebo-controlled study. Am J Gastroenterol 2003;98:412–9.
68. Cuoco L, Salvagnini M. Small intestine bacterial overgrowth in irritable bowel syndrome: a retrospective study with rifaximin. Minerva Gastroenterol Dietol 2006;52:89–95.
69. Majewski M, McCallum RW. Results of small intestinal bacterial overgrowth testing in irritable bowel syndrome patients: clinical profiles and effects of antibiotic trial. Adv Med Sci 2007;52:139–42.
70. Esposito I, de Leone A, Di Gregorio G, et al. Breath test for differential diagnosis between small intestinal bacterial overgrowth and irritable bowel disease: an observation on nonabsorbable antibiotics. World J Gastroenterol 2007;13: 6016–21.
71. Pimentel M, Park S, Mirocha J, et al. The effect of a nonabsorbed antibiotic (rifaximin) on the symptoms of the irritable bowel syndrome: a randomized trial. Ann Intern Med 2006;145:557–63.

72. Drossman DA. Treatment for bacterial overgrowth in the irritable bowel syndrome. Ann Intern Med 2006;145:626–8.

73. Lembo A, Zakko SF, Ferreira NL, et al. Rifaximin for the treatment of diarrhea-associated irritable bowel syndrome: short-term treatment leading to long-term sustained response. Gastroenterology 2008;134:A-545.

74. Ringel Y, Zakko SF, Ferreira NL, et al. Predictors of clinical response from a phase 2 multicenter efficacy trial using rifaximin, a gut-selective, nonabsorbed antibiotic for the treatment of diarrhea-associated irritable bowel syndrome. Gastroenterology 2008;134:A-550.

75. Pimentel M, Lembo A, Chey WD, et al. Rifaximin therapy for patients with irritable bowel syndrome without constipation. New Engl J Med 2011;364:22–32.

76. Dear KL, Elia M, Hunter JO. Do interventions which reduce colonic bacterial fermentation improve symptoms of irritable bowel syndrome? Dig Dis Sci 2005;50:758–66.

77. Sharara AI, Aoun E, Abdul-Baki H, et al. A randomized double-blind placebo-controlled trial of rifaximin in patients with abdominal bloating and flatulence. Am J Gastroenterol 2006;101:326–33.

78. Lauritano EC, Gabrielli M, Scarpellini E, et al. Small intestinal bacterial overgrowth recurrence after antibiotic therapy. Am J Gastroenterol 2008;103:2031–5.

79. Yang J, Lee HR, Low K, et al. Rifaximin versus other antibiotics in the primary treatment and retreatment of bacterial overgrowth in IBS. Dig Dis Sci 2008; 53(1):169–74.

80. Thabane M, Kottachchi DT, Marshall JK. Systematic review and meta-analysis: the incidence and prognosis of postinfectious irritable bowel syndrome. Aliment Pharmacol Ther 2007;26:535–44.

81. Spiller R, Garsed K. Postinfectious irritable bowel syndrome. Gastroenterology 2009;136:1979–88.

82. Villani AC, Lemire M, Thabane M, et al. Genetic risk factors for postinfectious irritable bowel syndrome following a waterborne outbreak of gastroenteritis. Gastroenterology 2010;138:1502–13.

83. Craig OF, Quigley EMM. Bacteria, genetics, and irritable bowel syndrome. Expert Rev Gastroenterol Hepatol 2010;4:271–6.

84. Dinan TG, Quigley EMM, Ahmed SMM, et al. Hypothalamic-pituitary-gut axis dysregulation in irritable bowel syndrome: plasma cytokines as a potential biomarker? Gastroenterology 2006;130:304–11.

85. Liebregts T, Adam B, Bredack C, et al. Immune activation in patients with irritable bowel syndrome. Gastroenterology 2007;132:913–20.

86. Scully P, McKernan DP, Keohane J, et al. Plasma cytokine profiles in females with irritable bowel syndrome and extraintestinal comorbidity. Am J Gastroenterol 2010;105:2235–43.

87. Barbara G, Stanghellini V, De Giorgio R, et al. Activated mast cells in proximity to colonic nerves correlate with abdominal pain in irritable bowel syndrome. Gastroenterology 2004;126:693–702.

88. Barbara G, Wang B, Stanghellini V, et al. Mast cell-dependent excitation of visceral–nociceptive sensory neurons in irritable bowel syndrome. Gastroenterology 2007;132:26–37.

89. Cenac N, Andrews CN, Holzhausen M, et al. Role for protease activity in visceral pain in irritable bowel syndrome. J Clin Invest 2007;117:636–47.

90. Guilarte M, Santos J, de Torres I, et al. Diarrhoea-predominant IBS patients show mast cell activation and hyperplasia in the jejunum. Gut 2007;56: 203–9.

91. Buhner S, Li Q, Vignali S, et al. Activation of human enteric neurons by superna-tants of colonic biopsy specimens from patients with irritable bowel syndrome. Gastroenterology 2009;137:1425–34.
92. Chadwick V, Chen W, Shu D, et al. Activation of the mucosal immune system in irritable bowel syndrome. Gastroenterology 2002;122:1778–83.
93. Holmen N, Isaksson S, Simren M, et al. CD4+CD25+ regulatory T cells in irritable bowel syndrome patients. Neurogastroenterol Motil 2007;19:119–25.
94. Ohman L, Isaksson S, Lundgren A, et al. A controlled study of colonic immune activity and beta7+ blood T lymphocytes in patients with irritable bowel syndrome. Clin Gastroenterol Hepatol 2005;3:980–6.
95. Cremon C, Gargano L, Morselli-Labate AM, et al. Mucosal immune activation in irritable bowel syndrome: gender-dependence and association with digestive symptoms. Am J Gastroenterol 2009;104:392–400.
96. Quigley E. Gut permeability in irritable bowel syndrome: more leaks add to slightly inflamed bowel syndrome conspiracy theory. Gastroenterology 2009; 137:728–30.
97. Barbara G. Mucosal barrier defects in irritable bowel syndrome. Who left the door open? Am J Gastroenterol 2006;101:1295–8.
98. MacSharry J, O'Mahony L, Fanning A, et al. Mucosal cytokine imbalance in irri-table bowel syndrome. Scand J Gastroenterol 2008;43:1467–76.
99. Aerssens J, Camilleri M, Talloen W, et al. Alterations in mucosal immunity iden-tified in the colon of patients with irritable bowel syndrome. Clin Gastroenterol Hepatol 2008;6.194–205.
100. Brint EK, MacSharry J, Fanning A, et al. Differential expression of Toll-like recep-tors (TLRs) in patients with irritable bowel syndrome. Am J Gastroenterol 2010. [Epub ahead of print].
101. Langhorst J, Junge A, Rueffer A, et al. Elevated human beta-defensin-2 levels indicate an activation of the innate immune system in patients with irritable bowel syndrome. Am J Gastroenterol 2009;104:404–10.
102. Kassinen A, Krogius-Kurikka L, Makivuokko H, et al. The fecal microbiota of irri-table bowel syndrome patients differs significantly from that of healthy subjects. Gastroenterology 2007;133:24–33.
103. Codling C, O'Mahony L, Shanahan F, et al. A molecular analysis of fecal and mucosal bacterial communities in irritable bowel syndrome. Dig Dis Sci 2010;55:392–7.
104. Dunlop SP, Jenkins D, Neal KR, et al. Randomized, double-blind, placebo-controlled trial of prednisolone in postinfectious irritable bowel syndrome. Aliment Pharmacol Ther 2003;18:77–84.
105. Corinaldesi R, Stanghellini V, Cremon C, et al. Effect of mesalazine on mucosal immune markers in irritable bowel syndrome: a randomized controlled proof-of-concept study. Aliment Pharmacol Ther 2009;30:245–52.
106. Klooker TK, Braak B, Koopman KE, et al. The mast cell stabilizer ketotifen decreases visceral hypersensitivity and improves intestinal symptoms in patients with irritable bowel syndrome. Gut 2010;59:1213–21.
107. Bolin TD. Use of oral disodium cromoglycate in persistent diarrhea. Gut 1980; 21:848–50.
108. Lunardi C, Bambara LM, Biasi D, et al. Double-blind crossover trial of oral sodium cromoglycate in patients with irritable bowel syndrome due to food intol-erance. Clin Exp Allergy 1991;21(5):569–72.
109. Stefanini GF, Saggioro A, Alvisi V, et al. Oral cromolyn sodium in comparison with elimination diet in the irritable bowel syndrome, diarrheic type. Multicenter study of 428 patients. Scand J Gastroenterol 1995;30:535–41.

110. Sanders ME, Akkermans LMA, Haller D, et al. Safety assessment of probiotics for human use. Gut Microbes 2010;1:164–85.
111. Quigley EMM. The future of probiotics. In: Michail S, Sherman P, editors. Probiotics in pediatric medicine. Totowa (NJ): Humana Press; 2008. p. 323–9.
112. Shanahan F. Gut microbes: from bugs to drugs. Am J Gastroenterol 2010;105: 275–9.

Emerging Pharmacological Therapies for the Irritable Bowel Syndrome

Monthira Maneerattanaporn, MD[a,b], Lin Chang, MD, AGAF[c,d], William D. Chey, MD, AGAF[a,*]

KEYWORDS

- Irritable bowel syndrome • Constipation • Diarrhea • Serotonin
- Guanylate cyclase C • Corticotropin-releasing hormone
- Tryptophan hydroxylase • Glucagon-like peptide

The irritable bowel syndrome (IBS) is a symptom-based disorder defined by the presence of abdominal pain and altered bowel habits.[1] Clinical presentations of IBS are diverse, with some patients reporting diarrhea, some constipation, and others a mixture of both. Like the varied clinical phenotypes, the pathogenesis of IBS is also diverse. IBS is not a single disease entity, but rather likely consists of several different disease states. This fact has important implications for the choices and efficacy of IBS treatment.

Traditional IBS therapies, such as fiber, antidiarrheals, laxatives, and antispasmodics, have tended to focus on individual symptoms, such as abdominal pain, stool frequency, or stool consistency. Recent drug development has attempted to take

Disclosure: Monthira Maneerattanaporn has nothing to disclose; Lin Chang has received grant support from Rose Pharma and Takeda, and is a consultant for Albireo, Ironwood, Movetis, Novo Nordisk, Rose Pharma, Prometheus, and Salix; William D. Chey is a consultant for Albireo, Ironwood, Movetis, and Salix.
[a] Division of Gastroenterology, University of Michigan Health System, 3912 Taubman Center, Ann Arbor, MI 48109-0362, USA
[b] Division of Gastroenterology, Department of Internal Medicine, Siriraj Hospital, Mahidol University, Bangkok 10170, Thailand
[c] UCLA Division of Digestive Diseases, UCLA Department of Medicine, VAGLAHS, at the David Geffen School of Medicine, UCLA, 10945 Le Conte Avenue, PVUB 2114, Los Angeles, CA 90095, USA
[d] UCLA Center for Neurovisceral Sciences and Women's Health (CNS/WH), Center for Neurobiology of Stress, 10945 Le Conte Avenue PVUB 2114, UCLA, Los Angeles, CA 90095, USA
* Corresponding author.
E-mail address: wchey@med.umich.edu

Gastroenterol Clin N Am 40 (2011) 223–243
doi:10.1016/j.gtc.2010.12.002
0889-8553/11/$ – see front matter © 2011 Elsevier Inc. All rights reserved.

better advantage of the increasing understanding of the pathogenesis of IBS, and therefore more comprehensively addresses the spectrum of symptoms reported by patients. Drugs such as alosetron, tegaserod, and lubiprostone represent the initial attempts. This article reviews the IBS drugs that have reached phase II or III clinical trials (**Table 1**).

EMERGING THERAPIES FOR CONSTIPATION-PREDOMINANT IBS

The overlap between constipation-predominant IBS (IBS-C) and chronic constipation (CC), both in terms of pathophysiology and clinical presentation, is well established.[2] This overlap undoubtedly contributes to why most drugs being developed for IBS-C are being codeveloped for CC. This section focuses on candidate drugs that have advanced to phase II or III of clinical development for patients with IBS-C or CC.

Serotonin Receptor Modulators

Serotonin (5-HT) plays an important role in gastrointestinal motility, intestinal secretion, and visceral sensation, and therefore modulation of 5-HT is an attractive target for drug development in patients with IBS-C and CC.[3,4] In normal subjects, 90% to 95% of the body's 5-HT is stored in enterochromaffin cells, which line the gastrointestinal tract.[5] Mechanical stimulation (ie, mucosal stroking from luminal contents) is a potent stimulus for enterochromaffin cells to release 5-HT into the intestinal lumen,[5,6] where it stimulates primary neurons to initiate peristalsis and secretory reflexes.[6] To date, seven families with 14 serotonin receptor subtypes have been identified. Of these receptor subtypes, $5-HT_{1p}$, $5-HT_3$, and $5-HT_4$ have the greatest evidence supporting a role in gastrointestinal and colonic function and sensation.[3,5]

Of great relevance to IBS-C and CC are the $5-HT_4$ receptors. $5-HT_4$ receptors can be found in the central nervous system, gastrointestinal tract, heart, and bladder. In the gastrointestinal tract, $5-HT_4$ receptors are found on enteric neurons and smooth muscle cells, and their stimulation leads to acetylcholine release causing prokinetic effects. Several $5-HT_4$ agonists have been developed as potential treatments for patients with IBS-C and CC. Based on biochemical structure, $5-HT_4$ agonists can be broadly categorized as benzamides (metoclopramide, cisapride, renzapride, mosapride, clebopride, and ATI-7505), carbazimidamides (tegaserod), benzofurancarboxamides (prucalopride), and other agonists such as velusetrag. $5-HT_4$ agonists vary greatly in their affinity and selectivity for the $5-HT_4$ receptor. Cisapride, a strong $5-HT_4$ agonist and weak $5-HT_3$ antagonist, and tegaserod, a partial $5-HT_4$ agonist, were once available in the United States,[7] but were removed from the market because of different and distinct cardiovascular safety concerns. $5-HT_3$ agonists are another interesting class of serotonin modulators with potential application in patients with IBS-C.

$5-HT_4$ agonists
Prucalopride Prucalopride is more selective for the $5-HT_4$ receptor than cisapride or tegaserod. Although all three agents have affinity for the $5-HT_4$ receptor and are similar in their prokinetic properties, cisapride and tegaserod interact with both human Ether-á-go-go-Related Gene potassium and $5-HT_{1b}$ channels, which are both postulated to be responsible for the development of adverse cardiovascular effects.[8,9] Thus, prucalopride's unique chemical structure is hypothesized to limit the development of these events.

Prucalopride's prokinetic activity has been confirmed in animals and humans.[10,11] In a placebo-controlled study in healthy volunteers, prucalopride accelerated total intestinal transit time and overall colonic transit time, particularly in the proximal colon.[12,13]

Clinical trials with prucalopride have focused on patients with CC. In the first of three large, multicenter, randomized, double-blind, placebo-controlled studies evaluating the safety and efficacy of prucalopride, Camilleri and colleagues[14] enrolled 620 patients who met criteria for CC. Participants were randomized to oral placebo or 2 or 4 mg once daily, of prucalopride for 12 weeks. The primary end point was the proportion of patients passing an average of three or more spontaneous complete bowel movements (SCBMs) per week during the 12 weeks of treatment. Various secondary end points were also assessed, including responses to the validated Patient Assessments of Constipation Symptoms (PAC-SYM) and Quality of Life (PAC-QOL) surveys. Statistically significant improvements in the primary end point were identified, with 28.4%, 30.9%, and 12.0% of patients taking 4 mg of prucalopride, 2 mg of prucalopride, or placebo, respectively, achieving the primary end point. Significant changes were also apparent in multiple secondary end points, including PAC-SYM and PAC-QOL scores. The most common adverse events were headaches, abdominal pain, and diarrhea, with most occurring within the first 24 hours of treatment. One cardiovascular event occurred, involving an episode of supraventricular tachycardia in a patient with a history of mitral valve prolapse and supraventricular tachycardia who took 2 mg of prucalopride. No significant differences in electrocardiographic findings were seen among the three groups and no deaths were reported.

Two additional phase III trials have been published (N = 713 patients, 641 with CC) using the same inclusion and exclusion criteria, trial design, and primary end point.[15] Both showed a 10% to 14% improvement in the primary end point in patients receiving prucalopride compared with those taking placebo. Side effects were similar in nature and frequency to those seen in the Camilleri[14] study. More patients who received prucalopride, 4 mg, discontinued treatment because of the drug than those receiving 2 mg or placebo. No differences were seen in hematologic changes, clinical chemistry, urinalysis, vital signs, or electrocardiogram parameters across the study groups.[14–16] A prolonged QT interval was identified in 0.5% to 1.5% of patients at 12 weeks among the three trials, with no differences identified between the placebo and prucalopride groups.

Recently, Camilleri and colleagues[17] presented data from a study assessing the safety of prucalopride compared with placebo in 89 elderly patients with a mean age of 82 years, 80% of whom had a prior history of cardiovascular disease. No differences in proarrhythmic effects or prolonged QTc intervals were identified between groups. Based on these studies, the European Medicines Agency approved prucalopride as a treatment for CC. Appropriately designed and powered studies evaluating the efficacy and safety of prucalopride in patients with IBS-C are eagerly awaited.

Mosapride Mosapride is a selective $5-HT_4$ receptor agonist that has documented stimulatory effects on gastric and colonic motility.[18] Unlike cisapride, mosapride does not bind to K^+ channels or D_2 dopaminergic receptors. Mosapride was primarily developed for upper gastrointestinal tract conditions, such as functional dyspepsia, gastroesophageal reflux disease, and nausea and vomiting and is available for these indications in several countries in Central and South America, Europe, and the Far East.[19–23] Pharmacodynamic studies in animals have shown that mosapride accelerates colonic transit time[24,25] and augments motility in the proximal and distal colon in a dose-dependent manner.[25,26] Furthermore, Kojima and colleagues[27,28] showed the stimulatory effect of mosapride on the defecatory reflex (intrinsic rectorectal contraction and rectoanal sphincter relaxation) post denervated lumbosacral plexus in guinea pigs.

No fully published studies have addressed the role of mosapride in the treatment of IBS-C or idiopathic CC. In 14 constipated patients with Parkinsonism or multiple

Table 1
Emerging therapies for irritable bowel syndrome

Drug Class	Name	Mechanism of Action	Treatment Effects
IBS-C			
Serotonin receptor modulator	Prucalopride, mosapride, pumosetrag	5-HT$_4$ and 5-HT$_3$ agonists accelerate gastrointestinal transit and may alter visceral sensation	Prucalopride: Three phase III trials in CC showed benefits for stool frequency and other constipation-related symptoms at doses of 2 and 4 mg[14] Mosapride: Phase III trial completed enrollment in the Middle East[30] Pumosetrag: Phase II trial, dose-escalation study in 14 patients with CC showed improvements in constipation symptoms and colonic transit[33]
Guanylate cyclase C receptor agonists	Linaclotide, plecanatide (SP-304)	Guanylate cyclase C agonist: Stimulates luminal chloride secretion with passive diffusion of sodium and water and secondary effects on peristalsis	Linaclotide: Phase III trials in IBS-C showed that linaclotide (266 μg once daily) for up to 26 weeks was superior to placebo for a composite responder end point encompassing abdominal pain and stool frequency, and multiple secondary constipation-related end points[44] Plecanatide: Phase IIa study in patients with CC improved constipation symptoms[47]
Bile acid modulators	Chenodeoxycholic acid (CDA), A3309	A3309 (intestinal bile acid transporter inhibitor): Bile acids accelerate colonic transit time, increase motility index, and increase secretion	CDA: Accelerated colon transit but up to 45% of patients developed abdominal cramps/pain[50] A3309: Phase IIb trial of A3309, 5, 10, and 15 mg/d, once daily showed dose-dependent effects on stool frequency and other constipation-related secondary outcomes[64]
Dopaminergic antagonist	Itopride	Dopaminergic antagonist leads to prokinetic effects	Phase II trial evaluating efficacy of itopride (50 and 100 mg) has been completed; results have not been reported[96]
IBS-D or nonconstipated IBS			
κ-opioid receptor agonist	Asimadoline	Activates opioid receptors, which may reduce visceral perception	Phase II study showed no overall effect in IBS but efficacy was shown in IBS-D with at least moderate severity and, to a lesser extent, in IBS-A[71]

Carbon-based adsorbent	AST-120	Adsorbs luminal substances, including serotonin and bile acids	Phase II trials showed that AST-120 was associated with a greater proportion of responders (percentage of patients reporting ≥50% reduction in days with pain) and greater reduction in bloating severity than placebo after 4 weeks[72]
Proanthocyanidin oligomer	Crofelemer	Reduces chloride ion secretion through CFTR and CaCC channels	Phase IIa showed that patients with IBS-D, particularly women, had more pain- and discomfort-free days, but no effect was seen on stool consistency or other IBS symptoms[82]
CRF antagonists	Pexacerfont, GW876008	Blocks CRF_1 receptors to decrease gastrointestinal motility and visceral sensitivity	Phase IIa study showed no significant effect on gastrointestinal transit or IBS symptoms[78] An initial clinical trial with GW876008 suggests that this drug is not effective in IBS, although the study may not have been appropriately designed to evaluate this effect[80]
2,3-Benzodiazepine modulator	Dextofisopam	Modulates autonomic responses	Phase IIb study showed significant benefit in patients with IBS-D/A in the first month of treatment, but less benefit in second and third months[85]
Tryptophan hydroxylase-1 inhibitor	LX1031	Reduces gastrointestinal levels of serotonin	Phase II trial showed that higher dose of LX1031 (1000 mg qid) significantly improved global IBS symptoms and stool consistency over a 4-week period in nonconstipating IBS Symptom improvement correlated with 24-hour urinary 5-HIAA levels[89]
$5HT_3$ antagonist	Ramosetron	Blocks $5\text{-}HT_3$ receptors to slow gastrointestinal transit and decrease visceral perception	Phase II trial showed significantly a higher proportion of responders reported global relief of IBS with ramosetron, 5 and 10 μg, versus placebo[91]
Abdominal pain			
Glucagon-like peptide-1 (GLP-1) analogue	ROSE-010	Inhibits small intestinal motility	A significantly higher proportion of patients reported >50% of the maximum total pain relief response after 100 and 300 μg of ROSE-010 treatments than after placebo[94]

Abbreviations: 5-HIAA, 5-hydroxyindoleacetic acid; $5\text{-}HT_3$, serotonin type 3 receptor; $5\text{-}HT_4$, serotonin type 4 receptor; CaCC, calcium-activated chloride channel; CFTR, cystic fibrosis transmembrane conductance regulator channel; CRF, corticotropin-releasing factor; IBS, irritable bowel syndrome; IBS-A, irritable bowel syndrome with alternating bowel habits; IBS-D, irritable bowel syndrome with diarrhea; κ-opioid, kappa opioid.

system atrophy, mosapride, 15 mg/d, for 3 months significantly accelerated colonic transit time by radio-opaque marker testing, blunted first sensation of rectal filling, increased the amplitude of rectal contractions, and decreased postdefecation residuals on video anorectal manometry. Mosapride also led to clinical improvements in bowel movement frequency and difficulty with defecation.[18] Another study found that 8 weeks of mosapride, 15 mg/d, improved the frequency of bowel movements in 20 patients with diabetes experiencing constipation.[29]

Mosapride is generally well tolerated. Side effects include diarrhea, dry mouth, and headache.[20] No QT abnormalities have been reported in association with mosapride treatment.[20,29] However, a single case of torsades de pointes was reported in a patient who had hypokalemia and was prescribed mosapride along with flecainine.[20]

A randomized, placebo-controlled phase III trial evaluating mosapride, 5 mg, three times daily for 8 weeks recently completed enrollment in the Middle East, and results are awaited.[30]

Partial 5-HT$_3$ agonist

Pumosetrag (MKC-733, DDP-733) Pumosetrag is a potent, partial 5-HT$_3$ agonist with prokinetic effects in animals and humans.[31] Three phase I trials (n = 40) have evaluated pumosetrag's pharmacodynamic effects on gastrointestinal transit and have attempted to identify an appropriate dose in humans. In a small, double-blind, crossover study conducted in healthy volunteers, pumosetrag (0.2, 1, and 4 mg) stimulated fasting antroduodenal migrating motor activity and delayed the gastric emptying of liquids but accelerated small bowel transit.[32]

Similar results were shown using echo planar MRI, in which 12 volunteers receiving pumosetrag developed slowing of gastric emptying and acceleration of small bowel transit.[6] A single-blind, dose-escalation study in which 14 constipated subjects sequentially received placebo (1 week) followed by pumosetrag, 0.2 and 0.5 mg, twice daily (2 weeks each), showed increases in stool frequency and improvements in straining, sensation of incomplete evacuation, and stool consistency among patients treated with pumosetrag.[33] Only pumosetrag, 0.5 mg, twice daily increased the elimination of radio-opaque markers, demonstrating its effects on colonic transit.

The most common side effects with pumosetrag across all studies were flushing, nausea, diarrhea, headache, and anorexia.[6,32,33] Mild, transient liver enzymes elevations were also reported, but no subjects were withdrawn from the study, nor were changes in QT interval reported. Whether further studies to evaluate pumosetrag in patients with IBS-C or CC are planned is unclear.

Guanylate Cyclase-C Receptor Agonists

The family of guanylin peptides comprise four members: guanylin, uroguanylin, lymphoguanylin, and renoguanylin.[34] They have similar structure to the heat-stable enterotoxin produced by *Escherichia coli* and other enteric bacteria that cause secretory diarrhea.[35]

These peptides, particularly guanylin and uroguanylin, have the conformation to bind with guanylate cyclase-C (GC-C) receptors, which are abundantly found on enterocytes lining the intestine.[36] Binding of GC-C receptors stimulates production of cyclic guanosine monophosphate, which triggers a cascade of intracellular events, including activation of the cystic fibrosis transmembrane conductance regulator channel. This function results in transepithelial chloride (Cl^-) and potassium (K^-) ion efflux from enterocytes, with secondary passive water secretion into the intestinal lumen.[37]

Linaclotide (MD-1100)

Linaclotide is a synthetic 14–amino acid peptide that avidly binds GC-C receptors. Linaclotide is believed to act locally, because systemic levels are not detectable after oral dosing. In mice, linaclotide stimulated intestinal electrolyte and fluid secretion and accelerated gastrointestinal transit time.[38] Of potential relevance to IBS, recent work has shown that linaclotide reduced or abolished visceral hyperalgesic responses through GC-C dependent activation in several different stress models: colorectal distension, water avoidance, acute partial restraint, and TNBS (2,4,6-trinitrobenzene-sulfonic acid)-induced colitis.[38] Although the degree of attenuation in hyperalgesia varied among the different models, these results raise some interesting questions about linaclotide's potential usefulness for treating pain associated with IBS.

Clinical studies have investigated linaclotide in patients with IBS-C and CC. In a phase IIa study of 36 women with IBS-C, a 5-day course of linaclotide, 1000 µg, but not 100 µg, significantly accelerated ascending colon ($P = .004$) and total colonic transit time at 48 hours ($P = .01$) measured by a validated scintigraphy protocol. Linaclotide at either dose had no effect on gastric emptying or small bowel transit time. Linaclotide accelerated the time to first bowel movement, decreased stool consistency, and enhanced ease of stool passage.[39] In a double-blind, placebo-controlled pilot study in 42 chronic constipation patients, linaclotide, 100, 300, or 1000 µg, once daily for 14 days improved stool consistency, stool frequency, and ease of stool passage. The clinical benefits of linaclotide were seen at all doses, with some degree of dose-dependence (except for ease of stool passage, which was effective only at the 300 and 1000 µg doses).[40]

Recently, Lembo and colleagues[41] reported results from a methodologically rigorous randomized, double-blind, placebo-controlled phase IIb trial in 310 patients with chronic constipation assessing the efficacy and safety of four dosages of linaclotide (75, 150, 300, and 600 µg/d). Linaclotide improved the primary end point of weekly spontaneous bowel movements (SBMs) and various other constipation-related clinical parameters, including stool consistency and straining in a dose-dependent fashion (not including the 75 µg/d dosage for straining and CSBM rate). In addition, patients treated with linaclotide experienced improvements in abdominal discomfort, bloating, and constipation severity. Linaclotide significantly improved disease-related quality of life (PAC-QOL) compared with placebo.[42] Constipation symptoms tended to return to baseline, without evidence of a rebound, after discontinuation of linaclotide.

The overall frequency of adverse events reported with linaclotide and placebo were similar,[41] with diarrhea the most common adverse event reported with linaclotide. In most cases, the diarrhea was mild to moderate in severity, occurred within the first week of therapy, and resolved without specific intervention. Although more patients treated with linaclotide discontinued trial participation because of diarrhea than those treated with placebo, there were no reports of dehydration or electrolyte imbalance.[39–41]

The results of the phase IIb trial were confirmed by two recently presented phase III clinical trials that randomized more than 1200 patients with CC to linaclotide, 133 µg or 266 µg, or placebo once daily for 12 weeks.[42,43] Of great relevance to IBS-C, a separate pair of phase III clinical trials that randomized more than 1600 patients with IBS-C also reported benefits for constipation-related complaints and abdominal pain with linaclotide, 266 µg, versus placebo for up to 26 weeks.[44] These studies showed that linaclotide significantly improved several prespecified primary end points, including a composite responder end point encompassing abdominal pain and CSBMs, and individual responder end points for abdominal pain and CSBMs ($P<.0001$). Linaclotide also significantly improved all prespecified secondary end points, including abdominal pain, abdominal discomfort, bloating, and bowel symptoms ($P<.001$). Based on these promising results, a new drug application for the indications of IBS-C and CC is expected to be submitted to the U.S. Food and Drug Administration (FDA) in the near future.

Plecanatide (SP-304)

Plecanatide is an orally administered, synthetic analog of uroguanylin that, like linaclotide, is a GC-C agonist. A distinct characteristic of uroguanylin is that it seems to work most effectively in acidic regions of the intestine, including the proximal duodenum, which is exposed to acidic gastric effluent, and the cecum, in which bacterial fermentation occurs.[45] The structure of plecanatide contains an NDE terminus that retains pH modulation capability. The pharmacologic and clinical relevance of this finding requires further elucidation.

A phase I, double-blind, placebo-controlled trial in healthy volunteers showed that plecanatide was well tolerated in the range of dosages tested, with little systemic absorption.[46] Data from a recently completed phase IIa study showed that oral plecanatide given at dosages of 0.3, 1.0, 3.0, and 9.0 mg once daily for 14 days improved stool frequency, straining, and abdominal discomfort in patients with chronic constipation. Plecanatide treatment was associated with no severe adverse events and, somewhat surprisingly, no patients reported diarrhea. Additionally, no systemic absorption of plecanatide was detected at any of the dose levels studied.[47] The status of plecanatide as a treatment for IBS-C is currently unknown.

Bile Acid Modulators

Bile acids have long been known to alter gut motility and secretion. Hydrophobic primary bile acids, including chenodeoxycholic acid (CDCA) and cholic acid, are derived from cholesterol through hepatic hydroxylation and conjugation, and enter the small intestine though the biliary tract. These primary bile acids are modified by intestinal commensal bacteria to become hydrophilic, secondary bile acids, including deoxycholic acid (DCA), lithocholic acid, and, to a lesser extent, ursodeoxycholic acid. Of all bile acids, 95% will eventually be reclaimed through active transport in the ileum and returned to the liver through the portal vein. Additionally, any bile acids that are not removed through active transport are subject to passive transport in the terminal ileum. Because of the efficiency of bile acid reclamation by the terminal ileum, only a small amount reaches the colon.[48,49]

In the setting of bile acid–related diarrhea after ileal resection,[50] high concentrations of bile acids decrease net colonic fluid and electrolyte absorption and induce secretion. This effect is inducible only if high concentrations (3–10 mM) of DCA and CDCA are present under optimal pH.[51–53] Keating and colleagues[54] recently showed that colonic epithelial chloride secretion could be acutely stimulated by a high concentration of DCA, but that chronic exposure to a low concentration of DCA inhibited colonic chloride secretion. Furthermore, instillation of bile acids directly into the colon increases intracolonic pressure and motility index[55] and may have effects on defecatory function.[56]

CDCA

Hepner and Hofmann[57] conducted the first controlled trial to explore the effect of bile acids for constipation in 1973. The study reported that five of six participants experienced a greater laxative effect with cholic acid compared with bisacodyl or placebo. Ten years later, Bazzoli and colleagues[58] reported on the benefits of CDCA for constipation in patients with cholesterol gallstones.

A more recent study in healthy volunteers showed that sodium chenodeoxycholate (CDC) at doses of 500 and 1000 mg significantly accelerated scintigraphically measured colonic transit compared with placebo. Dose-dependent differences from placebo were apparent at 24 hours ($P<.01$) and even more pronounced at 48 hours ($P<.001$). Acceleration of colon transit was accompanied by improvements in clinical outcomes, such as stool frequency, stool consistency, ease of stool passage, and sense of complete evacuation.[59]

Rao and colleagues[60] recently reported the main results from a study evaluating the effects of CDC on colonic transit and clinical parameters in women with IBS-C. CDC significantly accelerated overall colonic transit and improved clinical outcomes, including stool frequency and stool consistency, and facilitated the passage of stool. In contrast to colonic transit time, gastric emptying time was delayed in the CDC group compared with the placebo group. Furthermore, the investigators also found a correlation between fasting serum 7 alpha-hydroxy-4-cholesten-3-one ($7\alpha C_4$), a biomarker of bile acid synthesis, and colonic transit time in the placebo group: subjects with an increased $7\alpha C_4$ showed a faster overall colonic transit time. In the CDC group, $7\alpha C4$ showed a modest influence on colonic transit at 24 hours ($P = .055$) and 48 hours ($P = .019$). In another study, serum concentrations of $7\alpha C_4$ were greater in patients with IBS-C and CC whose oroanal transit time was delayed than in those whose transit time was normal.[61]

Gastrointestinal side effects were most common with CDC. Up to 45% of the CDC group reported development of lower abdominal cramping/pain, compared with none in the placebo group. Although not significantly different from placebo, larger numbers of patients in the CDC group reported diarrhea, nausea, gaseous sensation, and headache.[60] Other issues that have been raised include the potential impact of bile acids on gut immune function and colonic neoplasia.[48] In the dose range that has been tested, the side effect of abdominal cramping or pain may limit the practical application of CDC as a treatment for IBS-C.

Ileal bile acid transporter inhibitor: A3309

A3309 is a novel small molecule that inhibits ileal bile acid transporters. A3309 was initially evaluated for the treatment of dyslipidemia but is now being developed as a treatment of constipation and perhaps IBS-C. Through inhibiting bile acid reabsorption in the terminal ileum, A3309 leads to a greater delivery of bile acids to the right colon.

In a transgenic mouse model, oral A3309 showed a dose-dependent inhibitory effect on intestinal bile acid absorption and a dose-dependent reduction of plasma cholesterol. In a study using a meat-induced constipated dog model, A3309 (1.5, 5, 15, or 50 µmol/kg) or tegaserod (0.3, 1.0, 66 µmol/kg) dosed orally once daily for 3 days increased fecal output. In addition, A3309 led to higher levels of serum C_4 than placebo, reflecting an increase in bile acid synthesis.[62]

A phase I/IIa study evaluating the effects of A3309 (0.1, 0.3, 1.0, 3.0 and 10 mg) versus placebo for 14 days in 30 patients with CC was recently reported.[63] The higher dose of A3309 accelerated colonic transit, as measured with radio-opaque markers, and improved constipation complaints, including stool frequency and stool consistency. Adverse events were similar for the various dosages of A3309 and placebo.

Top-line data from a randomized, placebo-controlled phase IIb dose-range study in 190 patients with CC also recently became available.[64] A3309 once daily at dosages of 5, 10, and 15 mg/d showed dose-dependent effects on the primary outcome of weekly SBMs and several other constipation-related secondary outcomes. The two higher doses were most effective. No serious adverse events were reported. Modest reductions in serum cholesterol level were also noted. Phase III clinical trials in patients with CC are expected in the near future. Whether A3309 will be developed as a therapy for IBS-C remains unclear.

Dopaminergic Antagonist: Itopride

Itopride is a dopamine D_2 antagonist and acetylcholinesterase inhibitor that was primarily developed to treat upper gastrointestinal tract conditions, such as gastro-esophageal reflux disease, gastroparesis, and functional dyspepsia. Studies have suggested that itopride may impact lower gastrointestinal function. In a guinea pig model, itopride significantly accelerated the propagation velocity of ileal peristalsis and reduced colonic transit time.[65] Similar results were found in conscious dogs and rats, in which Itopride dose-dependently stimulated small bowel and colonic motility. Itopride also triggered giant migrating contractions, which resulted in defecation in some dogs.[66]

Generally, adverse effects of itopride have been mild. Studies in patients with functional dyspepsia showed that the most common adverse effects were abdominal pain, nausea, diarrhea, and constipation, which were not significantly different from those seen in the placebo group.[67] A distinct side effect from itopride is dose-dependent elevation of serum prolactin level, although recently reported trials noted no clinical consequences from this laboratory change.[67,68] No significant electrocardiographic changes, particularly in QT interval, were reported.

The efficacy of itopride (50 and 100 mg) is being investigated in a randomized, placebo-controlled study in patients with IBS-C.

EMERGING THERAPIES FOR DIARRHEA-PREDOMINANT IBS

Several drugs in development with novel mechanisms of action have shown efficacy in diarrhea-predominant IBS (IBS-D) and IBS with a mixed bowel pattern (IBS-M). These agents act on targets located along the brain–gut axis and include asimadoline (a κ-opioid receptor agonist), AST-100 (a carbon-based adsorbent), CRF-1R antagonists, crofelemer (blocks intestinal chloride secretion), dextofisopam (a 2,3-benzodiazepine modulator), LX1031 (a TPH-1 inhibitor), and ramosetron (a 5-HT$_3$ antagonist).

Opioid Receptor Agonist: Asimadoline

Kappa receptors are believed to modulate visceral perception through inhibiting visceral afferents in response to noxious stimuli.[69] Asimadoline is a selective, potent κ-opioid receptor agonist with a low permeability through the blood-brain barrier. In a crossover, placebo-controlled study in 20 patients with IBS and visceral hyperalgesia, a single dose of asimadoline, 0.5 mg, was associated with reduced pain-intensity ratings (measured using area under the curve but not thresholds).[70]

A randomized, placebo-controlled, dose-ranging study investigated the efficacy of 0.15, 0.5, and 1.0 mg doses of asimadoline over 12 weeks in 596 patients with IBS of varying subtypes.[71] The primary end point was the number of months a patient experienced adequate relief of pain. For each month, patients with adequate response were defined as those having a positive response to the weekly question "In the past 7 days have you had adequate relief of your IBS pain or discomfort?" for at least 3 of 4 weeks. No significant difference was seen between the active drug and placebo groups in the percentage of months with adequate relief (33.3%, 33.3%, 36.7%, 36.7% for placebo and asimadoline, 0.15, 0.5, and 1.0 mg, respectively). However, subgroup analyses showed that patients with IBS-D experienced significant benefit with the 0.5-mg dose of asimadoline (47% vs 20%; $P = .011$) and a trend toward significant benefit with the 1.0-mg dose (36.7% vs 20%; $P = .054$).

Patients with IBS-D with at least moderate pain at baseline also showed significant improvement in pain scores, pain-free days, urgency, and stool frequency with asimadoline compared with placebo, although sample sizes were relatively small.[71] Patients with IBS with alternating bowel habits (IBS-A) had a significantly higher response rate with the 1-mg dose compared with placebo (50% vs 27.6%; $P = .022$) but did not report significant improvement in other symptom end points. Asimadoline failed to show a benefit in IBS-C. Constipation and diarrhea were the most common side effects in this study. These results suggest that asimadoline may be an effective agent for treating IBS-D and, to a lesser extent, IBS-A. A phase III clinical trial evaluating the efficacy of asimadoline in IBS-D was initiated in 2010.

Oral Carbon Adsorbent: AST-120

AST-120 is a nonabsorbable, oral, carbon-based adsorbent with extensive porosity and adsorbing capability. It adsorbs ammonia, histamine, bacterial products, bile acids, serotonin, and other luminal mediators within the gastrointestinal tract. This compound reportedly has an excellent safety profile in more than 360,000 patients in Japan.[72]

A randomized, double-blind, placebo-controlled trial evaluated the efficacy of an 8-week treatment of AST-120 at a dosage of 2 g three times daily in 115 patients with nonconstipating IBS (AST-100, n = 56; placebo, n = 59).[72] The primary end point was the proportion of responders, defined as patients reporting a 50% or greater reduction in days with pain over a 2-week period compared with baseline. A significantly greater proportion of responders were taking AST-120 than placebo at week 4 (27% vs 10%; $P = .029$). Pain and bloating severity were measured using 100-mm visual analog scales. AST-120 was associated with a numerically greater reduction in mean pain severity compared with placebo (11 vs 6 mm). Reduction in bloating severity was significantly greater with AST-120 than with placebo after 4 weeks of treatment (14 vs −1 mm; $P = .002$). Fewer patients on AST-120 reported at least one adverse event than patients on placebo. Larger clinical trials are needed.

Corticotropin-Releasing Factor Receptor Type 1 Antagonist

Corticotropin-releasing factor (CRF) signaling pathways are involved in regulation of endocrine, autonomic, behavioral, and visceral responses to stress.[73] Extensive animal research has shown the relationship between activation of central and peripheral CRF receptors and increases in gastrointestinal motility, permeability, and visceral sensitivity.[74,75] Furthermore, CRF receptor type 1 (CRF-1R) antagonists have been shown to inhibit stress-induced stimulation of colonic motor function in animal models of stress.[76] Therefore, a CRF-1R antagonist has been identified as a potential target for treatment in IBS. The effect of a nonselective α-helical CRF receptor antagonist on sigmoid colonic motility, perceptual thresholds, and mood in response to rectal electrical stimulation was studied in 10 patients with IBS and 10 healthy controls, with equal numbers of men and women in each group.[77] Electrical stimulation increased colonic motility indices significantly more in patients with IBS than in healthy controls. This CRF antagonist blocked the increases in motility. Compared with baseline measurements, the CRF antagonist also decreased abdominal pain and anxiety ratings resulting from electrical stimulation in patients with IBS but did not decrease discomfort or pain thresholds.

In a recent placebo-controlled phase IIa trial, the pharmacodynamic effects of pexacerfont, a CRF-1R antagonist, on gastrointestinal and colonic transit and bowel symptoms were measured in 39 women with IBS-D.[78] Two doses of pexacerfont

(25 and 100 mg once daily) administered for 1 week showed no significant effects on overall colonic transit at 24 hours (primary end point), gastric emptying, orocecal transit, ascending colon emptying half-time, or colonic transit at 48 hours, nor did the treatment have any significant effects on stool frequency, stool consistency, and ease of stool passage scores. However, the average baseline stool frequency was only two stools per day, and average baseline stool form ranged from 4.1 to 4.7 on a seven-point Bristol stool form scale[79] in all three treatment groups. Thus, a significant treatment effect on bowel habits would not necessarily be expected in this group of patients with IBS-D. No safety issues were identified.

GW876008 is a selective, nonpeptide CRF-1R antagonist that crosses the blood–brain barrier and therefore can access both central and gastrointestinal sites. This medication did not alter hypothalamic-pituitary-adrenal (HPA) axis hormone levels to CRF stimulation and only modestly decreased HPA axis inhibition with metapyrone.[80] Preclinical animal models of IBS suggested that this agent would be effective.[80] In a 19-week, multicenter, randomized, placebo-controlled crossover design study, the efficacy of GW876008, 125 mg, once daily was assessed based on a weekly global improvement scale (seven-point Likert scale), a daily IBS pain/discomfort rating (five-point verbal scale), and individual lower gastrointestinal symptoms.[80] In this study, 132 patients with IBS (76% women) were randomized to receive either active drug (n = 67) or placebo (n = 65) in period 1 before crossover. Only data from this 6-week treatment period were analyzed to evaluate efficacy because a significantly different baseline pain severity was seen between the groups, which is a violation of crossover assumption. No significant differences in global improvement scale responder rate (0.27 vs 0.24), pain and discomfort responder rate (0.23 vs 0.19), or individual symptoms were seen between the GW876008 and placebo groups. In general, the medication was well tolerated, but the most frequent adverse events (>3%) were nasopharyngitis, headache, nausea, dizziness, abdominal pain, and fatigue.

Inhibitors of Chloride Secretion: Crofelemer

Crofelemer is a novel proanthocyanidin oligomer that has an antisecretory mechanism of action that reduces excess intestinal chloride ion secretion. Crofelemer was developed from sap extracted from the blood-bark latex of the South American plant *Croton lecheri* (dragon's blood).[81] For many years, this sap has been used to treat diarrhea (eg, caused by dysentery and cholera) and other gastrointestinal and lung conditions. Recent experimental studies showed that crofelemer exerts an antisecretory action on two distinct chloride channel targets on the luminal membrane of intestinal epithelial cells, namely the cystic fibrosis transmembrane regulator and calcium-activated chloride channel.[81] Crofelemer is being investigated for the treatment of acute infectious diarrhea, chronic diarrhea associated with HIV/AIDS, and IBS-D.

To evaluate the safety and efficacy of crofelemer in the treatment of IBS-D, a randomized, double-blind, placebo-controlled, phase IIa 12-week treatment study was conducted in 246 patients with IBS-D (75% women) randomized either to placebo or to crofelemer at dosages of 125, 250, or 500 mg twice daily.[82] The primary end point was improvement in stool consistency. The study found that none of the doses of crofelemer improved stool consistency, stool frequency, or urgency, or provided adequate relief of IBS symptoms. However, the 500-mg twice-daily dosage of crofelemer significantly increased pain- and discomfort-free days. This positive effect was largely driven by the strong effect (16% therapeutic gain) in women with IBS-D. Large clinical trials are needed.

Atypical Benzodiazepine: Dextofisopam

Dextofisopam is an autonomic modulator and the R-enantiomer of the drug tofisopam. Tofisopam is a benzodiazepine derivative that has anxiolytic properties but does not produce muscle-relaxant or sedative effects.[83] Unlike typical benzodiazepines, which have nitrogen atoms in the 1,4 or 1,5 position of their benzodiazepine ring, dextofisopam has nitrogen atoms in the 2,3 position. Dextofisopam binds to 2,3 benzodiazepine receptors located in subcortical regions of the brain but not in the gastrointestinal tract.[84] Dextofisopam's possible effect on decreasing motility has made it an agent of interest for the treatment of nonconstipating IBS.

In a randomized, double-blind, placebo-controlled phase IIb study, 140 adults (73% women) with IBS-D or IBS-A were randomized to either dextofisopam, 200 mg, twice daily or a placebo for 12 weeks.[85] The primary end point was the number of months patients reported adequate overall relief of IBS symptoms. A responder was defined as any individual who experienced adequate relief in 2 or more of 4 weekly assessments in 1 month. Patients with IBS taking dextofisopam experienced response for significantly more months than those taking placebo (1.7 vs 1.3 months; $P = .033$). Although dextofisopam was associated with a greater number of responders during the first month of treatment compared with placebo (73% vs 49%; $P = .002$), only a numerically higher responder rate was seen during the second month (56% vs 43%; $P = .084$) and no difference was seen during the third month (43% vs 38%; $P = .47$). Similarly, the initial significant benefit of dextofisopam on stool frequency seen in the first month of treatment diminished over the second and third months. A numerically, but not statistically, greater improvement was seen in stool consistency in the patients with IBS-D treated with dextofisopam than in those treated with placebo. The most common side effects associated with dextofisopam were abdominal pain, influenza, and nausea, but the occurrence rates were not significantly different from those for placebo. The study suggests that dextofisopam may be effective for treating IBS symptoms in patients with IBS-D and IBS-A, but that it may be more ideal in the setting of intermittent flares and on an as-needed basis. A phase III clinical trial has not yet been initiated.

Tryptophan Hydroxylase-1 Inhibitor: LX1031

The rate-limiting enzyme in the biosynthesis of 5-HT is tryptophan hydroxylase-1 (TPH-1). Serotonin signaling systems are important in the modulation of visceral sensation, gut motility, and secretion, and are believed to play a role in IBS pathophysiology.[86,87] Patients with IBS-D have increased platelet-depleted 5-HT concentrations during fasting and postprandial conditions compared with healthy volunteers and patients with IBS-C.[87] TPH-1 inhibitors that have the ability to selectively reduce 5-HT levels in the gastrointestinal tract but not in the brain are potential novel agents for the treatment of nonconstipating IBS.[88]

LX1031 is a novel TPH-1 inhibitor that decreases serotonin synthesis. Preclinical studies showed that LX1031 is a peripherally acting agent that reduces gastrointestinal 5-HT in a dose-dependent fashion. Phase I studies showed dose-dependent decreases in 24-hour urinary 5-hydroxyindoleacetic acid (5-HIAA) levels, supporting its inhibition of serotonin syntheses. In a randomized, placebo-controlled phase II study assessing the efficacy of LX1031 in nonconstipating IBS,[89] 155 patients with IBS-D or IBS-M were assigned to either 250 or 1000 mg of LX1031 four times daily or placebo for 28 days. The global relief of IBS symptoms over the 4-week treatment period was significantly improved with LX1031 given at 1000 mg four times daily, as was stool consistency. Symptom improvement correlated with a reduction in urinary

5-HIAA, a biomarker for serotonin synthesis. These findings must be confirmed in larger samples of patients with IBS.

5-HT$_3$ Antagonist: Ramosetron

5-HT$_3$ antagonists, such as alosetron and cilansetron, have been shown to be efficacious in the relief of IBS-D symptoms.[7] However, alosetron is currently only available in the United States on a risk-management program because of concerns about ischemic colitis and serious complications associated with constipation.[90] A double-blind, placebo-controlled phase II trial compared the efficacy of ramosetron at doses of 1 (n = 105), 5 (n = 103), and 10 μg (n = 101), and placebo (n = 109) given once daily for 12 weeks in patients with IBS-D.[91] The primary end point was the monthly responder rate of patient-reported global assessment of IBS symptom relief (0 = completely relieved to 4 = worsened) during the last month of treatment. A monthly responder was required to report "completely relieved" or "considerably relieved" for at least 2 of the 4 weeks that month. Patients taking ramosetron at doses of 5 and 10 μg had significantly higher responder rates than those taking placebo (42.57% [P = .027] and 43.01% [P = .026] vs 26.92%, respectively). Monthly responder rates were also significantly higher for these two doses than for placebo in months 1 and 2. In addition, ramosetron was associated with significantly greater responder rates for relief of "abdominal discomfort and/or pain" and relief of "abnormal bowel habits." A dose-related incidence of constipation and hard stools occurred, but no cases of ischemic colitis or serious complications of constipation were reported. This medication is approved for use in Japan but is not currently available in the United States.

EMERGING THERAPIES FOR ABDOMINAL PAIN IN IBS
Glucagon-Like Peptide-1 Analogue

Glucagon-like peptide-1 (GLP-1) is released after meals and stimulates insulin release and decreases gastric emptying and small intestinal motility.[92,93] GLP-1 analogues were initially developed to normalize blood glucose levels in patients with diabetes but are now being studied to treat abdominal pain attacks in patients with IBS because of the agent's inhibitory effect on small intestinal motility.[94]

A randomized, double-blind, placebo-controlled phase II study was conducted in Europe to assess the efficacy and tolerability of the GLP-1 analogue ROSE-010 in patients with IBS.[94] Patients who had a history of at least four abdominal pain attacks lasting 2 or more hours with an intensity of 40 mm or greater on a 100-mm visual analogue scale per month for at least 2 months were eligible for the study. In this crossover design study, patients were randomized to a single subcutaneous injection of 100 or 300 μg of ROSE-010 or placebo to treat a pain attack that began within 1 hour of administering the treatment intervention. The primary end point was the proportion of patients with a pain relief response defined as greater than 50% of the maximum possible response as measured using the area under the pain relief curve over 10 to 60 minutes after the administration of drug. Of the 166 (70% women) patients who were randomized, 99 received all three treatments (two different doses of ROSE-010 and placebo). Most of the patients who did not complete the study did not experience more pain attacks to receive subsequent treatment. A significantly higher proportion of patients reported greater than 50% of the maximum total pain relief response after 100 and 300 μg of ROSE-010 treatments than after placebo (23% and 24% vs 12%; P = .011 and P = .005, respectively). Times to meaningful and total pain relief were shorter for both doses of active drug versus placebo. Time to meaningful pain relief after study drug administration was defined as pain relief of greater than 50 mm on a visual analogue scale at more than two consecutive time points. More in-depth assessments of the IBS pain attack characteristics are ongoing and future clinical trials with ROSE-010 are being planned.

SUMMARY

A large number of candidate drugs are in various stages of development for IBS. Unfortunately, few drugs have found their way to the marketplace or met with commercial success because of various challenges in IBS drug development, including the heterogeneity of the patient populations, regulatory uncertainties (with regard to clinical trial design, outcome measures, and metrics for drug approval), a very low threshold for safety related issues, and a highly price sensitive market. One could argue that this lack of success is, at least partly, related to unrealistic expectations among industry, regulators, physicians, and patients. Because IBS is a symptom-based syndrome and not a disease, it is unrealistic to expect that a drug with a very specific mechanism of action will improve symptoms in more than a subgroup of patients with IBS. Therefore, unless a common, shared pathogenesis is found for all subgroups of IBS, individual drugs will continue to provide marginal therapeutic gains over placebo. Given this marginal therapeutic gain, and considering that IBS is a nonfatal condition, a high bar for safety would seem appropriate. However, a fine line exists between setting a high bar and creating barriers that impede new drug development. The reality is that IBS can be a serious, life-altering condition for more severely affected patients. A very fair question is whether the level of risk deemed acceptable should be the same for patients with mild IBS as for those more severely affected. Data suggest that patients are willing to accept very different levels of risk associated with drug therapy, depending on the severity of their symptoms.[95] This fact becomes relevant in a day and age when payors demand that patients with less-frequent, less-severe symptoms are managed with over-the-counter medications, thus relegating more expensive prescription medications to a "salvage" role, typically in patients who are more severely affected. These market trends have profound implications on the size of the patient pool for which prescription medications might be considered, clinical trial design, and the safety threshold deemed acceptable.

So what is the way forward for the development of novel therapies for IBS? Certainly efforts by regulatory agencies such as the FDA to identify and validate patient-reported outcome measures are commended, and offer the possibility of standardizing registration trial design and demystifying the drug approval process. However, true breakthroughs in IBS drug development are likely to only come with a better understanding of pathogenesis and the consequent development of robust and reproducible biomarkers. Until patients with IBS can be reliably subgrouped based on altered physiology, drug development will continue to be challenged by an overreliance on the imprecision of symptoms. In this age of super computers and globalization of knowledge, science continues to advance at a breathtaking pace, and the future of drug development for IBS is bright. For the foreseeable future, however, symptom-based criteria and patient reported end points will continue to dominate the landscape of new drug development.

REFERENCES

1. Longstreth GF, Thompson WG, Chey WD, et al. Functional bowel disorders. Gastroenterology 2006;130:1480–91.

2. Wong RK, Palsson OS, Turner MJ, et al. Inability of the Rome III criteria to distinguish functional constipation from constipation-subtype irritable bowel syndrome. Am J Gastroenterol 2010;105:2228–34.

3. Baker DE. Rationale for using serotonergic agents to treat irritable bowel syndrome. Am J Health Syst Pharm 2005;62:700–11.

4. Cash BD, Chey WD. Review article: the role of serotonergic agents in the treatment of patients with primary chronic constipation. Aliment Pharmacol Ther 2005;22:1047–60.

5. Hasler WL. Serotonin and the GI tract. Curr Gastroenterol Rep 2009;11:383–91.

6. Evangelista S. Drug evaluation: pumosetrag for the treatment of irritable bowel syndrome and gastroesophageal reflux disease. Curr Opin Investig Drugs 2007;8:416–22.

7. Ford AC, Brandt LJ, Young C, et al. Efficacy of 5-HT3 antagonists and 5-HT4 agonists in irritable bowel syndrome: systematic review and meta-analysis. Am J Gastroenterol 2009;104:1831–43.

8. Busti AJ, Murillo JR Jr, Cryer B. Tegaserod-induced myocardial infarction: case report and hypothesis. Pharmacotherapy 2004;24:526–31.

9. Potet F, Bouyssou T, Escande D, et al. Gastrointestinal prokinetic drugs have different affinity for the human cardiac human ether-a-gogo K(+) channel. J Pharmacol Exp Ther 2001;299:1007–12.

10. Briejer MR, Prins NH, Schuurkes JA. Effects of the enterokinetic prucalopride (R093877) on colonic motility in fasted dogs. Neurogastroenterol Motil 2001;13:465–72.

11. De Schryver AM, Andriesse GI, Samsom M, et al. The effects of the specific 5HT (4) receptor agonist, prucalopride, on colonic motility in healthy volunteers. Aliment Pharmacol Ther 2002;16:603–12.

12. Bouras EP, Camilleri M, Burton DD, et al. Selective stimulation of colonic transit by the benzofuran 5HT4 agonist, prucalopride, in healthy humans. Gut 1999;44:682–6.

13. Poen AC, Felt-Bersma RJ, Van Dongen PA, et al. Effect of prucalopride, a new enterokinetic agent, on gastrointestinal transit and anorectal function in healthy volunteers. Aliment Pharmacol Ther 1999;13:1493–7.

14. Camilleri M, Kerstens R, Rykx A, et al. A placebo-controlled trial of prucalopride for severe chronic constipation. N Engl J Med 2008;358:2344–54.

15. Tack J, van Outryve M, Beyens G, et al. Prucalopride (Resolor) in the treatment of severe chronic constipation in patients dissatisfied with laxatives. Gut 2009;58:357–65.

16. Quigley EM, Vandeplassche L, Kerstens R, et al. Clinical trial: the efficacy, impact on quality of life, and safety and tolerability of prucalopride in severe chronic constipation—a 12-week, randomized, double-blind, placebo-controlled study. Aliment Pharmacol Ther 2009;29:315–28.

17. Camilleri M, Kerstens R, Beyens G, et al. A Double-blind, placebo-controlled trial to evaluate the safety and tolerability of prucalopride oral solution in constipated elderly patients living in a nursing facility. Gastroenterology 2009;136:A46.

18. Liu Z, Sakakibara R, Odaka T, et al. Mosapride citrate, a novel 5-HT4 agonist and partial 5-HT3 antagonist, ameliorates constipation in parkinsonian patients. Mov Disord 2005;20:680–6.

19. Wei W, Ge ZZ, Lu H, et al. Effect of mosapride on gastrointestinal transit time and diagnostic yield of capsule endoscopy. J Gastroenterol Hepatol 2007;22:1605–8.

20. Curran MP, Robinson DM. Mosapride in gastrointestinal disorders. Drugs 2008; 68:981–91.
21. Ruth M, Hamelin B, Rohss K, et al. The effect of mosapride, a novel prokinetic, on acid reflux variables in patients with gastro-oesophageal reflux disease. Aliment Pharmacol Ther 1998;12:35–40.
22. Futagami S, Iwakiri K, Shindo T, et al. The prokinetic effect of mosapride citrate combined with omeprazole therapy improves clinical symptoms and gastric emptying in PPI-resistant NERD patients with delayed gastric emptying. J Gastroenterol 2009;45:413–21.
23. Jung IS, Kim JH, Lee HY, et al. Endoscopic evaluation of gastric emptying and effect of mosapride citrate on gastric emptying. Yonsei Med J 2010;51:33–8.
24. Ji SW, Park HJ, Cho JS, et al. Investigation into the effects of mosapride on motility of Guinea pig stomach, ileum, and colon. Yonsei Med J 2003;44:653–64.
25. Kim HS, Choi EJ, Park H. The effect of mosapride citrate on proximal and distal colonic motor function in the guinea-pig in vitro. Neurogastroenterol Motil 2008; 20:169–76.
26. Inui A, Yoshikawa T, Nagai R, et al. Effects of mosapride citrate, a 5-HT4 receptor agonist, on colonic motility in conscious guinea pigs. Jpn J Pharmacol 2002;90: 313–20.
27. Kojima Y, Fujii H, Katsui R, et al. Enhancement of the intrinsic defecation reflex by mosapride, a 5-HT4 agonist, in chronically lumbosacral denervated guinea pigs. J Smooth Muscle Res 2006;42:139–47.
28. Kojima Y, Nakagawa T, Katsui R, et al. A 5-HT4 agonist, mosapride, enhances intrinsic rectorectal and rectoanal reflexes after removal of extrinsic nerves in guinea pigs. Am J Physiol Gastrointest Liver Physiol 2005;289:G351–60.
29. Ueno N, Inui A, Satoh Y. The effect of mosapride citrate on constipation in patients with diabetes. Diabetes Res Clin Pract 2010;87:27–32.
30. Clinicaltrials.gov. Trial of mosapride versus placebo in the treatment of constipation-predominant irritable bowel syndrome. Available at: http://clinicaltrial.gov/ct2/show/NCT00742872?term=Mosapride&rank=3Randomized. Accessed December 2, 2010.
31. Chetty N, Irving HR, Coupar IM. Effects of the novel 5-HT3 agonist MKC-733 on the rat, mouse and guinea pig digestive tract. Pharmacology 2008;81:104–9.
32. Coleman NS, Marciani L, Blackshaw E, et al. Effect of a novel 5-HT3 receptor agonist MKC-733 on upper gastrointestinal motility in humans. Aliment Pharmacol Ther 2003;18:1039–48.
33. Fujita T, Yokota S, Sawada M, et al. Effect of MKC-733, a 5-HT receptor partial agonist, on bowel motility and symptoms in subjects with constipation: an exploratory study. J Clin Pharm Ther 2005;30:611–22.
34. Sindic A, Schlatter E. Renal electrolyte effects of guanylin and uroguanylin. Curr Opin Nephrol Hypertens 2007;16:10–5.
35. Forte LR, London RM, Freeman RH, et al. Guanylin peptides: renal actions mediated by cyclic GMP. Am J Physiol Renal Physiol 2000;278:F180–91.
36. Forte LR Jr. Uroguanylin and guanylin peptides: pharmacology and experimental therapeutics. Pharmacol Ther 2004;104:137–62.
37. Shailubhai K. Therapeutic applications of guanylate cyclase-C receptor agonists. Curr Opin Drug Discov Devel 2002;5:261–8.
38. Bryant AP, Busby RW, Bartolini WP, et al. Linaclotide is a potent and selective guanylate cyclase C agonist that elicits pharmacological effects locally in the gastrointestinal tract. Life Sci 2010;86:760–5.

39. Andresen V, Camilleri M, Busciglio IA, et al. Effect of 5 days linaclotide on transit and bowel function in females with constipation-predominant irritable bowel syndrome. Gastroenterology 2007;133:761–8.

40. Johnston JM, Kurtz CB, Drossman DA, et al. Pilot study on the effect of linaclotide in patients with chronic constipation. Am J Gastroenterol 2009;104:125–32.

41. Lembo AJ, Kurtz CB, Macdougall JE, et al. Efficacy of linaclotide for patients with chronic constipation. Gastroenterology 2010;138:886–95, e881.

42. Carson RT, Tourkodimitris S, MacDougall JE, et al. Effect of linaclotide on quality of life in adults with chronic constipation: results from 2 randomized, double-blind, placebo-controlled phase III trials. Gastroenterology 2010;139:e19.

43. Lembo AJ, Schneier H, Lavins BJ, et al. Efficacy and safety of once daily linaclotide administered orally for 12-weeks in patients with chronic constipation: results from 2 randomized, double-blind, placebo-controlled phase 3 trials [abstract #286]. Gastroenterology 2010;138:S53.

44. Forest Laboratories I, Ironwood Pharmaceuticals I. Ironwood and forest announce positive linaclotide results from second phase 3 trial in patients with irritable bowel syndrome with constipation. Available at: http://www.ironwoodpharma.com/newsPDF/IRWD.FRX.Ph3.MCP—103–302.11.01.10.pdf. Accessed December 2, 2010.

45. Joo NS, London RM, Kim HD, et al. Regulation of intestinal Cl- and HCO3- secretion by uroguanylin. Am J Physiol 1998;274:G633–44.

46. Shailubhai K, Gerson WA, Talluto C, et al. SP-304 to treat GI disorders—effects of a single, oral-dose of SP-304 on safety, tolerability, pharmacokinetics and pharmacodynamics in healthy volunteers. Gastroenterology 2009;136:A641.

47. Shailubhai K, Talluto C, Comiskey S, et al. Phase II clinical evaluation of SP-304, a guanylate cyclase-C agonist, for treatment of chronic constipation. Am J Gastroenterol 2010;105:S487.

48. Bajor A, Gillberg PG, Abrahamsson H. Bile acids: short and long term effects in the intestine. Scand J Gastroenterol 2010;45:645–64.

49. Pattni S, Walters JR. Recent advances in the understanding of bile acid malabsorption. Br Med Bull 2009;92:79–93.

50. Aldini R, Roda A, Festi D, et al. Bile acid malabsorption and bile acid diarrhea in intestinal resection. Dig Dis Sci 1982;27:495–502.

51. McJunkin B, Fromm H, Sarva RP, et al. Factors in the mechanism of diarrhea in bile acid malabsorption: fecal pH—a key determinant. Gastroenterology 1981; 80:1454–64.

52. Camilleri M, Murphy R, Chadwick VS. Dose-related effects of chenodeoxycholic acid in the rabbit colon. Dig Dis Sci 1980;25:433–8.

53. Mekjian HS, Phillips SF, Hofmann AF. Colonic secretion of water and electrolytes induced by bile acids: perfusion studies in man. J Clin Invest 1971;50:1569–77.

54. Keating N, Mroz MS, Scharl MM, et al. Physiological concentrations of bile acids down-regulate agonist induced secretion in colonic epithelial cells. J Cell Mol Med 2009;13:2293–303.

55. Kirwan WO, Smith AN, Mitchell WD, et al. Bile acids and colonic motility in the rabbit and the human. Gut 1975;16:894–902.

56. Edwards CA, Brown S, Baxter AJ, et al. Effect of bile acid on anorectal function in man. Gut 1989;30:383–6.

57. Hepner GW, Hofmann AF. Cholic acid therapy for constipation. A controlled study. Mayo Clin Proc 1973;48:56–8.

58. Bazzoli F, Malavolti M, Petronelli A, et al. Treatment of constipation with chenodeoxycholic acid. J Int Med Res 1983;11:120–3.

59. Odunsi–Shiyanbade ST, Camilleri M, McKinzie S, et al. Effects of chenodeoxycholate and a bile acid sequestrant, colesevelam, on intestinal transit and bowel function. Clin Gastroenterol Hepatol 2010;8:159–65.
60. Rao AS, Wong BS, Camilleri M, et al. Chenodeoxycholate in females with irritable bowel syndrome-constipation: a pharmacodynamic and pharmacogenetic analysis. Gastroenterology 2010;139:1549–58.
61. Abrahamsson H, Ostlund-Lindqvist AM, Nilsson R, et al. Altered bile acid metabolism in patients with constipation-predominant irritable bowel syndrome and functional constipation. Scand J Gastroenterol 2008;43:1483–8.
62. Gillberg PG, Dahlström M, Starke I, et al. The IBAT inhibition by A3309—a potential mechanism for the treatment of constipation. Gastroenterology 2010;138(Suppl): S-224.
63. Simren M, Abrahamsson H, Bajor A, et al. The IBAT inhibitor A3309—a promising treatment option for patients with chronic idiopathic constipation (Cic). Gastroenterology 2010;138(Suppl):S-223.
64. Albireo. Albireo announces positive results in patients with chronic idiopathic constipation from a phase IIb trial of A3309. Available at: http://www.albireopharma.com/News.aspx?PageID=232690. Accessed December 2, 2010.
65. Lim HC, Kim YG, Lim JH, et al. Effect of itopride hydrochloride on the ileal and colonic motility in guinea pig in vitro. Yonsei Med J 2008;49:472–8.
66. Tsubouchi T, Saito T, Mizutani F, et al. Stimulatory action of itopride hydrochloride on colonic motor activity in vitro and in vivo. J Pharmacol Exp Ther 2003;306:787–93.
67. Holtmann G, Talley NJ, Liebregts T, et al. A placebo-controlled trial of itopride in functional dyspepsia. N Engl J Med 2006;354:832–40.
68. Talley NJ, Tack J, Ptak T, et al. Itopride in functional dyspepsia: results of two phase III multicentre, randomised, double-blind, placebo-controlled trials. Gut 2008;57:740–6.
69. Camilleri M. Novel pharmacology: asimadoline, a kappa-opioid agonist, and visceral sensation. Neurogastroenterol Motil 2008;20:971–9.
70. Delvaux M, Beck A, Jacob J, et al. Effect of asimadoline, a kappa opioid agonist, on pain induced by colonic distension in patients with irritable bowel syndrome. Aliment Pharmacol Ther 2004;20:237–46.
71. Mangel AW, Bornstein JD, Hamm LR, et al. Clinical trial: asimadoline in the treatment of patients with irritable bowel syndrome. Aliment Pharmacol Ther 2008;28: 239–49.
72. Tack JF, Harris MS, Proksch S, et al. AST-120 (spherical carbon adsorbent) improves pain and bloating in a randomized, double-blind, placebo-controlled trial in patients with non-constipating irritable bowel syndrome (IBS). Gastroenterology 2010;138:S223.
73. Taché Y, Martinez V, Wang L, et al. CRF1 receptor signaling pathways are involved in stress-related alterations of colonic function and viscerosensitivity: implications for irritable bowel syndrome. Br J Pharmacol 2004;141:1321–30.
74. Taché Y, Martinez V, Million M, et al. Stress and the gastrointestinal tract III. Stress-related alterations of gut motor function: role of brain corticotropin-releasing factor receptors. Am J Physiol Gastrointest Liver Physiol 2001;280: G173–7.
75. Taché Y, Perdue MH. Role of peripheral CRF signalling pathways in stress-related alterations of gut motility and mucosal function. Neurogastroenterol Motil 2004; 16(Suppl 1):137–42.
76. Martinez V, Taché Y. CRF1 receptors as a therapeutic target for irritable bowel syndrome. Curr Pharm Des 2006;12:4071–88.

77. Sagami Y, Shimada Y, Tayama J, et al. Effect of a corticotropin releasing hormone receptor antagonist on colonic sensory and motor function in patients with irritable bowel syndrome. Gut 2004;53:958–64.

78. Sweetser S, Camilleri M, Linker Nord SJ, et al. Do corticotropin releasing factor-1 receptors influence colonic transit and bowel function in women with irritable bowel syndrome? Am J Physiol Gastrointest Liver Physiol 2009;296:G1299–306.

79. Lewis SJ, Heaton KW. Stool form scale as a useful guide to intestinal transit time. Scand J Gastroenterol 1997;32:920–4.

80. Dukes GE, Mayer E, Kelleher DL, et al. A randomised, double blind, placebo controlled, crossover study to evaluate the efficacy and safety of the CRF1 receptor antagonist GW876008 in patients with irritable bowel syndrome. Neurogastroenterol Motil 2009;21(Suppl):84.

81. Tradtrantip L, Namkung W, Verkman AS. Crofelemer, an antisecretory antidiarrheal proanthocyanidin oligomer extracted from Croton lechleri, targets two distinct intestinal chloride channels. Mol Pharmacol 2010;77:69–78.

82. Mangel AW, Chaturvedi P. Evaluation of crofelemer in the treatment of diarrhea-predominant irritable bowel syndrome patients. Digestion 2008;78:180–6.

83. Pellow S, File SE. Is tofisopam an atypical anxiolytic? Neurosci Biobehav Rev 1986;10:221–7.

84. Horvath EJ, Horvath K, Hamori T, et al. Anxiolytic 2,3-benzodiazepines, their specific binding to the basal ganglia. Prog Neurobiol 2000;60:309–42.

85. Leventer SM, Raudibaugh K, Frissora CL, et al. Clinical trial: dextofisopam in the treatment of patients with diarrhoea-predominant or alternating irritable bowel syndrome. Aliment Pharmacol Ther 2008;27:197–206.

86. Coates MD, Mahoney CR, Linden DR, et al. Molecular defects in mucosal serotonin content and decreased serotonin reuptake transporter in ulcerative colitis and irritable bowel syndrome. Gastroenterology 2004;126:1657–64.

87. Atkinson W, Lockhart S, Whorwell PJ, et al. Altered 5-hydroxytryptamine signaling in patients with constipation- and diarrhea-predominant irritable bowel syndrome. Gastroenterology 2006;130:34–43.

88. Liu Q, Yang Q, Sun W, et al. Discovery and characterization of novel tryptophan hydroxylase inhibitors that selectively inhibit serotonin synthesis in the gastrointestinal tract. J Pharmacol Exp Ther 2008;325:47–55.

89. Brown P, Riff DS, Jackson J, et al. LX1031, a novel locally-acting inhibitor of serotonin (5-HT) synthesis significantly improves symptoms in patients with IBS. Gastroenterology 2010;138:S129.

90. Chang L, Tong K, Ameen V. Ischemic colitis and complications of constipation associated with the use of alosetron under a risk management plan: clinical characteristics, outcomes, and incidences. Am J Gastroenterol 2010;105:866–75.

91. Matsueda K, Harasawa S, Hongo M, et al. A phase II trial of the novel serotonin type 3 receptor antagonist ramosetron in Japanese male and female patients with diarrhea-predominant irritable bowel syndrome. Digestion 2008;77:225–35.

92. Naslund E, Bogefors J, Skogar S, et al. GLP-1 slows solid gastric emptying and inhibits insulin, glucagon, and PYY release in humans. Am J Phys 1999;277: R910–6.

93. Tolessa T, Gutniak M, Holst JJ, et al. Glucagon-like peptide-1 retards gastric emptying and small bowel transit in the rat: effect mediated through central or enteric nervous mechanisms. Dig Dis Sci 1998;43:2284–90.

94. Hellstrom PM, Hein J, Bytzer P, et al. Clinical trial: the glucagon-like peptide-1 analogue ROSE-010 for management of acute pain in patients with irritable bowel

syndrome: a randomized, placebo-controlled, double-blind study. Aliment Pharmacol Ther 2009;29:198–206.

95. Lacy B, Everhart K, Weiser K, et al. Medication risk taking behavior in IBS patients. Am J Gastroenterol 2009;104:S489.

96. Clinicaltrials.gov. Study to evaluate the role of itopride HCl in patients with irritable bowel syndrome with predominant constipation. Available at: http://clinicaltrial.gov/ct2/show/NCT01027260?term=itopride&rank=2. Accessed December 2, 2010.

Complementary and Alternative Medicine for the Irritable Bowel Syndrome

Suma Magge, MD, Anthony Lembo, MD*

KEYWORDS

• CAM • IBS • Herbs • Acupuncture • Probiotics • Prebiotics

Irritable bowel syndrome (IBS) is a common chronic gastrointestinal disorder, characterized by bloating and chronic or recurrent abdominal pain associated with alterations in bowel habits.[1] IBS can be categorized based on the predominant bowel habit: constipation, diarrhea, or both (ie, alternating pattern of diarrhea and constipation). IBS affects between 10% and 15% of the North American population.[2,3] Because only a limited number of treatments are available for IBS, many patients choose complementary and alternative medicines (CAMs).[4]

CAM is a diverse group of medical treatments that are not commonly considered to be a part of conventional medicine yet frequently used together with conventional medicine. CAM is widely used particularly among patients who have chronic medical conditions that are difficult to treat. In 2002, it was estimated that approximately 35% of the population used CAM in the previous year.[5] A population-based study from Australia showed that approximately 21% of patients with IBS sought care from a CAM provider,[6] and a study from the United Kingdom found that approximately 50% of patients with IBS attending an outpatient gastrointestinal clinic had used CAM.[7] In the United States, a prospective 6-month study conducted in a large health maintenance organization setting found CAM use in 35% of patients with functional bowel disorders, including IBS, with an annual cost of $200. In this study, CAM use was highest in women and in those with higher education and anxiety.[8]

This article reviews current evidence supporting the use of CAM in IBS, with a focus on prebiotics, acupuncture, and herbal medicines.

Potential conflict of interest: Dr Lembo is a paid consultant for Ironwood, Salix, Prometheus, GSK, Astra-Zeneca, Ardelyx, Theravance. Dr Magge has no conflicts to report.
Division of Gastroenterology, Department of Medicine, Beth Israel Deaconess Medical Center, Rabb/Rose 1, 330 Brookline Avenue, Boston, MA 02215, USA
* Corresponding author.
E-mail address: alembo@bidmc.harvard.edu

Gastroenterol Clin N Am 40 (2011) 245–253
doi:10.1016/j.gtc.2010.12.005

PREBIOTICS

A prebiotic is considered to be a "non-digestible food ingredient that beneficially affects the host by selectively stimulating the growth and/or activity of one of a limited number of potentially health-promoting bacteria in the colon," most notably lactobacilli and bifidobacteria.[9] Stimulating the growth of probiotics such as *Lactobacillus* or *Bifidobacterium* results in an increase in the absorption of vitamin and minerals, improves digestion, and increases protection against harmful bacteria, fungi, and viruses.[10] Other mechanisms by which prebiotics modulate the immune system include increasing the number of lactic acid–producing bacteria, increasing the amount of short-chain fatty acids, and activating carbohydrate receptor immune cells.[11]

Prebiotics are most commonly carbohydrates. Fructo-oligosaccharides such as oligofructose and inulin are the best studied and meet the strict definition of a prebiotic put forth by Roberfroid. Other commonly used prebiotics include galacto-oligosaccharides (GOS), trans-GOS, soya oligosaccharides, xylo-oligosaccharides, pyrodextrins, isomalto-oligosaccharides, and lactulose. Prebiotics can be further classified into short-chain, long-chain, and full-spectrum prebiotics. Short-chain prebiotics, such as oligofructose, ferment more quickly in the colon, whereas long-chain prebiotics, such as inulin, ferment more slowly and therefore work predominantly in the. Full-spectrum prebiotics, such as oligofructose-enriched inulin, target the entire colon. Prebiotics can also be found in a variety of food sources such as bananas, garlic, wheat, rye, and asparagus.[9]

Only a few studies have been conducted on the role of prebiotics in patients with IBS. A clinical trial published in 2009 evaluated the effect of the prebiotic trans-GOS in changing the colonic microbiota and IBS symptoms.[12] A total of 44 patients with Rome II IBS-C (IBS with constipation), IBS-D (IBS with diarrhea), or IBS alternate criteria were enrolled in this 12-week trial. The patients were randomized to receive 3.5 g/d or 7.0 g/d of the prebiotic trans-GOS or 7.0 g/d placebo. IBS symptoms were assessed using the Bristol Stool Form Scale and an IBS-specific questionnaire developed and validated by Drossman and colleagues[13] on a weekly basis over the course of 12 weeks. In this study, the prebiotic trans-GOS significantly increased fecal bifidobacteria counts (3.5 g/d, $P<.005$; 7.0 g/d, $P<.001$) compared with placebo. The bacteriologic data suggested that the 7.0-g dose rather than 3.5-g dose had the best effect on increasing fecal bifidobacteria counts. The prebiotic trans-GOS also improved IBS symptoms, particularly at the 3.5-g/d dose, which resulted in significant improvement in stool consistency, flatulence, and bloating. This study suggests that prebiotics may serve as a therapeutic treatment of IBS. There were no adverse events in this study.

Other studies have analyzed the optimal dose of prebiotics. A study examined the dose-response effects of short-chain fructo-oligosaccharides (scFOS).[14] In this study, 40 healthy volunteers following their usual diets were randomized to 2.5, 5.0, 7.5, or 10 g/d of scFOS or placebo. The investigators concluded that 7 days of ingestion of scFOS at a dosage of 10 g/d resulted in an increase in fecal bifidobacteria counts and minimized side effects.[14]

For a discussion on the role of probiotics in the treatment of IBS, see the articles by Mark Pimentel and Eamonn Quigley elsewhere in this issue.

ACUPUNCTURE

Acupuncture, an ancient traditional Chinese medical practice, is becoming more widely accepted and used in the Western society. Acupuncture has been practiced in China for several thousand years, although this traditional healing art has become common in the United States only since the early 1970s. Traditional Chinese medicine is based on a theory of energy or life force (qi) that runs through the body in channels called meridians. Qi is essential to health, and disruptions of this energy flow, which are thought to contribute to symptoms and diseases, can be corrected at identifiable anatomic locations (acupoints) with acupuncture.[15] The acupuncture technique involves penetrating the skin with thin, solid, metallic needles that are manipulated by the hands or by electric stimulation. It has been used to treat gastrointestinal symptoms in functional and organ diseases and has been shown to influence visceral reflex activity, gastric emptying, and acid reflux.[16] In IBS, acupuncture is thought to alter visceral sensation and motility by stimulating the somatic nervous system and the vagus nerve.[9–11] Therefore, the brain-gut disturbances implicated in IBS make it reasonable to hypothesize that acupuncture might provide an effective treatment modality.

In 2006, a Cochrane database systematic review analyzed 6 randomized trials using acupuncture in IBS.[17] The studies were generally of poor quality, included relatively small numbers of patients, and differed significantly in the acupuncture method used. This systematic review found inconclusive evidence as to whether acupuncture is superior to sham acupuncture in treating IBS. Subsequently, several large well-conducted randomized studies have been published (**Table 1**). Schneider and colleagues[18] published the results of a study that included 43 patients with IBS who were randomized to acupuncture or sham acupuncture. Although patients in both groups improved significantly compared with baseline, there was no significant difference between the response rates in patients receiving acupuncture and sham acupuncture based on quality-of-life measurements.

More recently, a large clinical trial was published by Lembo and colleagues[19] from the Beth Israel Deaconess Medical Center in Boston, Massachusetts. This study tested the effect of acupuncture and sham acupuncture in relieving IBS symptoms compared with waiting-list control or no treatment. Following a run-in phase in which all patients except those in the no-treatment arm received sham acupuncture, a total of 230 adult patients with IBS were randomly assigned to 3 weeks of true or sham acupuncture (6 sessions) or continued no treatment. In addition, patients receiving true or sham acupuncture were also randomly assigned to either an augmented or limited patient-practitioner interaction. The primary end point of the study was the Global Improvement Scale, in which participants were asked about changes in their IBS symptoms during the course of the treatment. Secondary global end points included IBS Adequate Relief, IBS Symptom Severity Scale, and IBS Quality of Life Questionnaire. There was no significant difference in both primary and secondary outcomes between the groups that received acupuncture and sham. However, patients receiving acupuncture or sham acupuncture were more likely to be responders on the Global Improvement Scale than patients in the waiting-list control group (37% vs 4%, $P<.001$) (**Fig. 1**). Likewise, patients receiving acupuncture or sham acupuncture versus those on the waiting-list control were significantly more likely to be responders in regard to secondary outcomes. Three adverse events were reported during the acupuncture versus sham acupuncture phase of the study: (1) painful foot cramp following treatment (sham acupuncture), (2) nausea/hip pain (true acupuncture), and (3) rib pain after a fall (sham acupuncture). All these events were considered to be unrelated to the study procedure. The results demonstrated that, although there was a trend toward improvement with acupuncture, there was no statistically significant difference between acupuncture and sham acupuncture in improving the symptoms of IBS. Similar to the Schneider and colleagues[18] study, this study estimated that

Table 1
Selected randomized controlled trials of acupuncture vs sham acupuncture for IBS

Study	Design	Patients	Control	Outcome Measures	Main Results
Forbes et al,[30] 2005	DB, parallel group 10 sessions over 10 wk	59 patients with Rome I IBS	Sham	Primary: decrease in symptom score at week 13 Others: weekly assessments of 8 symptoms by Likert scales, HAD, EuroQoL	No difference between acupuncture and sham (40.7% vs 31.2%, $P>.05$) Both groups improved compared with baseline
Schneider et al,[18] 2006	DB, parallel group 10 sessions over 5 wk	43 patients with Rome II IBS. Study stopped early because of poor enrollment	Sham	Primary: improvement in QoL by FDDQL Others: BDQ, PHQ-D, SF-36 at baseline, at the end of therapy, and at 3 mo	No difference between acupuncture and sham (11% and 10% increase in global FDDQL score) Both groups improved compared with baseline No significant AEs
Lembo et al,[19] 2009	DB, parallel group 6 session over 3 wk	230 patients with Rome II IBS	Sham	Primary: IBS-GIS Others: IBS-AR, IBS-SSS, IBS-QoL	No difference between acupuncture and sham (41% vs 32%, $P = .25$) Both groups improved compared with waiting-list group (37% vs 4%, $P<.001$) No significant AEs

Abbreviations: AE, adverse event; BDQ, bowel disease questionnaire; DB, double-blind; EuroQoL, quality of life questionnaire; FDDQL, functional digestive disorders quality of life questionnaire; HAD, Hospital Anxiety and Depression Scale; IBS-AR, IBS Adequate Relief outcome measure; IBS-GIS, IBS Global Improvement Scale; IBS-QoL, IBS Quality of Life Questionnaire; IBS-SSS, IBS Symptom Severity Scale; PHQ-D, patient health questionnaire; SF-36, 36-Item Short Form Health Survey.

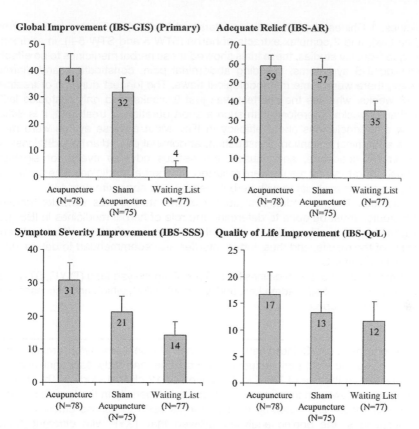

Fig. 1. Global response rates with acupuncture, sham acupuncture, and waiting-list control. Although there was a trend toward improvement with acupuncture compared with sham acupuncture, no statistically significant difference was present. Acupuncture and sham acupuncture were significantly different compared with waiting-list control for global measures except for IBS-QoL. IBS-AR, IBS Adequate Relief; IBS-GIS, IBS Global Improvement Scale; IBS-QoL, IBS Quality of Life Questionnaire; IBS-SSS, IBS Symptom Severity Scale.

more than 600 patients would be needed to properly power a study to show the superiority of acupuncture over sham acupuncture. This study showed that acupuncture and sham acupuncture were significantly better than no treatment, suggesting that either sham acupuncture is effective at relieving symptoms associated with IBS or the ritual of acupuncture (ie, nonspecific placebo effects) is effective.[20]

HERBAL MEDICINES

Herbal medicines are based on the use of plant and plant extracts as remedies to treat a variety of symptoms and diseases. Herbalism typically involves combining several herbs to obtain a desired effect. Many herbal medicines are used as the basis for prescription drugs in Western medicine.

A meta-analysis published in 2008 included 22 studies with 25 different herbal medicines.[21] However, only 4 of these studies were considered to be of good quality, whereas the remaining studies involving 17 Chinese herbal medicines were considered to be of poor quality. The 4 good-quality studies used the following herbal medicines: 1 Chinese herbal medicine (standard formula), 1 Tibetan herbal formula (Padma Lax), and 2 complex extracts of herbs (STW 5 and STW 5-II). In addition to being good-quality studies, these trials showed these herbal medicines to be effective in relieving IBS symptoms, including abdominal pain, constipation, and diarrhea. However, there were some methodological flaws. The longest duration of treatment was 18 weeks, whereas the shortest was just 2 weeks, and only 5 studies lasted more than 8 weeks. Therefore, with such a short duration of treatment, it is difficult to draw any conclusions about efficacy in IBS. Most adverse events were minor, such as abdominal distention, constipation, abdominal pain, diarrhea, dizziness and hypersomnia, headache, and nausea. No serious adverse events or significant abnormal laboratory test results were reported with herbal medicines. The percentage of adverse events associated with herbal therapy was approximately 4% in a total of 1279 subjects. The methodological quality of the studies was variable; therefore, further studies must be done to determine the role of herbal medicines in IBS. Even among the higher-quality studies, methodological issues affect the effect and generalizability of the results, and thus, further studies are recommended to determine the overall efficacy in IBS.

The best studied herbal medicines for IBS are Tong xie yao fang (TXYF), STW 5 and STW 5-II, peppermint oil, Padma Lax, and St John's Wort, which are discussed in the subsequent paragraphs.

TXYF

TXYF is composed of 4 Chinese herbal medicines: rhizoma atractylodis macrocephalae, radix paeoniae alba, pericarpium citri reticulatae, and radix saposhnikoviae.[22] A meta-analysis on the use of TXYF in IBS reviewed 12 clinical studies. The quality of the studies was low, and there was significant heterogeneity in the formulas, control, treatment duration, and outcome measurements used to assess efficacy. Despite these limitations, the pooled analyses showed that TXYF with different chinese herbal additions was better than conventional medicines. After the publication of the meta-analysis, a large study was conducted in China, involving 120 patients with IBS-D who were treated with TXYF (n = 80) or Miyarisan, a probiotic consisting of butyric acid bacteria, (n = 40) for 4 weeks.[23] TXYF was administered twice a day, whereas Miyarisan was administered 3 times a day. Efficacy was compared between the 2 groups based on symptoms before treatment and 2 and 4 weeks after treatment. This study also measured the number of activated mucosal mast cells in a subset of patients in each group. Although there was no significant difference between the 2 groups in regard to IBS symptoms, the number of activated mast cells decreased to a greater degree in the TXYF group compared with the Miyarisan group. Because this study was not placebo controlled, conclusions regarding the efficacy of TXYF could not be made. Therefore, further studies of its effect on IBS symptoms and mast cell numbers and function are warranted.

STW 5

STW 5 is composed of bitter candytuft, chamomile flower, peppermint leaves, caraway fruit, licorice root, lemon balm leaves, celandine herbs, angelica root, and milk thistle fruit. STW 5-II is similar to STW 5 except that it does not include angelica root and milk thistle fruit. A double-blind, placebo-controlled, multicenter trial from Germany evaluated the safety and cost-effectiveness of STW 5 and STW 5-II.[24] A total of 208 outpatients with IBS were randomly assigned to STW 5, STW 5-II, bitter candytuft monoextract (BCT), or placebo 3 times daily for 4 weeks. At the end of 4 weeks, STW 5 and STW 5-II were more effective than placebo. After 2 weeks of treatment, the IBS symptom score was significantly better for STW 5 and STW 5-II than for placebo ($P = .0085$ and $P = .0006$ vs placebo, respectively). After 4 weeks, the difference between STW 5/STW 5-II and placebo became more apparent ($P = .001$ and $P = .0003$ vs placebo, respectively). There were significant differences in the primary end points before and after treatment with STW 5 and STW 5-II but not with BCT. The tested herbal preparations were well tolerated, with a few adverse events. One patient reported headache and another reported constipation. This study suggests that both STW 5 and STW 5-II may be effective for the treatment of patients with IBS, although further trials are needed. The mechanism of action of these agents in patients with IBS remains to be fully elucidated.

Peppermint Oil

Peppermint oil is the major constituent of several over-the-counter remedies for symptoms of IBS.[25] Peppermint oil is obtained by steam distillation of the aerial parts of the flowering plant *Mentha piperita* L. The active principle of peppermint oil is menthol, a cyclic monoterpene with calcium channel blocking activity and a pharmacologic profile similar to that of dihydropyridine calcium antagonists. The plant is a cross between 2 types of mint, water mint and spearmint. A meta-analysis published in 1998 identified 8 trials that used peppermint in IBS. Of these 8 trials, 5 double-blind placebo-controlled trials were included for further analysis. The meta-analysis showed a significant ($P<.001$) global improvement of IBS symptoms in patients treated with peppermint oil compared with placebo. The placebo response in these trials ranged from 13% to 52%. A more recent randomized, double-blind, placebo-controlled study conducted in Taiwan randomized 110 patients with IBS symptoms[26] to an enteric-coated peppermint oil formulation or placebo 3 to 4 times daily for 1 month. Patients in the treatment arm had less abdominal distention, stool frequency, and flatulence than patients in the placebo arm. About 79% of the patients also had alleviation of abdominal pain. Two patients receiving peppermint oil reported adverse effects, heartburn and a transient skin rash.

These studies show that peppermint oil is effective and well tolerated in patients with IBS. Peppermint oil is also readily available at local health food stores and often sold at reasonable prices, making it appealing as a cost-efficient treatment of IBS. It is commonly enteric coated or contains a barrier that controls the location in the digestive system where the oil is released.

Padma Lax

Padma Lax is a complex Tibetan herbal formula composed of the dry extract of *Aloe*, calumba root, cascara, chebulic myrobalan fruit, condurango, elecampane, frangula bark, gentian root, ginger, heavy kaolin, long pepper, nux vomica, rhubarb, sodium hydrogen carbonate, and sodium sulfate. A double-blind randomized pilot study was conducted in Israel in patients with IBS-C.[27] Subjects were treated with either Padma Lax or placebo for 3 months. When compared with placebo, those receiving Padma Lax demonstrated significant improvement in constipation, severity of abdominal pain and its effect on daily activities, incomplete evacuation, abdominal distension, and flatus/flatulence. Side effects included loose stools in a small number of subjects, but they responded well after lowering the dosage. It was suggested that Padma Lax is a potential agent for the treatment of IBS-C, but further studies are needed.

St John's Wort

St John's wort is derived from the St John's wort plant and is commonly used for depression and several pain syndromes. Recently, a well-conducted trial by Saito and colleagues[28] randomized 70 patients with IBS (86% women) to either St John's wort, 450 mg, or placebo twice daily for 12 weeks. The primary end point was the overall self-reported composite score of different IBS symptoms (pain/discomfort, constipation, diarrhea, and overall severity). In this study, both groups reported an improvement in IBS symptoms, but a greater improvement was seen in the placebo group than in the St John's wort group.

JAPANESE HERBAL MEDICINES

Suzuki and colleagues[29] recently reviewed the published literature of Japanese herbal medicines such as Rikkunshi-to and Dai-Kenchu-to in functional bowel disorders. Rikkunshi-to, which is prepared from 8 crude herbs, was found to be possibly effective in reducing discomfort caused by functional dyspepsia. Likewise, Dai-Kenchu-to, a mixture of ginseng, ginger, and zanthoxylum fruit, was also found to be beneficial for constipation in children and patients with postoperative ileus. Nevertheless, given the paucity of randomized clinical trials and limitations in the standardization of the quality and quantity of herbs, particularly outside Japan, further studies are needed.

SUMMARY

CAMs are commonly used by patients with IBS, particularly, prebiotics, probiotics, acupuncture, and herbal medicines. Well-controlled clinical trials are lacking to support CAM use in IBS. Nevertheless, several treatments, particularly some probiotics and herbs (eg, peppermint oil), suggest that they may have a benefit in IBS. However, further study is still needed to definitely determine their role in managing patients with IBS.

REFERENCES

1. Agrawal A, Whorwell PJ. Irritable bowel syndrome: diagnosis and management. BMJ 2006;332:280–3.
2. Hungin AP, Chang L, Locke GR, et al. Irritable bowel syndrome in the United States: prevalence, symptom patterns and impact. Aliment Pharmacol Ther 2005;21:1365–75.
3. Saito YA, Schoenfeld P, Locke GR 3rd. The epidemiology of irritable bowel syndrome in North America: a systematic review. Am J Gastroenterol 2002;97: 1910–5.
4. Tillisch K. Complementary and alternative medicine for functional gastrointestinal disorders. Gut 2006;55:593–6.
5. Tindle HA, Davis RB, Phillips RS, et al. Trends in use of complementary and alternative medicine by US adults: 1997-2002. Altern Ther Health Med 2005;11:42–9.
6. Koloski NA, Talley NJ, Huskic SS, et al. Predictors of conventional and alternative health care seeking for irritable bowel syndrome and functional dyspepsia. Aliment Pharmacol Ther 2003;17:841–51.
7. Kong SC, Hurlstone DP, Pocock CY, et al. The incidence of self-prescribed oral complementary and alternative medicine use by patients with gastrointestinal diseases. J Clin Gastroenterol 2005;39:138–41.
8. van Tilburg MA, Palsson OS, Levy RL, et al. Complementary and alternative medicine use and cost in functional bowel disorders: a six month prospective study in a large HMO. BMC Complement Altern Med 2008;8:46.
9. Gibson GR, Roberfroid MB. Dietary modulation of the human colonic microbiota: introducing the concept of prebiotics. J Nutr 1995;125:1401–12.

10. Roberfroid M. Prebiotics: the concept revisited. J Nutr 2007;137:830S–7S.
11. Schley PD, Field CJ. The immune-enhancing effects of dietary fibres and prebiotics. Br J Nutr 2002;87(Suppl 2):S221–30.
12. Silk DB, Davis A, Vulevic J, et al. Clinical trial: the effects of a trans-galactooligosaccharide prebiotic on faecal microbiota and symptoms in irritable bowel syndrome. Aliment Pharmacol Ther 2009;29:508–18.
13. Drossman DA, Patrick DL, Whitehead WE, et al. Further validation of the IBS-QOL: a disease-specific quality-of-life questionnaire. Am J Gastroenterol 2000; 95:999–1007.
14. Bouhnik Y, Vahedi K, Achour L, et al. Short-chain fructo-oligosaccharide administration dose-dependently increases fecal bifidobacteria in healthy humans. J Nutr 1999;129:113–6.
15. Kaptchuk TJ. Acupuncture: theory, efficacy, and practice. Ann Intern Med 2002; 136:374–83.
16. Takahashi T. Acupuncture for functional gastrointestinal disorders. J Gastroenterol 2006;41:408–17.
17. Lim B, Manheimer E, Lao L, et al. Acupuncture for treatment of irritable bowel syndrome. Cochrane Database Syst Rev 2006;4:CD005111.
18. Schneider A, Enck P, Streitberger K, et al. Acupuncture treatment in irritable bowel syndrome. Gut 2006;55:649–54.
19. Lembo AJ, Conboy L, Kelley JM, et al. A treatment trial of acupuncture in IBS patients. Am J Gastroenterol 2009;104:1489–97.
20. Manocrattanaporn M, Chey WD. Acupuncture for irritable bowel syndrome: sham or the real deal? Gastroenterology 2010;139:348–50 [discussion: 350–1].
21. Shi J, Tong Y, Shen JG, et al. Effectiveness and safety of herbal medicines in the treatment of irritable bowel syndrome: a systematic review. World J Gastroenterol 2008;14:454–62.
22. Bian Z, Wu T, Liu L, et al. Effectiveness of the Chinese herbal formula TongXieYao-Fang for irritable bowel syndrome: a systematic review. J Altern Complement Med 2006;12:401–7.
23. Pan F, Zhang T, Zhang YH, et al. Effect of Tongxie Yaofang granule in treating diarrhea-predominate irritable bowel syndrome. Chin J Integr Med 2009;15: 216–9.
24. Madisch A, Holtmann G, Plein K, et al. Treatment of irritable bowel syndrome with herbal preparations: results of a double-blind, randomized, placebo-controlled, multi-centre trial. Aliment Pharmacol Ther 2004;19:271–9.
25. Pittler MH, Ernst E. Peppermint oil for irritable bowel syndrome: a critical review and meta-analysis. Am J Gastroenterol 1998;93:1131–5.
26. Liu JP, Yang M, Liu YX, et al. Herbal medicines for treatment of irritable bowel syndrome. Cochrane Database Syst Rev 2006;1:CD004116.
27. Sallon S, Ben-Arye E, Davidson R, et al. A novel treatment for constipation-predominant irritable bowel syndrome using Padma Lax, a Tibetan herbal formula. Digestion 2002;65:161–71.
28. Saito YA, Rey E, Almazar-Elder AE, et al. A randomized, double-blind, placebo-controlled trial of St John's wort for treating irritable bowel syndrome. Am J Gastroenterol 2010;105:170–7.
29. Suzuki H, Inadomi JM, Hibi T. Japanese herbal medicine in functional gastrointestinal disorders. Neurogastroenterol Motil 2009;21:688–96.
30. Forbes A, Jackson S, Walter C, et al. Acupuncture for irritable bowel syndrome: a blinded placebo-controlled trial. World J Gastroenterol 2005;260:4040–4.

Index

Note: Page numbers of article titles are in **boldface** type.

A

A3309 (ileal bile acid transporter inhibitor), 226, 231–232
Abdominal muscles, dysfunction of, 29
Abuse, 33, 50–51
Acupuncture, 246–249
ADRA genes, 59–60
Adrenergic pathway genes, 56, 58–60
Adverse life events, 51
Alarm features, 109
Allergy, food
    biomarkers of, 131–132
    in IBS, 146–148
    versus intolerance, 144–146
Allodynia, 24–27
Alosetron, 129, 169–171
Alternative medicine, **245–253**
Amitriptyline, 129, 187–188
Amygdala, gut interactions with, 29–32
Antibiotics, 214
    as biomarkers, 131
    microflora population and, 75–76
Antibody(ies), in celiac disease, 111
Anticholinergic agents, 167–169
Antidepressants, 185–188
Antidiarrheals, 166–167
Anti-inflammatory agents, 79, **207–222**
Antispasmodics, 167–169
Anxiety, 35
    genes of, 58
    overlap with, 5
Asimadoline, 128–129, 226, 232–233
AST-120 (carbon-based adsorbent), 227, 233
Autonomic nervous system dysfunction, 29, 129–130

B

Bacterial overgrowth, small intestinal, 72–74, 113–114
Bacteroides thetaiotamicron, 70
Barium enema, 112
Barostats, 124–125, 127–129
Behavioral therapy, 185–186, 189, 192–193
Belladonna, 167–169

Gastroenterol Clin N Am 40 (2011) 255–264
doi:10.1016/S0889-8553(11)00011-2
0889-8553/11/$ – see front matter © 2011 Elsevier Inc. All rights reserved.

gastro.theclinics.com

Moving?

Make sure your subscription moves with you!

To notify us of your new address, find your **Clinics Account Number** (located on your mailing label above your name), and contact customer service at:

Email: journalscustomerservice-usa@elsevier.com

800-654-2452 (subscribers in the U.S. & Canada)
314-447-8871 (subscribers outside of the U.S. & Canada)

Fax number: 314-447-8029

Elsevier Health Sciences Division
Subscription Customer Service
3251 Riverport Lane
Maryland Heights, MO 63043

*To ensure uninterrupted delivery of your subscription, please notify us at least 4 weeks in advance of move.

Printed and bound by CPI Group (UK) Ltd, Croydon, CR0 4YY

03/10/2024

01040461-0010